MEDICINE AND COLONIALISM: HISTORICAL PERSPECTIVES IN INDIA AND SOUTH AFRICA

EMPIRES IN PERSPECTIVE

Series Editor: Durba Ghosh
Advisory Editor: Masaie Matsumura

TITLES IN THIS SERIES

1 Between Empire and Revolution: A Life of Sidney Bunting, 1873–1936
Allison Drew

2 A Wider Patriotism: Alfred Milner and the British Empire
J. Lee Thompson

3 Missionary Education and Empire in Late Colonial India, 1860–1920
Hayden J. A. Bellenoit

4 Transoceanic Radical, William Duane: National
Identity and Empire, 1760–1835
Nigel Little

5 Natural Science and the Origins of the British Empire
Sarah Irving

6 Empire of Political Thought: Indigenous Australians
and the Language of Colonial Government
Bruce Buchan

7 The English Empire in America, 1602–1658: Beyond Jamestown
L. H. Roper

8 India in the French Imagination: Peripheral Voices, 1754–1815
Kate Marsh

9 British Narratives of Exploration: Case Studies on the Self and Other
Frédéric Regard (ed.)

10 Law and Imperialism: Criminality and Constitution in Colonial India
and Victorian England
Preeti Nijhar

11 Slaveholders in Jamaica: Colonial Society and Culture during the Era of
Abolition
Christer Petley

12 Australian Between Empires: The Life of Percy Spender
David Lowe

13 The Theatre of Empire: Frontier Performances in America, 1750–1860
Douglas S. Harvey

14 Anglo-Spanish Rivalry in Colonial South-East America, 1650–1725
Timothy Paul Grady

15 Royal Patronage, Power and Aesthetics in Princely India
Angma Dey Jhala

16 British Engineers and Africa, 1875–1914
Casper Andersen

17 Ireland and Empire, 1692–1770
Charles Ivar McGrath

18 Race and Identity in the Tasman World, 1769–1840
Rachel Standfield

19 The Quest for the Northwest Passage: Knowledge, Nation and Empire, 1576–1806
Frédéric Regard (ed.)

20 Arctic Exploration in the Nineteenth Century: Discovering the Northwest Passage
Frédéric Regard (ed.)

21 Baudin, Napoleon and the Exploration of Australia
Nicole Starbuck

FORTHCOMING TITLES

Class and Colonialism in Antarctic Exploration, 1750–1920
Ben Maddison

Mercurino di Gattinara and the Creation of the Spanish Empire
Rebecca Ard Boone

MEDICINE AND COLONIALISM: HISTORICAL PERSPECTIVES IN INDIA AND SOUTH AFRICA

EDITED BY

Poonam Bala

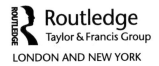

Routledge
Taylor & Francis Group

LONDON AND NEW YORK

First published 2014 by Pickering & Chatto (Publishers) Limited

Published 2016 by Routledge
2 Park Square, Milton Park, Abingdon, Oxfordshire OX14 4RN
711 Third Avenue, New York, NY 10017, USA

First issued in paperback 2015

Routledge is an imprint of the Taylor & Francis Group, an informa business

BRITISH LIBRARY CATALOGUING IN PUBLICATION DATA

Medicine and colonialism: historical perspectives in India and South Africa. –
(Empires in perspective)
1. Medical care – India – History – 19th century. 2. Medical care – India – His-
tory – 20th century. 3. Medical care – South Africa – History – 19th century. 4.
Medical care – South Africa – History – 20th century. 5. Medical care – Great
Britain – Colonies – History – 19th century. 6. Medical care – Great Britain
– Colonies – History – 20th century. 7. Traditional medicine – Great Britain
– Colonies – History – 19th century. 8. Traditional medicine – Great Britain –
Colonies – History – 20th century.
I. Series II. Bala, Poonam, 1958– editor of compilation.
362.1'091712'41-dc23

ISBN-13: 978-1-138-66313-8 (pbk)
ISBN-13: 978-1-8489-3465-8 (hbk)

Typeset by Pickering & Chatto (Publishers) Limited

CONTENTS

Acknowledgements   ix
List of Contributors   xi

Introduction – *Poonam Bala*   1
1 'Re-Constructing' Indian Medicine: The Role of Caste in Late
   Nineteenth- and Twentieth-Century India – *Poonam Bala*   11
2 The Resurgence of Indigenous Medicine in the Age of the HIV/AIDS
   Pandemic: South Africa Beyond the 'Miracle' – *Steve Phatlane*   25
3 Medicine, Medical Knowledge and Healing at the Cape of Good Hope:
   Khoikhoi, Slaves and Colonists – *Russel Viljoen*   41
4 Dealing with Disease: Epizootics, Veterinarians and Public Health in
   Colonial Bengal, 1850–1920 – *Samiparna Samanta*   61
5 Mahatma Gandhi under the Plague Spotlight – *Howard Phillips*   75
6 Plague Hits the Colonies: India and South Africa at the Turn of the
   Twentieth Century – *Natasha Sarkar*   85
7 The Blind Men and the Elephant: Imperial Medicine, Medieval
   Historians and the Role of Rats in the Historiography of Plague
   – *Katherine Royer*   99
8 Physicians, Forceps and Childbirth: Technological Intervention in
   Reproductive Health in Colonial Bengal – *Arabinda Samanta*   111
9 Not Fit for Punishment: Diagnosing Criminal Lunatics in Late
   Nineteenth-Century British India – *Jonathan Saha*   127
10 Multiple Voices and Plausible Claims: Historiography and Colonial
   Lunatic Asylum Archives – *Sally Swartz*   143
11 Death and Empire: Legal Medicine in the Colonization of India and
   Africa – *Jeffrey M. Jentzen*   159

Notes   175
Index   221

ACKNOWLEDGEMENTS

I would like to take this opportunity to thank the University of South Africa for providing all financial support and facilities for a visiting professorship; the idea for a India–South Africa project took shape during my visit to South Africa when several colleagues and friends made my first-time trip a memorable experience. I offer my special gratitude to Russel Viljoen for facilitating my visit and for his thoughtful discussions on the project. To Melanda and Anita, a special word of appreciation for being extremely helpful and kind during my stay.

The staff at the University of Delhi Library, Jawaharlal Nehru University, Lauren, Cheryl, Eric, Ron and Janet, and staff at Case Western Reserve University Library have been immensely helpful in procuring records for me – my thanks to them.

I would also like to make a note of thanks to the contributors to the volume whose unfailing co-operation and understanding enabled the smooth trajectory of this project.

I am grateful to the reviewers for their insightful comments, and to Durba Ghosh, the Series Editor, for her useful input in the early stages of the project. My thanks to Ruth Ireland for seeing this project through in its earlier stages, and to Stephina Clarke for her precision in overseeing the final edits. I also thank Sally Swartz for her collegial support.

Last, but not the least, and as always, I reserve a special place for my mother, whose love and support are always a blessing for me.

To my (late) father, Raghubir Narain, and my mother, Sharda,
for their love and support

LIST OF CONTRIBUTORS

Poonam Bala teaches sociology and is currently a visiting scholar at Cleveland State University in Ohio. A fellow in history at the University of South Africa, where she has been a visiting professor. She has authored several articles and books on pre-colonial and colonial India, including *Imperialism and Medicine in Bengal: A Socio-Historical Perspective* (1991) and *Medicine and Medical Policies in India: Social and Historical Perspectives* (2007), and edited *Biomedicine as a Contested Site: Some Revelations in Imperial Contexts* (2009) and *Contesting Colonial Authority: Medicine and Indigenous Responses in Nineteenth- and Twentieth-Century India* (2012). Her forthcoming book is titled, *Across Cultures: The 'Unheard' Voices of the Asian Indians in Ohio*, with projects on the Indian Medical Services and women in medicine in progress.

Jeffrey M. Jentzen is Professor of Pathology and Lecturer in the Department of History at the University of Michigan. He is the author or *Death Investigation in America: Coroners, Medical Examiners and the Quest for Medical Certainty* (2009) and is currently working on a book examining global perspectives and the transmission of death investigation practices, for the Harvard Press.

Stephens Ntsoakae Phatlane is a senior lecturer at the University of South Africa (UNISA) where he teaches post-colonial African and modern South African history. Steve is also the author of *Poverty, Medicine and Disease in South Africa: The Era of High Apartheid, 1948 to 1976* (2008). He has published several articles in accredited journals, including 'Poverty and HIV/AIDS in Apartheid South Africa' (*Social Identities: Journal for the Study of Race, Nation and Culture*).

Howard Phillips is a professor in the Department of Historical Studies at the University of Cape Town where he pioneered the teaching of the social history of health, disease and medicine. He is the author or co-author of numerous articles and books in this field, including *'Black October': The Impact of the Spanish Flu Epidemic on South Africa* (1990), *The Spanish Influenza Pandemic of 1918–1919: New Perspectives* (2003), *The Cape Doctor in the Nineteenth Century: A*

Social History (2004), *At the Heart of Healing: Groote Schuur Hospital 1938–2008* (2008) and *Plague, Pox and Pandemic: A History of Epidemics in South Africa* (2012).

Katherine Royer is a physician and professor of history at California State University Stanislaus where she teaches courses on disease and world societies as well as the history capital punishment and specializes in the history of the body set in the *longue durée*. She is Board Certified in Internal Medicine and a Member of the American College of Physicians and has published in medicine, as well as history, most recently on the role of the body in rituals of punishment. Her forthcoming book, *The English Execution Narrative: 1200–1700*, will be published by Pickering & Chatto.

Jonathan Saha is a lecturer in modern history at the University of Bristol where he teaches Asian history. He is author of *Law, Disorder and the Colonial State: Corruption in Burma c. 1900* (2013) and has also published a number of articles on the history of madness, medicine and misconduct in late nineteenth-century colonial Burma.

Arabinda Samanta is Professor in History at the University of Burdwan, West Bengal, India. He has written extensively on various aspects of social history of Bengal and has authored *Malarial Fever in Colonial Bengal: Social History of an Epidemic* (2002), *Sahityer Itihaas Kimba Itihaaser Sahitya* (2002), *Praakritik Biparjay O Manush* (2003), *Rog, Rogi, Raastra* (2004), and co-edited *The Revolt of 1857: Memory, Identity, History* (2009), *Life and Culture in Bengal: Colonial and Post-colonial Experiences* (2011).

Samiparna Samanta is an assistant professor of history at Georgia College and State University, Milledgeville, Georgia, USA. As part of her own research, Samiparna focuses on South Asia predominantly in the areas of history of science and medicine, socio-cultural, environmental history; colonialism, British Empire, human–animal interactions. She has published articles on imperialism and inequality; masculinity and violence in Indian films. She teaches a wide variety of topics including modern Asia, world civilizations, Indo-Islam, history of disease and epidemics. She is currently working on a book project that uses the lens of animal cruelty and protection to write a social history of Bengal from 1850 to 1920.

Natasha Sarkar is Junior Faculty Fellow at the Center for Historical Research, Ohio State University, USA. She has published several articles on the modern plague pandemic and the social history of medicine in South Asia, exploring questions related to gender and disease, alternative medicine and cultural response to disease. Her forthcoming articles include 'Ayurvedic Revivalism: Appropriating a Sense of "National" Identity through Modernity' (*International Journal of Science in Society*) and 'Ethical Dilemmas in Stem Cell Research: Questioning the Moral Status of the Embryo in India' (*Science, Technology and Society*).

Sally Swartz is Associate Professor in the Psychology Department at the University of Cape Town. She is a practising clinical psychologist and psychoanalytic psychotherapist, and provides training for postgraduate students in the area of adult psychotherapy. She has published extensively in the areas of psychoanalytic psychotherapy in South Africa, approaches to clinical psychology training, and the history of colonial psychiatry. She has published widely on insanity and psychiatric practices in the Cape Colony in the *Journal of Southern African Studies, History of the Human Sciences, Feminism and Psychology, International Journal of Mental Health, Theory and Psychology, History of Psychology*, 13 (2010), pp. 160–77; and with H. Laurenson, 'The Professionalization of Psychology within the Apartheid State, 1948–1978', *History of Psychology*, 14 (2011), pp. 249–63.

Russel Viljoen is Professor of History at the University of South Africa. His main research area is eighteenth-century colonial South Africa with reference to Khoikhoi studies. He is the author of *Jan Paerl: A Khoikhoi in Cape Colonial Society, 1761–1851* (2006). He has published articles and book chapters on smallpox in eighteenth- and nineteenth-century South Africa with reference to colonial and indigenous societies.

INTRODUCTION

Poonam Bala

While studies in the history of medicine over the previous two decades have alluded to developmental trajectories of colonial and indigenous medicines, they have projected these against a broad canvas of engagement and alienation processes over a period of time. This volume moves beyond these presentations to explore new perspectives in understanding the dynamism and engagements between colonialism and medicine in India and South Africa. It examines the nature of medicine, medical practices, strategies, and knowledge 'transfers' and exchange between the two regions.

In gauging the nature of imperial control in India and South Africa, Dagmar Engels and Shula Marks, in their path-breaking study *Contesting Colonial Hegemony: State and Society in Africa and India* (1994), address issues of 'coercion' and 'consent' through the application of Antonio Gramsci's theories to the colonial state.[1] Equally significant and influential in unravelling this dynamic is *De-centering Empire: Britain, India and the Transcolonial World* (2006) in which Durba Ghosh and Dane Kennedy present new perspectives in understanding the power of imperialism beyond the 'imperial center and colonial periphery' dichotomy of relationships between the 'ruler and the ruled'; it also highlights significant issues in the historiography of understanding the British empire and their impact on the colonies, paving the way for further studies in examining the impact of the empire in specific contexts.[2]

In recent years, several studies have focused on the history of dynamics of interaction between racial discrimination and the prevalence of hierarchy and inequalities within the medical profession.[3] They have portrayed the historical trajectories in terms of medical institutions, policies and medical practices. Going beyond the earlier analytical frameworks, Harriet Deacon portrays the need to look at the distinction between 'racist medicine and medical racism'.[4] Focusing on the Cape Colony, she makes a persuasive argument demonstrating that 'legislation, class, institutional settings and popular stereotypes could influence the form, timing and degree of racism in the medical profession and in the medical theory and practices'.[5] Yet, doctors in the Cape Colony were indispensable to imperial control, and were 'agents of empire' playing 'the role as healers, educators, and rulers'.[6] In understanding the politics of medicine in the Cape Colony, Anne Digby's recent study, examining the interplay between 'colonial or western medicine, missionary medicine and indigenous healing', is noteworthy.[7] Portraying a rich and comprehensive history of the dynamics of health, health care providers and indigenous healing practices in South Africa, Digby's study brings to light resistance and adaptation as distinct facets of the dynamics of indigenous African medical practitioners and the 'pluralistic' choices adopted by patients.[8]

While the character of colonial rule has been central to all studies on colonialism and their engagement with colonized societies and their institutions, some of these have been noteworthy in their contribution to the emerging discourses on colonialism in Africa. Perhaps the first major comprehensive historical study that portrays the growth and influence of various medical institutions in South Africa was that by Edmund H. Burrows in which he traces the development of the medical profession alongside scientific and medical progress as a result of the great epidemics of Cape Town.[9] Although within African colonial historiography, eurocentric perspectives have largely dominated discourses on African history, some more recent works provide new interpretations and African perspectives on these. Needless to say, the African interpretation of the Scramble or Partition has gone unnoticed in African history – at least, until the historical first International Congress of African Historians in 1965 that focused on the emerging themes in African history. Recognized as one of the pioneers of twentieth-century African history, Albert. A. Boahen's work bridges the void in understanding the colonial experience of the colonized by providing a persuasive discussion in which he remarks on the 'suddenness and unpredictability' of colonial rule in Africa.[10] The 'sudden' and 'unpredictable' imposition of imperial powers, as Boahen perceives them, became apparent within a short span of two decades – from 1880 to 1900 – when 'all of Africa', he argues, 'except Liberia and Ethiopia, was seized and occupied by the European imperial powers of Britian, France, Germany, Belgium, Portugal, Spain and Italy'.[11] From this emerged approximately forty artificially created colonies such that, by 1910, Africa was entirely under the colonial system. While Africa, especially sub-Saharan Africa, 'occupies a prominent place in Atlantic history and its indispensability in making the Americas and Europe since the fifteenth century',[12] the historiography of the Indian Ocean offers insights into the historical importance of trade, merchant communities and exchange of commodities along the trading coast lanes between AD 700 and 1750, prior to European intrusions. Kirti N.Chaudhuri's *Trade and Civilisation in the Indian Ocean* has, by far, been one of the most influential and comprehensive studies echoing such interconnections.[13]

In recent years, there also has been a growing interest in transnational history which seems to have been inspired by a revived enthusiasm for British imperial history and an understanding of the impact of imperialism in metropolitan societies. In the words of Antoinette Burton, this marks a 'critical return to the connections between metropole and colony, race and nation'[14] – connections through which imperial powers were to be shaped and redefined during their colonising experience. Similarly, Marshall G. S. Hodgson, in his powerful critique of defining 'progress' in terms of the 'modern West', deployed the concept of 'Afro-Eurasia' as a paradigm to unravel the historical developments 'underpinned by complex inter-regional connections and the gradual growth of a common store of human knowledge'.[15]

The essays in this collection offer different aspects of transnational perspectives and the interconnectedness of historical realities in specific contexts of European colonialism, political movements and ideas. The issues in each essay portray not so much the African or Indian 'adaptation' or 'resistance' to colonial initiatives as the policies of European adaptation and resistance to the initiatives of the colonized. They also reveal similar 'processes' employed by the colonial administration, in their colonizing trajectories. With a common theme of the intellectual engagements of medicine with indigenous populations and their already existing institutional paradigms, the essays included here enable an understanding of medicine as providing 'mobility in modernity' as perceived through new structural formations, institutional set ups, the emergence of national and social reform movements, resistance from the colonizer as much as from the colonized and the role of indigenous elites in enabling socio-political cultural connections within colonial modernity. Underlying these negotiations, medicine can thus be seen as 'purveying solutions required by the imperial governments',[16] and in so doing, it became equally powerful in establishing 'new institutions of knowledge'.[17] In this context, Mark Harrison's study identifies the role played by colonialism in shaping British medicine.[18] For instance, the development of colonial hospitals facilitated pathological anatomy and the emergence of new forms of medical knowledge through regulated procedures of testing which were later added to the practice of British medicine – for colonial practitioners, according to Harrison, used new medicines from the colonies in their civilian practices in Britain. While David Arnold substantiates the notion of the 'coercive power' of western medicine in colonial India which, he argues,

> was a colonial science and not simply an extension of western science to a colonial output. To this effect, medicine was not only seen as powerful but an equally penetrating part of the colonizing process in India as well as in Africa, and Latin America.[19]

In maintaining that the 'technological reconfiguration' remained paramount in the colonial administration in British India, the role of medicine as a 'vehement apparatus'[20] in allowing a deeper engagement with the colonized can hardly be gainsaid. While the 'concern' for the use of biomedicine as a tool of cultural domination has been vividly expressed in some major scholarly works, it is about using biomedicine 'as an extension of racist and imperialist projects', as also the 'use of Africa, as a safe place to conduct experiments and engage in coercive action that would have been unethical and unenforceable in Europe'.[21]

The historiography of disease and medicine in colonial India has, in recent years, focused on epidemic diseases which have been understood as a means of unravelling the social and political dynamics of colonial practices and the medical profession and its practitioners.[22] The evolution of public health measures, these studies indicate, has been a marker of the new trends and approaches in medicine alongside medical and scientific progress. Explaining public health issues, colonial attitudes and Indian resistance, thus, has been the pivot of analysis for medicine and its engagements in colonial India. Public health has also been seen as a 'window' though which decisions on providing health to the civilian population could be instituted, albeit with underlying limitations. It therefore existed as a significant paradigm in understanding the response and attitudes to state medicine and outbreaks of epidemics, while also enabling an understanding of the attitudes of the imperial government towards epidemics. Radhika Ramasubban, for instance, discusses public health and sanitary measures as 'tools' used to dominate the Indian population,[23] and Ira Klein refers to them "as 'ugly ducklings' of a civil service which rewarded political and military competence, for example, far more highly" under imperial rule.[24]

South Africa played an important role in the formation of Africa's image in Europe during the eighteenth century; an image that can be deciphered from several early accounts of South Africa written by exploratory expeditions of travellers, most of whom were employed by the Dutch East India Company (VOC) to explore the economic potentials of the interiors of the Cape.[25] The 'new' knowledge gained from the scientific accounts of travellers facilitated colonial expansion and at the same time secured credibility and place within European science. The interconnections between science and the colonial state, generally, became more meaningful as encounters and engagements with the Indian and African populations gained prominence.

In understanding these engagements, it is important to recognize that while new ideas of European science and medicine, with their incipient hegemony, may have been 'enforced', they were socially and culturally 're-constituted.' In doing so, thus, colonial medicine was shaped by the very nature of these processes of reception and assimilation in India and South Africa. In view of this, thus, bodies were seen as sites on which colonial expressions of health and medical prerogatives could be dictated to and enforced upon. While issues of coercive power and modernity remain embedded in these expressions, they existed in various forms as discussed in individual essays in the volume. Equally significant were the results of transfer of ideas and knowledge in mutual engagements. In one fairly uncommon situation, these 'transfers' led to an unusual syncretism of knowledge systems which entailed a mutual form of interaction and influence between white and African medical practitioners[26] when the latter chose to adopt the healing practices of Indian Ayurveda medicine that bore parallels with Zulu medical practices.

In a recent study on the rise of the middle classes in a global context, Abel Ricardo Lopez and Barbara Weinstein seek to assess the 'historical understandings of modernity and middle class formation' in Australia, America and Britain.[27] Historicizing this development in colonial India, in Chapter 1 of this volume Poonam Bala focuses on the role of the urban-educated, middle-class elites and the members of higher social echelons in engaging issues of modernity in a form akin to a 'fractured modernity'.[28] It is argued that these elites remained instrumental in renegotiating the very same project of modernity of which they were a product. This was the project that engaged revisiting Indian medical science, facilitated by the rising national movement which also witnessed the emergence of Ayurveda[29] as a political and national symbol. In engaging encounters with imperial imperatives and western biomedicine, the existence of indigenous medical systems (including Ayurveda and Unani) and medical pluralism led to the emergence of new forms of institutional and structural paradigms.

In Chapter 2, Steve Phatlane traces the trajectory of the acceptance and rejection of indigenous medical knowledge by colonial administrators and in the post-apartheid government. Hence within these initial two chapters tensions and conflicts between knowledge formation and proponents of western biomedicine are evident.

In Chapter 3, Russel Viljoen reflects on the emerging colonial identities as a result of the transmission and influence of indigenous and colonial medical knowledge and healing practices at the Cape of Good Hope under the colonial conquest of the VOC. Because of its focus on indigenous knowledge, as possessed by the Khoikhoi, this essay covers an earlier period of colonial rule, that of the Dutch conquest in the seventeenth century. It also offers useful comparisons with Poonam Bala's and Steve Phatlane's discussions on the conflicts and tensions, punctuated by periods of resistance and acceptance, between colonial and indigenous medical encounters.

In Chapter 4, Samiparna Samanta goes beyond the established historical underpinnings of understanding the human–animal relations under colonialism to identify processes of knowledge formation as seen in the cattle plague. While disciplining the indigenous farmers as much as the diseased animal formed part of the policy dictates, for the Bengali *bhadralok*, who exhibited receptivity to colonial ideas of modernizing traditional forms of knowledge, the animal–human association was defined by them in terms of European ideas of science and rationality. In this chapter, as well as Bala's, the role of the influential patrons and elites in appropriating indigenous knowledge as well as the formation of new knowledge forms as a result of their engagements with the colonial authorities, remains paramount.

The significant historical events, changing medical paradigms, structural transformations and new institutional frameworks under the exigencies of the British empire reveal various aspects of interconnected histories in India and South Africa. The interconnected histories and the social and cultural transformations underlying them have been portrayed in Myron Echenberg's analysis of the third plague pandemic in British colonial ports across the globe.[30] Echenberg documents the challenges posed by the onset of the third plague epidemic – challenges that also dictated, or sometimes reinforced, unequal relations between hegemonic structures and ruling ideologies. The challenges became noticeable when at the turn of the twentieth century, the new paradigm of public health measures revealed new encounters with different cultures in the port cities. Thus, while Alexandria and Sydney were more successful in containing the epidemic thorough 'consensus' and 'cooperation', in India (as also in Hong Kong), imposition and 'enforced' ways often fuelled social conflicts between the colonial imperatives and the Indian population which, in turn, was aggravated by nationalist politics and political movements, thus limiting the public health initiatives. In Chapter 5, in gauging the consequences of the plague pandemic in South Africa, Howard Phillips portrays these connections through an analysis of Gandhi's autobiographic writings written during his stay in South Africa. Seen against a political backdrop when nationalistic feelings were rife in India, if race was not an issue, there was much to decipher in terms of caste and class attitude from Gandhi's *Autobiography*. Along the same tenets, with a comparative approach, Natasha Sarkar's chapter explores the trajectories of colonial medical intervention in managing plague in India and South Africa where, besides its impact on the social and cultural lives of indigenous populations, the character of colonial medicine was shaped by the very nature of its reception and assimilation. In both, elements of social and political transformations facilitated by the plague epidemic as well as its management take precedence.

While the science of bacteriology opened up new vistas for colonial medicine in the late nineteenth century, it created a wide gulf between scientific ideas in Europe and the imperial prerogatives in the tropical colonies.[31] Despite the revolutionary progress in biomedicine, sanitary practices and public health measures, infectious diseases were often seen as a threat to the economy and political stability of the colonial government. Arguably, thus, as Echenberg argues, 'the scramble for territory in Africa and Asia and the American takeover of much of what remained of Spain's old empire in the Caribbean and the Pacific had placed a heavy burden on newly subject peoples'.[32]

While scientific and medical explanations of communicable diseases have dominated medical paradigms, understanding the role of animals as vectors has provided a framework for the medical community since the late nineteenth century. Yet, in India, the role of rats in the transmission of plague did not find an easy acceptance and recognition within the international scientific community. The trajectory of initial rejection and a hesitant acceptance of rat as a vector, and the role of the Plague Research Commission in maintaining a subtle balance between colonial expectations, scientific mandates and their possible consequences on the colonized is discussed by Katherine Royer in Chapter 7. She highlights interesting debates around assigning 'rat' an important place within the historiography. In a recent and enriching study, Martha Few and Zeb Tortorici portray significant contributions of animal–human to 'histories and cultures', with new interpretations on the role of animals as 'social actors' in the colonizing attempts in Latin America.[33]

Among the several colonial initiatives undertaken as part of the colonial project to 'reform' and 'modernize' indigenous traditions, those aimed at the management of childbirth remained paramount. Throughout much of the nineteenth century, and later, the Indian tradition of *dai*, or midwifery, has been subject to scrutiny in debates and reforms on childbirth as part of the discourses on health in colonial India. Understanding the social construction of *dais*, or midwives, thus entails tracing the dynamics of the changing socio-cultural context; and Bengal, owing to its socio-cultural, political and administrative significance, is a site that has enabled this. As Krishna Soman argues, 'Colonial attempts at "modernising" the established practices in midwifery were often met with resistance, as management of childbirth became an agenda of intervention in favour of establishing western medicine by the British.'[34] Arabinda Samanta's discussion, in engaging issues in reproductive health and childbirth and the socio-cultural implications of new medical technologies as opposed to natural body processes, raises new perspectives of the manner in which public and private domains gradually merged at the behest of local elites, practitioners and medical establishments. Seen as interfering with Indian traditions, arguably the Indian indifference to childbirth and maternal health, and social and cultural reforms and nationalistic engagements in keeping the cultural traditions with the western paradigm, allude to the 'enforced modernity' in colonial India.[35]

In the late nineteenth century, African psychiatry unravelled the manner in which colonial psychiatry existed as an 'indispensable' part of colonial control. As Harriet Deacon puts it, 'in the Cape Colony, the concept of the "African insane," a violent, criminal, incurable group more affected by physical than psychological therapy, was consolidated during the latter part of the nineteenth century'.[36] In any case, ideas of the universality of medical knowledge about madness and racism remained deeply entrenched in the Cape, 'because of the need to embrace both white and black insanity in lunacy legislation and medical discourse (and thus protect the profession), while differentiating between them on grounds of diagnosis, prognosis and treatment'.[37] While asylum management was based on class and racial divisions in the Cape, it also gave rise to a universal psychiatry theory that continued well into the late twentieth century.[38] Drawing upon these changes, in Chapter 9 Jonathan Saha describes parallels in India and sub-Saharan Africa where issues of race, gender, criminality and insanity dominated colonial attempts at implementing disciplinary measures for criminals and convicts; at the same time, colonial prisons were used as a site of expression for resistance and disruption by the indigenous populations. Psychiatry and disciplinary practices in India were, thus, more punitive than reformatory. On a similar note, Sally Swartz illustrates a 'colonial psychiatry-oppression' relationship as being definitive in colonial expressions in the Cape colony, while the psychiatry and psychiatric practices were still being shaped by these relationships. She brings out the debates that go into the making of histories of colonial psychiatry in Africa with a unifying theme of 'the relationship of colonial psychiatry (and psychiatric institutions) to racism and oppression'. While the late nineteenth century saw the emergence of new scientific and medical paradigms, with ideas of race and racial differences entwined with issues of morality, when 'a theory of politics and rights was transformed into an argument about nature; equality … was taken to be matter not of ethics, but of anatomy'.[39]

Yet another tool deployed to discipline the colonized was seen in the development of medico-legal methods and disciplinary institutions for the administration of justice and legality in issues of criminality and public health, as discussed by Jeffrey M. Jentzen in the final contribution to this collection. More importantly, the same practices were employed by the indigenous people to protect themselves against the perceived oppressive measures of the colonial government.

The nature of encounters presented in this volume alludes to an important set of outcomes. It exhibits elements of extreme conflict and tensions between colonizers, their initiatives and the colonized. If enforced modernity was on the agenda of western hegemonic ideals, then resistance, and a hesitant, somewhat total rejection of colonial values was also widespread, even though, as indicated earlier, the encounter was not confined to processes of 'adaptation' and 'resistance'. However, given that both India and South Africa exhibited similarities and parallels in both social structure and political processes, their histories have been shaped by the shifting nature of these processes; more importantly, the existence of medical pluralism allowed the simultaneous existence of several knowledge structures,[40] while the boundaries between the encountering paradigms of knowledge have remained 'flexible'. To this effect, 'flexibility' can be gauged in terms of 'allowing each agency to interpret and re-interpret' the boundaries of the paradigms within which these negotiations are taking place, often characterized by the emergence of new structural formations. Besides, despite being punctuated by unsettling moments, the 'flexible' boundaries facilitated assimilation of medical ideas and paradigms with ideas that drew from 'tradition' but were promoted and facilitated by 'innovation'. In seeking to understand the outcomes of mutual assimilation, thus, it may be significant to note that the capacity to 'assimilate new technologies is as significant as inventiveness itself',[41] which then becomes 'a history of transmission through social, cultural and political engagements' so that these trajectories represent histories *within* the region.

In sum, the essays presented in this volume attempt to unravel an important area of scholarly interest – that of understanding 'medicine–empire–people' relations in a broader and comparative context of *histories within* the region which, I hope, will usefully elicit further interest in similar studies in a global perspective and in other regions.

1 'RE-CONSTRUCTING' INDIAN MEDICINE: THE ROLE OF CASTE IN LATE NINETEENTH- AND TWENTIETH-CENTURY INDIA

Poonam Bala

The history of medicine in India represents a significant trajectory of both resistance and accommodation of various medical forms of knowledge, often associated with changes in the ruling state, its ideologies and imperatives. In this context, it is not surprising that nineteenth- and twentieth-century India was marked by a series of major challenges faced by protagonists of Indian medicine,[1] nationalists, reformers, and influential patrons and elites. What these challenges were, who they were managed by and how they were best managed are some of the questions that often loom large in debates on medicine in colonial India. In discussing Indian medicine under British rule, thus, two main themes emerge: first, the existence of influential local elites, intellectuals, nationalists and reformers, as patrons supporting the medical system; and second, the challenges posed as a result of shifting policies, especially following the implementation of the Montague-Chelmsford Reforms in 1919.[2] While indigenous patrons, although initially hesitant, appropriated indigenous medical knowledge, sometimes reconstructing and reassessing it, power and authority remained issues of concern for protagonists of both Indian and western systems in relation to the Reforms, for the new system of governance allowed more freedom in the hands of Indian ministers to take charge of health issues.

The late nineteenth century witnessed the deployment of science and medicine as signifying cultural authority, forging new alliances alongside the emergence of new associations that enabled the reinforcement of scientific activities, through a small section of western-educated Indians. With their high social status in Indian society, indigenous patrons represented the best-educated social echelon and, hence, were quick in responding to British calls for new medical policies. While the existence of high-caste Hindus facilitated and reinforced ideas of reconstructing traditional Indian medicine, it also reveals an interplay of power, hegemony and monopoly between Indian and western medical sciences, through existing elements of authority and hegemony of biomedicine. Concerned primarily with various social reforms, they 'published tracts on science with or without government patronage', for which reason religious and social reforms came to be seen through science's authoritative 'second sight'.[3] Much of the twentieth century witnessed the emergence of the Indian State accompanied by new caste identities and varying levels of patronage which shaped the very nature of medical practice in colonial India through a specific trajectory of conflict, acceptance and eventual accommodation of indigenous and western systems of knowledge. Indicative of a process of mutual interaction and encounter, the dynamics of engagement with science, medicine and authority is best understood in terms of the processes that underlie these prerogatives. The curious phase of conflict and resistance, and possible acceptance and convergence, was manifest in the culture of Indian medicine, the protagonists of which were high caste Hindus, intellectuals and elites. Prior to the advent of the British in India, both 'technological and political factors imposed limitations on the horizontal stretch of castes, while caste-wise division of labour favoured the cooperation of households from different castes'.[4] Medicine was one area where caste boundaries of the traditional hierarchical order became less distinct as one moves into late nineteenth- and early twentieth-century India. The political strength that has often been defined by the occupational specialization of the caste and has enabled an understanding of inter-caste relations, also became flexible in these matters.

More recently, the limits of Western biomedicine in terms of its authority have been projected in terms of the nature of conflicting situations to medical power in colonial contexts.[5] Likewise, Ayurveda medicine became a site not only representing a rich cultural medical heritage of India but a site through which these new transformations and the dynamics of Ayurveda–biomedicine were visible. Discussed in recent works,[6] visions of transformations in Indian medical knowledge have been understood in terms of a new form of Ayurveda that came into being 'as a reaction to the introduction and patronage of a new medical system by the British colonialists'.[7] Initial reaction to, and later an understanding of, a system of knowledge has also been a central topic of interest in the sociological study of the nature of modernity. Indeed, despite the 'differences' between Ayurveda and Western medicine, attempts at appropriating medical knowledge by the East India Company (hereafter EIC) authorities as well as indigenous patrons, continued unabated. Initially, indigenous medicine received support from the EIC administrators in the early part of its rule, in 1832, in the form of the Native Medical Institution[8] (hereafter NMI), often claimed as an EIC establishment with simultaneous instructions in indigenous and Western medicine. Established with the purpose of training Indians to fill the positions of native doctors in the civil and military establishments of the Bengal Presidency, the NMI ceased to exist in 1835 after a decision to assess medical education at the NMI as fairly 'inadequate' in training quality practitioners was unanimously accepted.[9] Issues of lack of anatomical practices was also a guiding force behind this decision. This was, perhaps, the start of an unsettling 'professional encounter', which was reinforced in later years. Even in England, a formal medical education system was virtually non-existent well into the second decade of the nineteenth century, when the Apothecaries Act of 1815 initiated formalization of medical education; the tangible amendments came much later, with the need to reform medical education and to regulate medical practice. Henry Warburton,[10] Chairman of the Select Committee on Anatomy, pioneered the transformation of medical practice in the early decades of the nineteenth century; he drafted the Anatomy Bill in 1828 to monitor schools' supply of and access to unclaimed bodies of people who died in workhouses and hospitals. With the reporting of unprecedented murders by the *Lancet* and the *British Medical Journal*, a new Anatomy Bill was introduced and promulgated as an Act in 1832.[11] While the Anatomy Act of 1832 did much to stop the unlawful acquisition of human bodies by granting licenses for anatomical purposes to any person qualified to practise, fear and suspicion continued to loom large in the minds of the public.[12] Several policy initiatives were seen to maintain links with the regulations governing Britain at the time; this is also seen in concerns over anatomical practices followed in the medical curriculum in India and Britain. These trepidations become more pertinent as one looks at the narrative trajectory of anatomy and surgery in nineteenth-century England together with legalization after the Anatomy Act of 1834. This Act not only gave medicine a new professional status but also remained indispensable to early medical policies in India.[13]

The reforms in medical education were an important part of educational policies in the nineteenth century. The abolition of the NMI provided an impetus to reforms in medical education in the years to follow, for several of these policy dictates followed from those in the metropole during the early years of a new and reforming medical profession. The demise of the NMI did not, however, affect the practise of Ayurveda as medicine continued to be practised at the village and family levels, 'while having little to do with larger state structures'.[14]

By the middle of the nineteenth century, the implementation of Thomas Babington Macaulay's idea to introduce English as the medium of instruction as well as the arts and sciences of Europe in India, influenced the way in which the Calcutta elite were to envision India. This may have been the start of nationalism at its best, for

> Indians not only intensified their search of inspirational models within their own heritage but felt compelled to appropriate the scholarly models of the Orientalists and infuse them with heightened feelings of national pride.[15]

Perhaps, this may have been the precursor to later ideas of self-legitimation and cultural identity. Besides, a new intellectual tradition was nurtured as a legacy of the Hindu College[16] when Henry Louis Vivian Derozio[17] was appointed as an instructor of English literature. By the mid-eighteenth century, Calcutta had flourished into a viable urban centre where the educated and prominent Bengali elites made fortunes with their commercial associations with the British.[18] Although initially not inclined towards literary activities, their successors embraced literary engagements.[19]

The Medical Registration Act of 1858 and the establishment of the General Medical Council, for instance, were two major landmarks in this direction. By the late nineteenth century, medical education had almost become 'the greatest power in the profession'.[20] The role of caste in relation to medical knowledge in colonial India is exemplary of the modernizing approach that involved the adaptation of traditional structures – a transition that is sometimes seen as 'not being autonomous but part of a process which affected both the metropolis and the colony'.[21] While much of late nineteenth- and early twentieth-century India was marked by efforts at 'protecting' indigenous knowledge, the elites and the influentials were active participants of a new vision of Ayurveda. Their long history of an unsettling association with the colonial authorities, punctuated by phases of conflict, appropriation and convergence, and possible 'modification' of Indian medical knowledge contributed to this vision and re-examination of the Ayurvedic essentials. Although initially troubled and occasionally paused by moments of mutual acceptance, much of the middle and late nineteenth century witnessed an obdurate relation between the colonial policy dictates and the requirements of the indigenous population.

Throughout much of the late nineteenth and twentieth century, medicine served as an important site through which the colonial regime could be legitimated. Issues around the authority of medicine were first visible in the elite discourse in Bengal, although they later spread to other provinces. Known as the 'most canonical of all literary of nineteenth-century Bengal, Bankim Chandra Chattopadhyaya is known for promoting science as the superior form of knowledge'.[22] The Bengali literati formed the Bengal Social Science Association in 1867 which later became a 'centre for excellence in research on sociology of science'.[23] While political voices and opinions of high caste Hindus were significant factors in negotiating a new and 'modern' status of Ayurveda, travel, contact and the proliferation of women's medical discourses were equally exemplary of the emergence of new ideas of identity and space. In addition, the 'gender-segregated forms of medical practice and hospital care could be achieved through the establishment of clinical institutions – hospitals and dispensaries exclusively for women and children'.[24]

Convincingly demonstrated in her recent study, Narin Hassan discusses how women travellers facilitated a shift 'to the "new" Indian woman in the late nineteenth century as a figure shaped by and imagined to support colonial and medical reform from within India itself',[25] further stating that representations of reform and cultural progress became a focal point within a number of texts produced by British and Indian women in colonial India during the 1880s and 1890s at the same time as the Dufferin Fund expanded medical focus on the management of bodies and empire as intertwined.[26]

While 'women's medical discourses' could be seen as 'central conditions of the empire',[27] it was through them that women travellers could negotiate their identity.[28] In India, these negotiations were reinforced by the establishment of the Countess of Dufferin's Fund in 1880 to provide medical aid to women in India; for it forged new alliances resulting from an interaction between British female doctors and native women. Thus, in the context of British medical women practising in India, they 'were colonizing women because they brought Indian women within the purview of the "medical gaze" which was at the same time an imperial gaze'.[29]

Dr Francis Hoggan's[30] seminal article, 'Medical Women for India', started a new chapter in providing health and medical care to Indian women. Influenced by her, George Kittredge (an American business resident in Bombay) and Sorabjee Shapurji Bengali (a prominent member of the Parsi community), who were among the most prominent influential patrons, set up the Medical Women for India Fund of Bombay in 1882 with the idea of establishing a hospital and a dispensary exclusively for women in Bombay; with the same motivation, the Dufferin Fund was also set up by colonial administrators, with support from the rich and influential local patrons.

Besides the involvement of and efforts by various high caste groups, nationalists and proponents of indigenous medicine, several women were also at the helm of the move towards a new vision of Indian medicine, most prominent of whom was Krupabai Satthianadhan in whose writings reform and moving from the past old traditions are obvious. Hailed as a 'figure of late nineteenth-century colonial representation',[31] pioneering the reform activities of the late nineteenth century, through her *Miscellaneous Writings*, Krupabai Satthianadhan could easily 'articulate models of domestic management that borrowed, and sometimes reshaped, such a tradition in Britain'.[32] Not surprisingly, by this time, the progress of literary activities and journalistic enterprise were seen as a sure marker of the impact and spread of English education.[33] Besides, the proliferation of indigenous medical literature also added to the spur in literary activities at the time with the proliferation of Urdu literature and the 'formation of gentlemanly societies of *Unani* doctors from the 1880s'.[34] Significantly, several journals and pamphlets produced by the middle-class, educated elite contributed to the move to establish Indian thoughts as part of the country's cultural heritage. Prafulla Chandra Ray's seminal work on the history of Hindu chemistry bears testimony to this. In addition, his nationalist ideas found expression in his article, 'India Before and After Mutiny' which he wrote in 1885.[35]

The rise of the printing press also aided the effective communication of cultural thoughts on self-preservation as well as on personal care and health. Although the 'middle class constituted the social-base of reform movements and participated energetically in the development of the new print culture', it was the 'prominent *bhadralok* intellectuals who received support from "some of the city's great *nouveau riche* upper class Indian families".[36] Under these circumstances, a 'second look' at the past meant a lucid projection of Indian science and medicine as vital to cultural tradition. Notable among the new visions was the projection of Vedas[37] as validating the advanced level of medical knowledge of Indian medicine. Kissory Chandra Mitra, a *bhadralok* intellectual, was instrumental in promoting this image of India's traditional past.[38] With an appreciation for Indian medicine and the armamentarium of drugs it could offer, Prafulla Chandra Ray[39] founded the Bengal Chemical and Pharmaceutical Works in 1893 to enable the manufacture and sales of indigenous drugs. Defending the scientific claims of Ayurveda, several journals disseminating its scientific essentials were brought out; notable among them was *Arogya-Jiwan*, a Hindi journal focusing on women's health launched in 1893. Over issues of specific drugs for treatment, thus, 'claims to an essential composition theme treatable only by the medicine available indigenously was a common theme among those writing medical books for popular consumption in the early twentieth century'.[40]

Prior to this, the foundation of the Indian Association for the Cultivation of Science in 1876 by Mahendralal Sircar was a new chapter in the Indian assertion of indigenous sciences and medicine. He founded the *Calcutta Journal of Medicine* in 1868 with the idea of increasing Indian engagements in medical and scientific activities.[41] Dismayed by the 'functionalist approach' of colonial sciences, as David Arnold puts it,[42] Mahendralal Sircar remained instrumental in reinforcing an awareness of the need to bring scientific and medical education under 'native management and control'.[43]

The impact of Western scientific and medical progress has been understood as a process of 'mutual learning' – a process from which Britain and her colonies were to benefit. Hassan identifies 'travel' and transactions of women overseas as contributing to this exchange which led to circulation of medical knowledge, ideas and objects.[44] Overall, this was more than a mere diffusion of medical ideas, for the encounter led to the emergence of new forms of institutions and structures at the periphery as well as the core.[45] While the indigenous population remained engaged with casting a new vision for India's medical heritage through education and literary activities, an important policy change and a landmark in the dynamics of the events that would later shape perceptions of Indian society, its caste composition and cultural heritage came with the 1901 Census. Acclaimed as the most 'crucial' policy imperative guiding colonial ideas concerning public appointments in the services of the empire, the Census created 'social consciousness' and reinforced caste divisions and religious identities that were deployed by the colonial administrators to explain 'caste-disease' association in India; more so, the manner in which the Census explained and defined specific disease situations within caste categories fuelled nationalistic tensions in the Indian. Thus, reifying caste from its social context, the Census classified the Indian population on the basis of social standing and social precedence. Viewing this as 'a more dramatic illustration of the use of "caste" rhetoric and the activities of "caste" publicists', L. Carroll identifies these as adopted by the English-educated 'who aspired after jobs and political place, who were hurt by "caste" ratios and by "low caste" classifications, who needed communal constituencies to prove their "leadership" role and qualify for nomination to political post'.[46] In the aftermath of a statistical grouping of the Indian society, new policy initiatives were undertaken with new aspects of political and administrative control of the Indian population.

Policy Changes, Indigenous Engagements and Medicine

The late nineteenth and early decades of the twentieth century were marked by several changes in the nature of the political state – changes that would eventually alter the way in which Indian medicine was to be practised and perceived in later years. Seen as an administrative expression of 'the colonial definition of Indian society',[47] certain local associations actively responded to caste-consciousness policy of the colonial government, for this affected the employment of Indians in the colonial bureaucracy. Results of this became apparent. For instance, the Nadar Mahajana Sangam educational and charitable institution came into being in response to the colonial government's interest in supporting diverse sections of the Indian society in public appointments and political representations. The revival of indigenous medicine was a historic result of these changes, for it unfolded the engagements between indigenous medicine, colonial imperatives and policy initiatives. Over the course of a few years, the Ayurvedic movement became a major revivalist movement in Indian history. Expressed in terms of textual authority through translation of Sanskrit texts into English, aided by the printing press that popularized Ayurvedic knowledge, as well as creating a new institutional support through various dispensaries, the movement had far reaching impact on the indigenous population.[48] I see the engagement of the Ayurvedic movement with Western medicine in terms of institutional and organizational alliances expressed in the late nineteenth and early twentieth centuries which found expression in the establishment of the first Ayurvedic dispensary in Calcutta in 1878 by Kaviraj Chandra Kishore Sen and the foundation of the Arya Vaidya Samajam[49] in 1902 by P. S.Varier, both of whom were ardent patrons of Ayurvedic knowledge, and hence of the Ayurvedic movement.

Linked with similar activities, other medical practitioners participated in the movement, incorporating Unani medicine in the process. Acclaimed as addressing the issues of vaids,[50] the Arya Vaidya Samajam provided them new directions for preparing drugs purely on Ayurvedic principles for more effective treatments; supported by local princes and professional middle classes, the Arya Vaidya Samajam eventually became a hallmark of professionalism in Indian medicine, much like its western counterpart.[51] The partition of Bengal in 1905 marked another event that intensified country-wide and nationalistic visions of colonial attitudes. It sparked off protests and political unrest at a time when nationalistic feelings and anti-colonial sentiments were strong. Ideas of conceptualizations of nationhood in the form of *swadeshi*, or self-rule, followed.[52] It also intensified the growing nationalist campaigns that would, henceforth, include new educational and technological realignments. Continued agitation, punctuated by occasional violent reactions and administrative pressure from the elites and medical practitioners alike, compelled its annulment in 1911. This marked the beginnings of a nation-state when 'initial attempts to "relocate colonial power unleashed a political struggle to establish a nation-state that would institute the logic of rational aritifice more fully and efficiently."'[53]

As the nationalist sentiments grew stronger, *swadeshi* came to be recognized as a nationalist ideology through which ideas and visions of 'modern' India as expressions of India's cultural heritage could be articulated. Drawing on traditions and cultural identity with an inspiration to legitimize and reform became the ultimate aim of these articulated ideas. Arguably, claims to the existence of scientific traditions in India continued to be made by the Hindu intellectuals. In this scenario, valorization of ancient Hindu texts over contemporary texts acquired prominence.[54] This also meant that 'Hindu texts could be projected as the basis of unitary modern community of Indians'.[55] Members of the urban educated class became increasingly engaged as advocates of Hindu cultural nationalism.

The period between 1920 and 1940 was one marked by mass movements across the country, which made imperative some kind of allegiance and mutual cooperation between princely states and the colonial state.[56]

In this essay, the role of scientific knowledge, institutions and colonialism in mutually co-producing each other has been analysed. Under the overarching rubric of colonial structures and imperatives, amateur scientists often sought to deploy scientific expertise to expand the empire while at the same time seeking to take advantage of the opportunities to develop their careers as 'scientists'. To this effect, scientific collaborations with India, although minimal in the initial phases of British rule, were punctuated by noticeable 'eclectic exchanges and syncretic interface between western and Indian medicine' in the nineteenth century.[57]

Amidst an intense political situation emerged a new landmark in the history of medical engagements in colonial India. The All India Ayurvedic Mahasammelan (hereafter, Mahasammelan) was formed in 1907; hailed as the first organised effort by the Ayurvedic community and nationalist leaders, a vision for a new India was one of its objectives.[58] Following this, much of the second decade of the twentieth century witnessed not only the negotiation of changes and relocation of colonial power but equally significant repercussions of these negotiations that were manifested in social consciousness in Indian society. More so, during the interwar years, 'Ayurveda came to be increasingly linked with nationalist politics',[59] aided by the scholarly reappraisals of India's medical past and heritage. Notable among these works was that of P. C. Ray's *History of Hindu Chemistry* (1932) for which he was often lauded as a nationalist scientist.[60] Besides, the emergence of a medical market, 'depicting an epitome of colonial engagements with India, going beyond the commercial interests to embody intellectual and sensual interests as well', perhaps, enabled these efforts.[61] The defence for Indian science and medicine had become apparent by this time. Popular journals on Ayurveda added to these claims. Shaukat Rai Chaudhary's *Ayurveda Ka Vaigyanik Swaroop* (1918) promoted notes on Ayurvedic pathology and physiology.[62]

It can be argued that in colonial India, medicine and policies were closely intertwined which meant that every policy change resulted in a new medical transformation that perhaps, closely or not so closely, related to its predecessor. Needless to say, this appears to have continued in postcolonial India talking, of which Alavi remarks, 'the structure of the contemporary Indian society has been shaped by 200 years of the colonial experience and cannot be grasped without fully understanding the nature of colonial transformation.'[63]

In this context, it is important to note that these colonial transformations were a move towards assertions of authoritative cultural representations in which a modern nation could be visualized. The introduction of Montague-Chelmsford Reforms of 1919 increased the nationalist pressure, and hence to 'protect' indigenous knowledge. The Reforms were instrumental in bringing about a consciousness of new negotiations between the indigenous population and colonial authorities; representing the first step in the decentralization of health administration in India, they were equally noted for extending political power and autonomy to local governments which meant that the establishment of a dual government-central and provincial, or *dyarchy*, created two major categories of 'reserved' and 'transferred'; while the former included issues of finance, police and revenue, tax among others, public health and education came under the charge of elected Indian ministers as a 'transferred' category. They also alluded to a new form of political and civic responsibility assigned to the Indian elite as well as to new health policies that henceforth would be subject to accountability in terms of allocation and health expenditures. Seen as an institutionalization of health and physical well-being of the population, the new form of governance also revealed the manner in which political power was to be implemented in later years. Thus, 'the disposition of society as a milieu of physical well-being, which figured as an important political objective in which the "police" of the social body must ensure along with those of economic regulations and the needs of order'.[64]

In the aftermath of this policy change, and continuing from the previous decades, religious reformers, medical practitioners and educated elites sought to valorize India's cultural heritage through translations of ancient canonical texts and claims of medical knowledge as part of India's pristine heritage. Their intentions were to revisit indigenous knowledge and to modify it, partly to bring it in par with the advancing western forms of knowledge and partly to challenge the policy dictates that demanded this change.

The Reforms gave power and autonomy to elected minsters and local governments, allowing an increasing entry of Indians in the bureaucratic services, the medical services saw for the first time a rapid 'Indianisation' and a deeper association of elected ministers with issues of public health and indigenous medicine. The Government of India Act 1935 provided further autonomy to provincial governments with the establishment of the Central Advisory Board of Health in 1937 allocating public health activities to the newly appointed Public Health Commissioner.[65] Not surprisingly, when new ideas of a 'population problem' dominated the thinking of the public health officials, in the interwar period, Indian intellectuals and other influential patrons and protagonists of western science and medicine, including economists, eugenicists, women social reformers and birth controllers quickly responded to this new 'concern'.[66]

Thus, by the late nineteenth and early twentieth centuries, the 'undisputed' authority of western medicine had found expressions in the various reforms undertaken at the time. Continuing into the twentieth century, and paused by several turns in the political events, it became evident by the 1930s that Indian nationalists were more concerned with dealing with issues of public health, while still maintaining that power and authority were no less significant. In his examination of the history of the connection between India and Europe, Wilhelm Halbfass claims that 'the encounter with modern science and technology was the momentous part of its encounter with the West'.[67] In the same light, at the inaugural session of the Indian Science Congress in the year 1914, the immeasurable worth of science and its indispensability in industrial regeneration was highlighted.[68] Although the initial realization to institutionalize science and to fulfil the 'early visions of Asia as the "nurse of sciences" and the "inventress of delightful and useful arts", was attained through the establishment in 1784 of the Asiatic Society by William Jones, the Society'[69] almost became anachronistic towards the late nineteenth century, remembered as a precursor to 'introducing and institutionalizing modern "western science" and stimulating new research in colonial India'.[70] In identifying issues of power and authority, Nicholas B. Dirks sees colonialism as 'a hegemonic structure, which articulated its own particular impact and influence through a variety of institutional and ideological forms'.[71] These structures, it may be argued, were expressed when, in their attempts to bring Indian intellectualism and the cultural manifestations of developed arts and sciences close to a meaningful relationship with western knowledge, the British sought to search for 'correspondences and connections' that would suitably place India within the cultural context of Europe,[72] and hence make it more easily fathomable. Thus, while 'Indians assimilated and adapted western doctrines and technologies, so western scholars and administrators embarked on a protracted intellectual engagement with Indian epistemologies that lasted well into the nineteenth century'.[73]

While Indian nationalism functioned as a paradigm within which nationalistic sentiments and claims for Hindu science and medicine were expressed, it also witnessed tensions as it sought to interact with colonial power and imperatives. This was best seen in the late nineteenth and early twentieth centuries when several years of encounter and engagements with British authorities and their policy dictates witnessed a powerful resurgence of new modalities of understanding indigenous sciences. While association of Ayurveda with nationalist politics remained paramount in these efforts, its encounters with advocates of western medicine resulted in noticeable changes in the way Ayurveda was perceived, as the 'revelation' of its scientific essentials became intense. In the years following the Reforms, management of indigenous medicine became the stated goal of provincial governments with full support from the Indian National Congress as the leading voice of political and nationalist opinions favouring religious and cultural reforms while also voicing demands for state support and recognition. As nationalist voices grew in strength and number, so did the defence of Ayurveda. At a time when Ayurveda and its canonical texts came under increasing attack, the role of the educated and influential elite in its defences, undoubtedly, remained imperative. For instance, G. Srinivasa Murti,[74] although educated in western medicine, provided a strong defence for Ayurveda in his report on the state of indigenous medicine in 1921.[75] About the same time, 1921, Shyamadas Vacaspati, an Ayurvedic scholar of repute, founded a national university of Bengal, the Gaudiya Saravidyayatana which was later expanded to accommodate an Ayurvedic wing. Several other educational institutions were established in a move to protest against the increasing and popular notions of colonial 'intrusions'. This, however, did not mean the end of the association of Indian and western thoughts, nor did it deter perceptions of 'mutual' engagements from being implemented. The formation of the Ayurvedic Committee in 1923, promote Ayurvedic learning through a central Ayurvedic College;[76] The college was an amalgamation of the extant Ayurvedic Colleges – Astanga Ayurvedic College, Baidyashastrapith and the Govinda Sundari Ayurvedic College – and adopted an integrated course of teaching Indian and western medical sciences that proves this point. Most of these developments and encounters were a feature of the Bengal Presidency, with Calcutta as the capital city and the seat of all administrative activities. As a historically important city, Calcutta speaks of the start of a long trajectory of EIC rule and colonial rule; it was also important in unravelling the encounters of Indian and western cultures. Thus, the developments in Calcutta can be seen as 'a two-sided process of acculturation, or the merging of interests and identities by representatives of civilizations in encounter'.[77]

The rise of the medical community, the emergence of institutional networks the intellectual and literary engagements, social and religious reforms, and nationalism coupled with a vision of Ayurveda as a 'nationalist' symbol, were all manifestations of public perception of medical and scientific knowledge. Situating these developments within sociological approaches to the public understanding of science and medicine presents useful explanations of the dilemma of science, scientific authority and modernity.[78] Locke sees this dilemma as one that would attempt to 'deconstruct scientific statements by localizing them as the particular products of particular scientists', which is specific 'to competent members within modernity'.[79] Thus, while the Reforms ensured responsibility to Indian ministers in crucial aspects of health and education, they also created new capacities for medical men to appropriate as well as 'oppose' the overarching western medical paradigm as per their requirements. The real change in the colonial transformations and indigenous structures, however, came with new medical engagements during the outbreak of epidemics, initiating new sanitary practices and implementing preventive measures at the popular level. Links between medicine and colonial power became evident by then. While sanitation was seen as a 'new order of knowledge and power'[80] epidemics too ushered in a new mode of handling public health issues. It also justified a more focused need to address them, for it was seen as a threat to colonial security.[81] Issues on protecting the colonial population came to the fore when quarantine measures adopted by them were looked upon unfavourably. As Sarkar argues in her essay in this volume, any attempts to segregate plague victims was met with opposition from various caste communities that rejected any intermingling owing to fear of 'pollution'.[82]

To conclude, although initially limiting and constrained, the impact of medical policies in British India was significantly enhanced as a result of an increasing involvement of the indigenous population including medical practitioners, elites and other influential people. Clearly, new interactions and social engagements paved the way for attempts to defend, understand, valorise, reform and rationalise Indian medicine. Made possible by the rich and the powerful, medical practitioners and the local population, notable political changes at the turn of the twentieth century provided the much-needed framework for indigenous political activities, as claims to indigenous traditions and knowledge were integrated within the nationalist paradigms; unimpeded by the growth of western medical profession, elements of power, authority and agency were expressed through the new paradigm which also witnessed social and public reactions to colonial policies. In the process, and intercepted by ideas of modernity and claims to professional power, the encounter also reveals the limitations to medical power imposed by the 'appropriation and opposition' to western medicine.

2 THE RESURGENCE OF INDIGENOUS MEDICINE IN THE AGE OF THE HIV/AIDS PANDEMIC: SOUTH AFRICA BEYOND THE 'MIRACLE'

Steve Phatlane

Introduction

The inauguration of Nelson Mandela as the first democratically elected president of South Africa brought down the final curtain on decades of apartheid misrule, marking the beginning of a new chapter of hope for the 'rainbow nation'. This was an achievement hailed by the international community as the political miracle of the 1990s.[1] But to dampen the euphoria, it soon became evident that in the area of health care, the infant democracy had inherited an expensive, hospital-based, high-tech medicine that was not only inappropriate for the health needs of the majority of rural black South Africans, but also reflected a highly fragmented health system that would need more than just the defeat of apartheid to correct.

While it was generally anticipated that a major feature of South Africa's new challenge would revolve around issues of poverty eradication, job creation, crime prevention and new directions in historical writing, academic debate and public comment became increasingly dominated by the centrality of a new struggle of global proportions – the fight against HIV/AIDS.[2] In the mid-twentieth century, cancer was the disease which carried the awe, symbolism and threat that tuberculosis possessed a hundred years before. Yet the arrival of HIV/AIDS in the second half of the century has since introduced a sinister new contestant for cancer's crown with an epidemic that poses an even greater demographic danger than tuberculosis and cancer combined. This is what prompted Desmond Tutu's observation,

> The end of apartheid was a historic and momentous moment in the life of South Africa. But our suffering has not ended. Just as we were bringing to a close a terrible chapter in our history, another crisis was just beginning.[3]

As if to concur with Tutu, Alan Whiteside and Clem Sunter have also remarked: 'Fate has dealt South Africa a cruel blow by replacing apartheid with HIV as public enemy number one'.[4] Indeed, not since the polio epidemic of the 1950s did people fear infection to the extent that they did with the emergence of AIDS in the early 1980s. Unlike earlier epidemics, AIDS appeared in the era of modern antibiotics, when it was thought that the risk of transmissible infection was a thing of the past. It rudely fractured society's false sense of security and medical confidence.[5] Since its arrival, individuals have been called upon to take responsibility for their bodies and to limit their potential to harm others. Available evidence suggests that despite South Africa's political miracle, millions of ex-victims of the apartheid era still live precariously on the margins of poverty. Outside the urban areas, very few black people have access to biomedicine, and the limited services available are decidedly inferior to those enjoyed by urban dwellers. Indeed, the health-care service infrastructure inherited in 1994 was highly unsuitable for mounting the effective, mass-based intervention that is critical for managing the HIV/AIDS pandemic.

For the post-apartheid government, the best way to reverse this picture was not merely to channel inappropriate health-care services and expensive technology to the rural areas where need was greatest. Instead, it opted to make health care more responsive to the consumer's health needs. To this end, it mobilized all health-care role players, including the historically marginalized indigenous healers, in a concerted national effort to mitigate the impact of the global pandemic. There was general consensus that the AIDS crisis should be addressed from multiple fronts. It was Thabo Mbeki, the then president, who set the tone for the new approach when he said, 'all of the information that has been communicated points to the reality that we are faced with a catastrophe, and you can't respond to a catastrophe merely by saying, I will do what is routine'.[6] Concurring with his statement, Alan Jeeves argued, 'research on disease that stops at the laboratory door is inadequate ... when matters as central to culture, society, and individual well-being as human sexuality and reproductive health are involved, the need for a plural approach is particularly evident'.[7] These arguments support the view held by Marisa Jacobs that, 'If there is to be any improvement in the health of the under-served population of the world, there will have to be full utilization of all available resources both human and material'.[8] Besides prompting a re-evaluation of theory in those branches of the social sciences concerned with health, the HIV/AIDS pandemic has also opened up critical inquiry into areas once anathema to mainstream scholarly inquiry, such as sex, sexuality and sexually transmitted infections. In this way, researchers were called upon to remove their gaze from the immediacy of the epidemic and to reflect in more abstract terms upon the ways in which it can be comprehended, analysed and eventually combated.[9] Part of the paradigm shift was a focus on the centuries-old African alternatives of managing affliction. Inherent in the concept of African Renaissance is the implication that Africans should find solutions to Africa's problems and part of doing this is to return to the roots of African culture. On 31 August 2003, the World Health Organization (WHO) called on African governments to formally recognize indigenous medicine and to integrate it into their national health systems.[10] Irrespective of one's views about indigenous healing, the basic question remains: why do many Africans still turn to them in spite of demonstrable advances in biomedicine? This chapter attempts to answer this question by exploring the factors underlying the resurgence of indigenous medicine in South Africa in spite of concerted attempts by the colonial and apartheid governments to undermine its significance. Partly on the basis of an agreement on scientific and technological co-operation signed on 9 July 1995 between the governments of South Africa and India, two former British colonies and members of BRICS (Brazil, Russia, India, China and South Africa), I will also refer, albeit very briefly, to Indian experiences of the impact of colonialism on indigenous medicine. It was, perhaps, not a coincidence that Mahatma Gandhi, who spent twenty-one years in South Africa fighting unjust laws that discriminated against indigenous people, also spent time fighting against British colonial rule in his mother country, India. Brief as it was in India's long history, the colonial period left a legacy of cultural changes surpassing those of other times. The same may be said of the colonial and apartheid periods in South Africa.[11]

Varying Perceptions of the Cause of Disease

Illness is a universal human condition; all societies have developed strategies of coping with it. Over the aeons, Africans have used an array of therapies to keep healthy and prevent debilitating illness. In an effort to explain illness and cope with its ramifications, beliefs and practices have evolved that are deeply enmeshed with African culture. As a multi-ethnic and multicultural society, South Africa has a multiplicity of overlapping and competing beliefs and value systems.[12] The country's social and economic structures are rooted in western culture, reflecting a highly technological worldview. Historically, these western value systems are rooted in the scientific revolution; the scientific view of reality, it is claimed, is the only valid approach to knowledge.[13] The medical system that emerged from this worldview is based on the 'germ theory' of disease causation referred to in this study as biomedicine. This widely accepted microbial explanation sees illness as the result of the invasion of the human body by germs. Illness is thus assumed to be an area of scientific investigation whose elimination requires the intervention of a university-trained medical practitioner using drugs, often administered within a highly sophisticated technological environment.

On the other hand, the vast majority of South Africans are of non-western origin; their worldview differs significantly. Although historically, the country's health-care system has been constructed around the scientific model, and not-withstanding its enormous contribution in reducing mortality from infectious diseases, biomedicine is not accepted by everyone as the only health resource. Besides, in South Africa, medicine was not introduced into a vacuum. For centuries, indigenous healers were the sole custodians of health care for the majority of Africans where illness has always been explained on issues other than those sanctioned by science. According to this model, western microbial explanations are often perceived as irrelevant to an African 'traditionalist' who ascribes some illnesses to the clandestine actions of malevolent persons who are capable of afflicting their victims by deployment of magic.[14] In terms of this perspective, human beings have the capacity to mobilize the power that exists in the universe and are themselves vulnerable to attacks by others using that power.[15] Hence, serious illness is often attributable either to witchcraft or ancestral wrath.[16]

Closely analysed, the above argument does not imply that African explanations of the cause of disease deny the existence of microbial cases of infection. But contrary to how disease is conceptualized in western cultures, Africans often blame their misfortune on other human beings. In the words of an indigenous healer, a typical African traditionalist often fails to understand why a minute virus (HIV) should want to harm an individual with whom it has absolutely nothing in common. 'If the creature is said to have caused the illness', so runs the argument, 'then it must have been manipulated by someone who is probably envious of the victim's well-being'.[17] In seeking an explanation for his tuberculosis, such an individual might have great difficulty accepting the scientific explanation that a tiny organism (*tubercle bacillus*) has invaded his body. Instead, he would hypothesize that the problem must be related to some metaphysical force, if not an indication of the displeasure of ancestral spirits, as possible punishment for the omission of a ritual.[18] These views have shaped the nature and attitudes of the biomedical profession towards indigenous medicine.

Although natural causes are not completely excluded, a broad outline of indigenous medical systems illustrates that supernatural causes are often invoked to explain the origin of disease and misfortune. Thus, exclusive reliance on bio-medicine may mean that the patient believes (rightly or wrongly) that there is more to the malaise than a single aetiological factor. In reality, no single factor can cause illness and no magic drug can single-handedly reverse illness. Multiple factors contribute to illness and thus multi-faceted interventions should work together to promote healing.[19] If, indeed, the therapies found in every society stem largely from prevailing causality beliefs, which in turn form the rationale for treatment, then the strength of indigenous medicine lies in its ability to offer both the social and mystical explanations for disease and its treatment. Existing evidence suggests that it is not only difficult to alter one's beliefs and prejudices, but almost impossible to lose them all.[20]

Colonialism and the Suppression of Indigenous Medicine

No continent has been so discredited, negatively stereotyped and nonchalantly dismissed as Africa, its people and their cultures. Presented in history books as people with no past beyond their contact with the white man, reduced to the status of colonial subjects and ruled by people with pronounced racist attitudes, Africans have suffered the indignity and the humiliation of being told by others what components of their own cultures should be retained and which ones should be summarily discarded. It was largely in this hostile colonial environment that indigenous healers came to be viewed as inimical to social and cultural progress.[21] Perhaps even more tragic is the fact that this distortion of African history and the tendency to discredit African cultures became so entrenched that it took on a dimension of truth for many unsuspecting individuals, including Africans themselves. This is clearly illustrated by one medical practitioner in Soweto, Dr Nthato Motlana's disparaging assault on the suggestion that regardless of their known shortcomings, some indigenous medical therapies might be of value. He argues that they are 'based on superstition, meaningless pseudo-psychological mumbo-jumbo which is positively harmful'.[22] Such denigration of indigenous cultures cannot be separated from the oppression of indigenous people during colonial times. Admittedly, for most people, quick and effective relief from pain is understandably preferable. The strength of biomedicine lies in its ability to offer this quick relief for most categories of illnesses and to provide scientific and logical explanations for aetiology and treatment.[23] However, the brickbat against indigenous medicine arises from attempts to use biomedicine to establish validity – to use it as a yardstick to measure the worth of all therapies. For example, in his celebrated study of Zande witchcraft, Edward Evans Pritchard assessed the worth of the therapeutic magic of the Zande as a system of natural observation and prediction. He then abstracted chains of causal reasoning, which he found to be flawed when evaluated according to scientific, logical standards. He concluded that Zande theory was false because it contradicted the account of the world as delivered by science.[24] Similarly, it has been argued that African folk-reasoning about disease cannot be validated. Traditional African discourse has been described as 'closed' because it denies accepted causal explanations – in contrast to science, which has been described as 'open'.[25] Such dogmatic views may well have changed today, but the core scientific comparison still persists and indigenous healing methods continue to face social suppression.

Historical scholarship on medicine during the colonial period in India reveals that colonialism worked against the indigenous healing traditions by depriving the practitioners of elite patronage.[26] According to Poonam Bala, however, unlike in South Africa, initial contact between the two medical systems in India resulted in acceptance and cooperation, which gave way to a conflict of interests only when western medical science became professionalized.[27] Both India and South Africa exhibited features of a strained relation between indigenous and western medicine, punctuated by colonialism undermining the legitimacy of the only health resource that the larger population had access to. It is, however, difficult to assess the health conditions of black South Africans prior to the advent of colonialism owing to the lack of documented evidence of indigenous medical practice, except that the latter dominated health care for most of the period. The available oral evidence suggests that Africans as a group, like all pre-industrial populations bore the brunt of periodic famine, while their infant and maternal mortality rates were much higher than those of settler populations. In his contribution to the present volume, Russel Viljoen rejects the view that medical knowledge was brought to the Cape by Europeans. Instead, certain indigenous medical practices were rooted in Khoikhoi society centuries before Jan Van Riebeeck set foot on South African soil.[28] The fact that biomedicine in both India and South Africa was introduced as an aspect of colonial conquest suggests that it was mainly designed to meet the health needs of the colonizers.[29] Until 1880, as agents of the empire the medical doctors at the Cape were more functional to the imperialists and all indigenous forms of healing were kept at bay.

Not even the Calcutta Native Medical Institution in India had as its objective the promotion of indigenous medicine as an equal or alternative to the western system. For example, by offering instruction in Ayurveda and Unani (indigenous systems of healing as practised in India) medicine, the intention was merely to attract recruits from the Vaidyas (practitioners of Ayurvedic medicine) and other communities with a tradition of medical practice, and once recruited, it was hoped, they would come to recognize the superiority of western medicine. In David Arnold's view, 'the British saw science, technology and medicine as exemplary attributes of their "civilising mission", clear evidence of their own superiority over, and imperial responsibility for, a land they identified as superstitious and backward'.[30] This was a form of enforced modernity not dissimilar to what transpired in South Africa, as evident in a government publication:

> Persuading the Bantu peoples of South Africa to accept modern medicine has been a big task, involving a painstaking campaign ... The real struggle has been against ignorance, superstition, mistrust, fear and witch-doctors. Gradually, however, the Bantu is being weaned away from the centuries-old superstitions and belief in witch-doctors, and the future is hopeful.[31]

Similarly, when the experiment of trying to combine elements of different medical traditions proved unworkable, the Calcutta Native Medical Institution came under serious criticism and was eventually abolished in 1835 and replaced by a new college to teach exclusively western medicine.[32] In Arnold's words, western medicine 'was taken as a hallmark of a superior civilization, a sign of the progressive intentions and moral legitimacy of colonial rule in India and the corresponding backwardness and barbarity of indigenous practice'.[33]

In South Africa, a historical scholarship reveals that the practice of indigenous healing was declared illegal by the Cape Medical Act of 1891. Although in terms of the Native Code of 1928, indigenous healers were given a measure of recognition in Natal and Zululand, where they were trained, licensed and expected to pay an annual fee of three pounds and one pound, respectively, no such formal recognition was extended to the more than 2,000 others throughout the country at the time.[34] As the influence of missionary teaching spread countrywide, indigenous healing came under severe pressure. In fact, during the colonial period, to engage in 'witchcraft' in other provinces rendered the healer liable to criminal prosecution.[35] In the long run, a form of government-sponsored conflict of interests developed between indigenous and biomedical practitioners which sets up an interesting comparison with the developments in India, as explained above. As the secretary of Public Health pompously proclaimed:

> The continued activity of Native 'witchdoctors' and herbalists means that the policy of utilising hospitals, doctors and nurses as a civilising agency and to bring the benefits of European medicine to the Native peoples is not being successful.[36]

Indeed, officialdom made no attempt to hide its displeasure that the majority of Africans still patronized indigenous healers despite government and missionary efforts to halt the practice. The hostility towards indigenous healers continued unabated, with the Public Health Secretary declaring that 'so far as preventing and curing diseases is concerned, the Native peoples would be much better off without them'.[37] Thus, under pressure from both colonial agents and Christian teachings, the power base of indigenous healers was gradually eroded; biomedicine gained a strong foothold in the recognized treatment of disease throughout the country. Indigenous healers were forced to practise their craft discreetly, fearing both social stigma and the legal sanctions which could result from public exposure. Notwithstanding this official attitude and the lack of statutory provision protecting indigenous medicine, its use continued until well into the post-apartheid period. Africans continued to consult indigenous healers, often prior to and after treatment at a health-care facility or a biomedical practitioner. Interestingly, neither the degree of westernization, nor the level of education significantly influenced patterns of utilization of healers, except that such visits were kept a secret and were often denied as they would interfere with the image of the educated African. As Ntuli, an attorney whose father was an indigenous healer, has observed 'publicly, most educated Africans cast aspersions on anything germane to indigenous medicine and yet they consult indigenous healers surreptitiously'.[38]

In colonial India, the Indian Medical Service which owed its institutional origins out of the medical and military requirements of early colonial rule, represented direct intervention of colonial imperatives in the social, cultural and material lives of the Indian people. However, one explanation for the slow emergence of an independent western medical profession in India, as in South Africa, was the continuous availability and perceived efficacy of indigenous medicine.[39] For this reason, the British felt obliged to recognize the existence of such culturally entrenched therapeutic beliefs and practices, though it cannot be denied that the medical intervention was always driven by the scientific interests of the colonial state.

Most arguments justifying the marginalization of indigenous healers in South Africa focus on the ill effects of their procedures. A typical example is the administration of renal enemas on children with infectious diarrhoea, which was often fatal following excessive dehydration. Edward Green and Lydia Makhubu, have also warned against the dangers of induced vomiting after taking indigenous healers' herbal mixtures.[40] Traditional vaccination and reusing razor blades during blood-letting ceremonies and circumcision rites without sterilizing the cutting edges has also come in for criticism. In view of such valid concerns, the proponents of integration of indigenous and western medicine argue that the government has the duty, indeed the obligation, to protect the public against potentially harmful practices, such as these, by regulating indigenous medicine rather than suppressing it or even pretending that it does not exist. Attitudes such as these often rest on an irrational belief that one could overcome reality by simply refusing to admit its existence. On the other hand, the health professionals continue to argue that the practice of indigenous healing lacks a scientific base. As Heyl puts it:

> We just do not know enough about the practice of the traditional healer to really assess his value ... Council [SAMDC] steeped as it is in the scientific method and a quest for more knowledge and better skills to create a sound basis for medical practice, cannot condone such haphazard and unscientific procedures.[41]

A counter-argument to this, presumably well-intentioned criticism, is that by Heyl's own admission, the South African Medical and Dental Council (SAMDC) knew little about indigenous healing; as a SAMDC member he was, thus, unqualified to pass judgement on the worth of the craft. One might well argue that the SAMDC should have investigated this form of health practice before discarding it as an alternative health resource. It would, however, appear that reasons other than considerations of efficacy were behind the decision taken by the SAMDC to work towards invalidating this particular aspect of indigenous knowledge systems.[42] This is not to deny the existence of charlatans and 'quacks' among indigenous healers. It is conceded that the so-called 'magicians' from whose acts the bona fide healers and their organizations have distanced themselves, have often been found guilty of complicity in cases of ritual homicide, when human body parts are required for 'powerful magic'.[43] Because the mutilated corpses of victims are seldom buried, many incidents of muti-related murders have gone unreported. Judging from court records, some indigenous healers have indeed been found guilty of identifying the required body parts as well as the type of victim whose flesh would yield the best results.[44] It is here that both healers and their clients are equally responsible for the effects of unethical medical practice; for the healer supplies his distinctive services only when there is a demand for them.

Admittedly, such practices have not only undermined the historical contribution of indigenous healers to health and healing but have also provided useful ammunition for critics of indigenous medicine in general, thereby undermining public acceptance of its potential role in the current age of the AIDS pandemic. More recently, indigenous medicine faced bad reviews in the media mainly because of the Health Ministry's insistence on the role of nutrition including garlic, olive oil, African potatoes and beetroot in the management of AIDS as substitutes for antiretroviral drugs.[45] In 2009, there were an estimated 185,500 practitioners of indigenous medicine in contrast to only 34,000 biomedical doctors and 68,000 full-time herbalists as compared to only 11,000 pharmacists.[46] Arguably, the critical question is whether indigenous medicine has a role to play in the battle against HIV/AIDS; if so, what is this role? To provide an answer to this requires reflection on a related question: Historically, have indigenous healers made a significant contribution to the fight against disease in general and sexually transmitted infections in particular? For surely, 'if the past has been an obstacle and a burden, knowledge of the past is the safest emancipation'.[47]

Sexually Transmitted Infections in Retrospect and HIV/AIDS in Prospect

Some research has been conducted on the nature of diseases commonly dealt with by indigenous healers and the potential benefits of their collaboration with biomedical practitioners within the context of primary health care.[48] However, reliable information on sexually transmitted infections, particularly among black South Africans prior to 1994, is difficult to come by. Although syphilis had been identified as the country's major health problem in the 1930s and 1940s,[49] negative stereotypes about Africans' sexuality and sexually transmitted infections have led to a taboo of silence. Most literature on these infections, written primarily by whites, makes the direct inference that Africans are by nature promiscuous and predisposed to immorality. The medical officer of health for Pretoria went as far as to suggest that more than half the African population in 1946 had sexually transmitted diseases.[50] Thus, underlying the anti-miscegenation legislation of the apartheid period, which practically created an official divide between the races, was the desire to protect whites from the perceived dangers of sexual contact

with Africans.[51] However, given the dearth of clinical health services for most
rural Africans until the late twentieth century, there can be no doubt that the
majority of sexually related infections were treated by indigenous healers, who
unfortunately did not keep records of their patients.

So far there can be no question that indigenous healers treated a variety of
conditions including impotence, infertility and mental illness. The fact that
Africans know of and have specific names for several sexually transmitted infections implies that they have also developed their own strategies to cope with
them. For example, the Bapedi speak of *makgoma* as a condition that arises when
a man has sexual intercourse with a widow before she is ritually cleansed. To
kgoma is a Sepedi word meaning 'to touch' or 'come in contact with'.[52] In African
culture, a widow or widower must not have sexual contact with anyone before
undergoing a cleansing ritual using indigenous herbs. This has been the competence of indigenous healers from time immemorial. In her study *Women and
Sexually Transmitted Diseases* among the Vhavenda, Fhumulani Mavis Mulaudzi
also found that like many African tribes, the Venda speak of *dorobo* (drop) as a
sexually transmitted infection caused by dirt.[53] In Sepedi, when a man has contracted this infection it is said *monna o tsamaile selege or ba mo lomile* (man has
erred) when he oozes a thick, purulent discharge through his penis.[54] This has a
striking similarity with the Sepedi word, *toropo* for the same condition.[55] A com-
plication of this condition is that an infected woman may not fall pregnant and
if she does, she is likely to deliver a sick baby.[56] The Vhavenda also speak of *divhu*
as a disease which a man contracts by having sexual intercourse with a woman
who has not been ritually cleansed after an abortion.[57]

Some of these infections have symptoms similar to those of contemporary
AIDS patients. This explains why initially AIDS was perceived as a new name for
known diseases and was often mistakenly defined as *makgoma*. Indigenous healer
Ngaka Tsiane concedes that most young men who consult him on a daily basis
suffer from an STI of one kind or another and that he is able to treat them with
spectacularly good results.[58] Indeed, the majority of indigenous healers claim
that depending on the appropriate herbal mixture, and proper consumption, the
enemas that are so unpopular in biomedical circles are the most effective in this
area of disease control. Concurring with Tsiane, Ngaka Hlathikhulu Ngobeni
claims that STIs are the most common problems indigenous healers deal with
on a regular basis. Because of the stigma attached to such infections (and despite
the availability of cheap and effective biomedical treatment), many still opt to
consult indigenous healers. Over the years, indigenous healers have been treating sexually transmitted infections with tremendous success and may therefore
make a significant contribution in the management of the contemporary AIDS
pandemic – management, not cure, because the majority of credible indigenous
healers readily admit that they have no magic cure for AIDS.

Against this background, it may be argued that since the main obstacle in curbing the spread of the pandemic is mainly cultural rather than technical, harnessing the expertise of indigenous healers and securing their co-operation is critical to addressing the denial, taboos and myths associated with AIDS. For example, the alarming escalation of paedophilia is clearly the result of charlatans masquerading as healers who advise their patients that having sex with a virgin cures AIDS. Then too, AIDS is often concealed by the fact that death is caused by the body's failure to resist other infections such as TB. Collaboration between health-care systems could mean that such opportunistic infections could be effectively curbed. For example, Tsiane has been at the forefront of the initiative to establish the Directly Observed Treatment Strategy (DOTS) training programme for indigenous healers in partnership with the Mmamethlake district of Moretele in the Mpumalanga Department of Health. DOTS is an effective primary health-care initiative of the WHO; it uses non-medical personnel to monitor out-patient TB treatment.[59]

The establishment of the Indigenous Knowledge Systems Centre (IKSC) as an offshoot of the Medical Research Council (MRC) confirms the resurgence of indigenous medicine in the post-apartheid period. Part of IKSC's brief is to evaluate indigenous therapies and prevent unscrupulous conduct by unqualified practitioners.[60] This was prompted by many untested claims that a 'cure' for AIDS had been found, such as Olga Mokoena's *somhlolo* (miracle) mixture,[61] and Siphiwe Hadebe's *umbimbi* herbal mixture.[62] In 2003, Cyril Khanyile, who had practised medicine in New York, established the Second Chance Clinic and began using herbal remedies which he claimed inhibited the spread of the HIV in the body and increased the CD4 count.[63] These claims were, however, refuted by the national Co-ordinating Committee for Traditional Health Practitioners (CCTHP).[64] With limited resources available to conduct clinical trials, a working relationship has been forged between indigenous healers and botanists and this has led to the emergence of an immune-boosting drug which apparently improved the quality of life of some rural Kwazulu-Natal people living with the virus. Anecdotal evidence shows that a weight gain of up to 15 kg and renewed vigour was experienced by people at Ngwelezane Hospital in Empangeni.[65] According to an indigenous healer, Credo Mutwa, the drug was developed from *sutherlandia frutescens*, an indigenous shrub whose medical qualities were recognized centuries ago by the Khoi, San and Zulu healers.[66] Almost concurring with van Rijn that, 'applying western-based research to African setting presents its own problems, and challenges the universality of scientific findings and highlighting the relevance of history of apartheid and colonial rule'[67] a multi-disciplinary team of botanists and herbalists, investigated and confirmed the medicinal value of this plant for viral infections, immune boosting and depression. According to Mutwa, although indigenous healers cannot cure AIDS, they can indeed treat illnesses like diarrhoea and lung infections that attack immune systems shattered by HIV, since it is the disease not the virus that often kills AIDS patients and that *sutherlandia frutescens* is also effective in combating AIDS-related wasting.[68]

Creating an Enabling Environment for Collaboration

The African National Congress (ANC) went into the 1994 elections on a political platform promising a better life for all, including better health care. It was, therefore, anticipated that the post-apartheid government would address the HIV/AIDS pandemic. Not surprisingly, even before it assumed control, the ANC recommended in its National Health Plan for South Africa (NHPSA) and the Reconstruction and Development Programme (RDP), that indigenous medicine be utilized in the provision of health care. The AIDS pandemic called for a disease-focus approach to health that led many social and behavioural scientists worldwide to rethink health-care delivery.[69] Medical beliefs and practices once deemed 'superstitious' and 'irrelevant' were reassessed and given fresh interpretation. By 1977, the World Health Assembly (WHA) of the WHO had passed a resolution promoting training and research on indigenous medicine. And a year later, most developing countries endorsed the concept of Primary Health Care (PHC) the provision of appropriate care at grassroots level and a search for alternative models of health-care delivery. This was partly prompted by financial constraints and the shortage of medical personnel and equipment to meet the exacting standards of biomedicine. A decade later, the WHO again urged member states to explore how indigenous healers could be utilized to extend health-care coverage. In its Traditional Medicines Strategy 2002–5, the WHO recommended that indigenous medicines be evaluated for quality and efficacy before inclusion in national health policies. Despite these international moves, it was not until the pandemic was firmly entrenched in South Africa that the political leadership devoted due attention to combating HIV/AIDS. This lack of urgency was not unrelated to the failure of previous governments to act decisively on critical health issues.[70] The apartheid regime had clearly lost the battle against the pandemic when the health ministry admitted as early as 1992 that it was already too late to contain the AIDS threat. The initial conceptualization of AIDS as an exclusively homosexual problem may also have influenced official urgency (or lack thereof) in responding to the crisis. The government's priorities at the time also come to the fore; the defence budget of the beleaguered apartheid regime far outstripped that of health.[71]

When the ANC government came to power, there was a clear limit to what a cash-strapped government in transition could do for a health service already groaning under the burden of the global pandemic, hence the search for accessible indigenous alternatives. However, despite Mandela's declared commitment to make the fight against HIV/AIDS one of his priorities, the pandemic was apparently not yet perceived as an urgent matter. Mandela was more preoccupied with efforts to lift the nation out of its spiral of violence and to establish international confidence in the 'rainbow nation', than he was with initiatives to limit the impact of the pandemic.[72]

Mandela's successor, Thabo Mbeki, also failed to provide leadership on the pandemic, attributing AIDS to poverty. Mbeki's controversial statements should be understood within the context of a country still in the throes of transformation; a call for African solutions to African problems embodied in his ideal of an African renaissance. Thanks to the debate he generated, the social, historical, cultural and economic contexts of AIDS are now regarded as vital to an understanding of the epidemic in sub-Saharan Africa. Regardless of the role of HIV, these non-biological factors have created a very different epidemic in Africa than in Europe and America. Henceforth, a broad-based strategy addressing not only the peculiarities of the virus but also many intersecting concerns have become necessary.[73] Historically, in terms of the Homeopaths, Naturopaths, Osteopaths and Herbalists Act of 1974, South Africa did have a licensing programme which recognized indigenous medicine and herbalists. The Act paved the way for future policies on indigenous medicine.

In recognition of the potential of indigenous medicine in the fight against AIDS, South Africa made medical history with the opening on 5 October 1998 of Samuel Kwadi Traditional Hospital, near Kwamhlanga in the Mpumalanga Province.[74] However, due to lack of funding, the institution was forced to close down shortly thereafter, although other institutions were established, foremost among which was the Traditional Healing Clinic in Kwazulu-Natal, staffed by members of the Kwazulu-Natal Traditional Healers Council and the Professional Herbal Preparations Association.[75]

There are issues when practitioners of indigenous medicine are incorporated into mainstream delivery of health care alongside biomedical practitioners with the idea of 'modernizing' health care. Often their knowledge and practices are abruptly transformed due to the enforcement of standardization and conformity with practice regulations, as a result of which, their experiential knowledge is devalued and their personal approach to patients is replaced by a de-contextualized objectivity which is characteristic of biomedicine; this also violates the epistemiological basis of indigenous medicine.[76]

Conclusion

An important observation emerging from this chapter is that indigenous medicine represents the largest resource base for meeting the health needs of most black South Africans. Although many traditional medical beliefs and practices are at odds with the conventional biomedicine, they should not be dismissed as mere superstition. Psychological research reveals that the effectiveness of the healer is largely based upon the extent to which his value system matches that of the patient. In the final analysis, the success of any system of medicine, modern or indigenous, has to be assessed in terms of the criteria of availability, accessibility, affordability and acceptability. In this respect, De Beer, suggests that health services should be accessible to a minimum of 80 per cent of the total population and should be relevant to meet the specific health needs of a cultural group within the constraints of the country's resources.[77] With a large clientele base and popularity of indigenous medicine, South Africa can use indigenous healers to alleviate the shortage of medical caregivers and, thus, increase health-care coverage, thus bridging the cultural divide in conceptual appreciation of health problems. It would be strategic for biomedical practitioners to work closely with indigenous healers, because it is often they who are the first port of call for many rural dwellers suffering from sexually transmitted infections. As Mankazana put it,

> It is important to delegate duties for which the present day medical graduate is not competent ... those involving trans-cultural psychiatry. Refusal of such delegation usually comes from unwillingness to trust others.[78]

In South Africa, venereal disease and other issues of reproductive health have been matters of political controversy for centuries. In both the colonial and apartheid periods, indigenous healing was marginalized, often with the aid of legislation, largely for reasons that had little to do with efficacy. It is primarily a lack of recognition and proper technical support that has hindered the development and refinement of indigenous therapeutic procedures and remedies. In the light of this discussion, there is a need to examine and understand the cultural health beliefs of indigenous communities – for health and social practices are usually the manifestations of cultural beliefs and individual experiences.

The post-apartheid government's declared integrated approach seeks to ensure the efficacy, safety and quality of indigenous therapies by creating an enabling environment for collaboration. The benefits of collaboration were understood more clearly by a modern medical doctor, Tolani Asuni:

> The question of cooperation of traditional and modern healing practice does not pose a great problem to the consumer. He will use both facilities with or without the knowledge or approval of either. His concept of disease allows for this. While modern medicine can procure a cure, it does not deal with what is regarded as the basic cause of his illness which may be a curse, the vengeance of a god, the evil machinations of another person, etc. The objective of traditional healing practice in this situation is to counteract the basic cause, thereby making modern medicine effective and lasting in its cure. In other words the traditional system complements the modern system.[79]

On the whole, the importance of indigenous medicine, not as a rival of but as a complementary health resource, cannot be overemphasized. Modern medicine alone in both India and South Africa had fallen far behind Europe and North America and had failed to cope with the health problems produced by rural poverty. While in India this space could be said to have been closed by Ayurveda, which has been transformed into health products for middle-class consumers in modern Indian society, in South Africa, this is the gap that could potentially be filled by African indigenous medicine. It is clear that continuities from the past played a very crucial role in the social and cultural changes experienced in both India and South Africa in the post-colonial periods and such changes would not have occurred as they did without the context and impact of colonialism itself and the respective responses of Indians and South Africans. This study concurs with Arnold, that any uncritical acceptance of modernity as presented by Europeans would confine indigenous people to a state of permanent tutelage and subordination and thus leave them one step behind, which would result in them being second best or imperfect copies of a European ideal. With regards to South Africa, almost synonymous with apartheid for forty years and now notorious for HIV/AIDS, it remains to be seen whether integration in the National Health Service (NHS) will be the key to the effective management of the devastating effects of the pandemic. There is no question that unless there is state-sanctioned collaboration between the two systems, the fundamental human right of a maximum degree of health will remain an elusive prospect for rural Africans, and health as defined by the WHO will continue to be a privilege enjoyed by the affluent few.

Acknowledgements

This chapter is a revised version of the paper I presented at an International Conference on 'Ten Years of Democracy in Southern Africa', at Queen's University, Canada, in May 2004. I would like to thank the University of South Africa for a travel grant which facilitated research for this paper and conference attendance.

3 MEDICINE, MEDICAL KNOWLEDGE AND HEALING AT THE CAPE OF GOOD HOPE: KHOIKHOI, SLAVES AND COLONISTS

Russel Viljoen

Introduction

Based on published travel accounts and archival material, this chapter recounts the existence, transmission and influence of indigenous and colonial medical knowledge and healing practices at the Cape of Good Hope, South Africa since colonial conquest in 1652 to the end of the eighteenth century. It examines what impact colonial conquest and colonial medicine had on existing and emerging colonial identities at the Cape – namely the Khoikhoi, slaves and colonists – and with it, marks the 300th anniversary of smallpox first introduced to South Africa in 1713. By reflecting on colonial disease and medicine in twenty-first-century South Africa, this chapter reasserts that medical knowledge *per se* was not brought to the Cape by Europeans, but maintains that certain indigenous medical practices and indigenous knowledge systems were rooted in the everyday life of the indigenous Khoikhoi people, centuries before Jan van Riebeeck and others set foot on South African soil.[1]

The Cape of Good Hope was officially occupied by the Dutch East India Company (VOC) in April 1652, in an effort to reach the Far East, notably the spice-producing countries, including mainly India and Sri Lanka (Ceylon). However, the presence of Dutch settlers posed no immediate threat to the existence of the original inhabitants of the Cape, the San and Khoikhoi. Similarly, ideas of western medicine, however, were not immediately imposed on the local indigenous people, even though, the VOC authorities had erected one poorly equipped and staffed hospital to provide medical care to Company employees and sick sailors. Commenting on the poor state of the hospital, O. F. Mentzel, a German observer, said that 'conditions at the hospital more often send a person to his grave than the ravages of his disease itself'.[2] Decades later, Carl Thunberg, a German physician who later started a medical practice in Cape Town, noted that the same 'ruinous' building was still in use during the 1770s.[3] Since the Cape had initially been regarded only as a refreshment post to nourish mariners en route to the East, trade with the local stock-owning Khoikhoi population was paramount. Ironically though, it was through trade that colonial medicine eventually permeated Khoikhoi society.

For most part of the late seventeenth and early eighteenth centuries, colonial medical facilities, the quantity and quality of medicine remained poor. Medical supplies were not only expensive, but also scarce. Soon after taking up his post as Commander of the Cape colony, Jan van Riebeeck, who was also a surgeon, was the first one to complain about insufficient medical supplies. In 1659, he wrote to Amsterdam complaining that they received 'no medicines for two years'.[4] A year later, he again informed his superiors in Holland how sparse the medical supplies had become compared to the previous shipment.[5] The only time medicine and medical supplies were imported were when ships docked. Even then, there was no guarantee that it would be brought ashore, or destined for the Cape. In 1676, Governor Isbrand Goske authorized two doctors to board a ship named *De Vryheyt* to inspect its medicine-chest for drugs and medicine that could be used ashore.[6] In her study of ship's surgeons employed by the VOC, Iris Bruijn has shown that the Cape had a Dispensary where medicines were stored that arrived from the Netherlands. The medical policy adopted by the VOC during the course of the seventeenth century outlined that ships bound for the East Indies must employ a ship's surgeon and that sufficient medicines and medical supplies be taken onboard in medical chests.[7] Medicines were at first only manufactured in the Netherlands, and shipped to the Batavia Castle where it was stored and dispensed to VOC-controlled regions that included the Cape and India. However, by the late 1660s, a separate pharmaceutical company was established in Batavia under the leadership of H. Cruijs, a trained pharmacist who had to swear under oath that the manufactured medicines were of a high quality and mixed in accordance to the *Amstelodamensis Pharmacopeia* specifications. Ships and hospitals in the region were henceforth supplied with medicine manufactured in both Amsterdam and Batavia.[8] Hospitals that formed part of the trading network, located in Sri Lanka, China, the Cape and Bengal, India, where a hospital was constructed in Chinsurah in 1728, were supplied with medicines from Batavia or Amsterdam.[9] The establishment of hospitals in both the Cape and India were not civilian hospitals but in fact military hospitals to care for sick soldiers, VOC officials and sick sailors. These colonial hospitals were effectively 'private institutions' exclusively reserved for VOC personnel.

By the 1680s, colonial medicine and pharmaceutical knowledge were boosted with the arrival of the French refugees, Huguenots, several of whom had some medical training.[10] Several years later, a few German immigrants,[11] together with the French-speaking doctors, monopolized the medical 'profession' at the Cape. According to C. Price, emphasis was not placed on surgery but rather on medicine.[12] Despite the presence of a few doctors, 'private' practice hardly developed to its full potential and remained an unrewarding venture for the most part of the eighteenth century.

The social structure of Cape society with its developing class divisions allowed only the urban 'wealthy' access to the few available medical facilities at that time. The majority of colonists were generally poor and could not afford even the most basic form of medicine. The shortage of doctors, the lack of medical supplies and medical care eventually led to the emergence of self-medication even though the sick would have preferred the services of a doctor. One rheumatic sufferer told a European observer that the service of doctors was expensive, but 'thought it very comfortable for a person to have access to a physician in case of sickness'.[13] This, however, was a worldwide trend. In Europe, and elsewhere in the western world, 'the demographic impact of the profession of medicine remained negligible'.[14]

Yet, despite the lack of adequate medical knowledge, some Cape governors saw the exchange of medical knowledge as a means to initiate and establish trade relations with Khoikhoi pastoralists. For example, in 1654, following a request of a certain Khoikhoi captain, a VOC medical practitioner was told by his superiors 'to exert his utmost skill to cure him ... that they become more accustomed, attached, and well affectioned towards us'.[15] Medicine or medical assistance offered by colonists to local Khoikhoi during the formative years of conquest was, thus, essentially confined to establishing and fortifying trade relations.[16] Since the practice of western medicine remained largely rudimentary in Cape society, this arguably generated the need for an exchange of healing practices. Some seafarers often preferred Khoikhoi herbal medicine to western medicine. As the medical facilities at the Cape, like in Europe, found itself in an appalling state, it was often left to the coastal Khoikhoi communities to doctor sick sailors. Not only could sailors depend on local Cape Khoikhoi to supply them with livestock and fresh water as they rounded Table Bay en route to the East, but also in some instances on the provision of indigenous medicine and medical care as well. As a result, European seafarers often recognized the advantages of Khoikhoi herbal remedies after spending months at sea. Many European seafarers testified of such encounters with the Cape Khoikhoi. The French sailor, Jean-Baptiste Tavernier, was one example. In 1660, praising Khoikhoi medicine, he wrote the following:

> however beastly they are, yet [they] have a special knowledge of herbs, which they know to use against the sickness from which they suffer, as the Dutch have proved. If they are bitten by any poisonous beasts, or suffer from any ulcers, they can bring about a cure in a short time by means of the herbs which they know how to select.[17]

Years later, in 1698, another explorer, Francois Leguat, chronicled a similar account, lauding the healing powers of Khoikhoi medicine. He wrote that they

> administer the remedy with greater success than what we oftentimes do ours. The
> sick that have been brought a-shoar [*sic*] at the Cape have often experienced this, and
> those wounds that very skilful surgeons have given over, have in a short time been
> cur'd [*sic*] by these people.[18]

These are but two accounts which show how European sailors in times of need accepted indigenous herbal medicine to cure their ills. It seems evident, thus, that for the Khoikhoi to have medicated European mariners for at least a century, they would have had thriving medical practices in place at the time of colonial conquest. In Khoikhoi society, healers were ordinary men and women, recognized only by the trinkets and small horns that adorned their necks. Drawn from the sages of the community, these men were skilled in botany, surgery and medicine. Each Khoikhoi hut (*kraal*) had healers and midwives who performed an array of duties ranging from doctoring ailments to delivering infants. Indigenous healers were generally appointed by the leaders of the clan, while midwives were selected by women. Herbal medicine and remedies occupied a special place in Khoikhoi medical hierarchy. Herbal remedies were essentially of vegetable origin, and were mixed and prepared to cure a specific type of ailment. Surgery, compared to herbal medicine, constituted a relatively minor part of Khoikhoi medicine but still proved effective when applied. A variety of surgical operations such as bloodletting, cupping, cauterization and scarification were performed on a fairly regular basis, or when required.[19]

As the majority of Khoikhoi captains still wielded power over their followers during the seventeenth century and early part of the eighteenth century and since medical practices fell partially under their control, outsiders at the time of conquest, found it generally difficult to penetrate Khoikhoi society. Although one captain of the Saldanha Khoikhoi[20] accepted western methods of healing to cure his crooked knee which he injured years ago, other captains simply barred western medicine from their *kraals*. Soon after conquest, Oedasoa, an influential chief of the Cochoqua Khoikhoi, rejected western medicine and preferred consulting his own physician.[21] Even ordinary Khoikhoi individuals at the time of conquest, were not easily impressed with western medicine and saw it as a curse rather than cure. For example, when a Khoikhoi youth was hospitalized in the Fort following a freak accident, he was removed that same night by his family, as they believed 'their native skill … can cure him better'.[22]

The latter years of the seventeenth and early eighteenth century saw little changes with regard to the use of western medicine in Khoikhoi society. As contact between Khoikhoi and white settlers was not as yet commonplace, it created very few opportunities for either group influencing the other. But as the demand for livestock increased and trading expeditions to Khoikhoi *kraals* became routine, the situation began to change. The exchange of liquor, tobacco, beads and trinkets for livestock effectively allowed for the gradual introduction of western medicine into Khoikhoi society. Many Europeans reckoned it was only a matter of time when colonial medicine could be used to sway the Khoikhoi to trade more freely. By paying regular visits to Khoikhoi *kraals* ostensibly to befriend Khoikhoi leaders in order to enhance trade relations, Europeans hardly made the task of protective captains any easier. In order to make the refreshment station a profitable venture, those in charge of the colony utilized every means available to enhance trade relations with the Khoikhoi. Basic medicine which consisted largely of bottled medicine, brandy and medical instruments to treat basic injuries, carried along by VOC traders for personal use, was regularly offered to local Khoikhoi whom they encountered. In 1677, a Dutch surgeon, who for some reason had led a trading expedition into the interior, received three rams from the Hessequa Khoikhoi for medical services rendered.[23] A clear pattern seems to have emerged towards the end of the seventeenth century whereby western medicine was seen by the colonial authorities as a viable medium, and one through which trading relations with the Khoikhoi could be expedited. While successful treatment invariably led to favourable trading links, the opposite, presumably, resulted in strained relations. Thus, despite the chronic shortages of medical supplies and the difficulties that Cape governors experienced in obtaining these supplies from their superiors in Holland,[24] they still regarded medicine as an important ploy in fostering friendly relations with the Khoikhoi.

The period between 1500 and 1700 was an era in which several indigenous societies in North and South America, Africa, Australia and those located in the Indian Ocean were exposed to a host of western epidemic diseases.[25] The French historian, Emmanuel LeRoy Ladurie, calls this era, 'the unification of the globe by disease'.[26] From the outset of colonial conquest, European diseases rather than European medicine have affected Khoikhoi society the most. Since conquest, several transmittable diseases of western origin, to which the Khoikhoi had little or no immunities, were gradually introduced by sailors and white immigrants.[27] Frequent interaction with seafarers and traders created more than ample opportunities to disseminate western diseases. For example, two major diseases in the form of dysentery erupted in September 1661 and again in 1662, claiming the lives of Khoikhoi, including several of its leaders.[28] Grevenbroek[29] argued that impetigo,[30] a skin disorder, was introduced by the colonists soon after their arrival. Subsequently, a variety of diseases were brought to the Cape. Typhus, commonly known as the 'disease of the poor',[31] appeared as early as 1666,[32] and by the time smallpox struck for a second time in 1755, jaundice and bilious fever were also diagnosed.[33] Swellendam, a former densely populated Khoikhoi region, was found almost completely deserted by the 1770s. According to one survivor, many of his contemporaries had died of ulcers.[34] Following this minor outbreak, a more serious bilious fever epidemic erupted in 1775, claiming the lives of hundreds of Khoikhoi.[35] A skin disease frequently identified among the elderly after colonial conquest was erysipelas.[36] According to Thunberg, an aged Khoikhoi woman suffered from this infection in her legs which were marked by the disease's symptoms of redness and swelling.[37] Both leprosy and tuberculosis were diagnosed much later and were said to have been particularly rife among the Khoikhoi during the nineteenth century.[38]

Smallpox, which struck for the first time in 1713, was unquestionably the most lethal of all European-introduced diseases. The outbreak of the first smallpox epidemic brought by European sailors quickly exposed the Cape Colony's poor medical facilities. When smallpox struck, no civilian hospital existed, which cast the town in a state of total disarray. In the absence of proper medical facilities and scientific knowledge, there was little that the few under qualified colonial doctors and apothecaries could do to combat the epidemic and cure sufferers.

The outbreak of the series of smallpox epidemics affected Cape colonial society in many different ways. At the very least, it transformed the perceptions of colonized population on issues regarding public health. Prior to the series of outbreaks, the authorities and Cape settler population paid little attention to public health as concerted efforts, it seems, were made only when major disasters struck.[39] Even though no civilian hospital existed when the second major epidemic erupted in 1755, the authorities decreed far-reaching precautionary measures by way of public notices, to prevent the spread of smallpox. The first major colonial public health programme was thus embarked upon stipulating that houses and slave lodges be fumigated, all cases of smallpox had to be reported, social gatherings were prohibited, corpses could no longer be transported to Cape Town but be buried on farms, and that drinking water was not to be contaminated.[40] Despite these decreed precautionary measures, a third epidemic in 1767 was not prevented. However, the authorities and colonial practitioners were slightly better prepared to contain the virus after *inenting* (inoculation) was introduced to the Cape.[41] There is no evidence to suggest whether or not the Khoikhoi and slaves were among those inoculated against smallpox; we do, however, know that they were quarantined and isolated in makeshift colonial hospitals outside Cape Town, and were cared for by slave and Khoikhoi. Other colonial society offers equally interesting parallels with the Cape colony. It is thus useful to recognize how other colonial powers reacted towards epidemics and how colonial medicine was administered in times of crisis, particularly among the indigenous people. In Spanish America, efforts to protect local Indians against smallpox were delayed until an approved method against the virus came to be recognized in Spain itself. This, according to William McNeill, happened shortly after 1798 when Edward Jenner discovered a vaccination against smallpox.[42]

The onset and spread of smallpox weakened Khoikhoi society in various ways affecting all levels of their society.[43] Bewitchment was one sentiment expressed at the time when smallpox carried off 'hundreds' of Khoikhoi people. The colonial traveller, Francois Valentijn for example, chronicled how Khoikhoi cursed 'the Dutch whom they said had bewitched them'.[44] Others again, attached a spiritual connotation to the virus, by calling it an 'evil sickness'.[45] These remarks were presumably made by *kraal* healers or captains who knew how smallpox had ruined and dislodged their communities. The outbreak of smallpox was so severe, sometimes beyond control, that it caught many by surprise and gave Khoikhoi healers very little opportunity to devise some kind of medical cure. Not only did the 1713 outbreak result in the loss of hundreds of lives of individuals prematurely, but it also affected the hierarchical and political structures of certain Khoikhoi communities posing new challenges as far as succession was concerned. Loss of leadership forced survivors to secure outside help proving that their society was effectively in decline. In February 1714, for instance, months after smallpox struck in Cape Town, four captains and their immediate successors of the Piketberg Khoikhoi died after contracting smallpox. Shortly thereafter, their relatives and followers arrived at the Castle requesting the Governor to appoint new captains to stabilize their unsettled community.[46] The appointment of new captains by the colonial authorities shows not only the weakened state of certain Khoikhoi communities as far as leadership was concerned, but reveals how a colonial disease – smallpox – a side-effect of colonial conquest, redefined their status as an independent indigenous community. The trouble taken by the Piketberg Khoikhoi, of whom many were presumably women and children, to travel to Cape Town is moreover indicative of how desperate they were to rebuild and reorganize their political structures which had been devastated by smallpox.

In other colonial societies, notably colonial America, the British embarked upon a much more serious campaign to conquer indigenous peoples by deliberately spreading the virus among them.[47] In colonial America, smallpox was used in some kind of 'germ warfare' against the indigenous Indian populations. In 1763, a certain Lords Jeffrey Amherst 'ordered that blankets infected with smallpox be distributed among' Indian communities.[48]

Unlike the Khoikhoi that were exposed to smallpox for the first time in 1713, the people of India had been exposed to smallpox for centuries, pre-dating the Christian era. So engraved was smallpox in the medical history of India that a smallpox deity, known as the Hindu goddess, Shitala Mata was brought into existence.[49] Believers thought that she possessed curative powers and, therefore, worthwhile worshipping in the likely event when smallpox struck. Donald R. Hopkins shows how throughout the centuries, smallpox visited India periodically until it became more frequent during the seventeenth and eighteenth centuries leaving widespread devastation in its wake. By the 1750s and 1760s three major epidemics struck in Bengal killing thousands of people.[50] As the inhabitants of colonial India dealt with recurring outbreaks of smallpox throughout the eighteenth century, so too did the colonial and indigenous population of the Cape.

Recurring smallpox outbreaks local Khoikhoi populations and settlers believed to have appeared periodically since 1713 undoubtedly posed a host of new challenges to colonial authorities and the Khoikhoi people.[51] Unlike the formalized public health measures which white Cape Town instituted in 1755, rural Khoikhoi communities of the south-western Cape devised their own strategy to prevent possible contamination. Among the rural Khoikhoi, escape, by leaving their huts, was seen as a natural means of protection against possible infection. Once the news reached the interior that smallpox had broken out in Cape Town in May 1755, Khoikhoi immediately deserted their *kraals* and fled into the interior leaving behind many of their possessions, including their livestock.[52] It seemed that fleeing from their *kraals* only exacerbated matters as the virus was dispersed to other African communities, notably the Xhosa of the Eastern Cape. Jeff Peires writes that Xhosa people in the middle of eighteenth century were struck 'by a terrible smallpox epidemic'[53] which, in essence, meant colonial diseases, particularly smallpox, not only affected the Cape Khoikhoi, but several African societies who came into contact with Khoikhoi smallpox sufferers. This, in turn, often led to resentment towards the Khoikhoi, who found themselves barred from joining autonomous African societies in the interior. Fleeing their *kraals* also led to the immediate de-population of certain areas in the south-western Cape which was soon occupied by trekboers. With this mass movement dislocation, it is little surprise that in 1769, two years after the 1767 eruption, Backleij Plaats near Swellendam, an area occupied by the Hessequa Khoikhoi for centuries, was found deserted.[54]

Although the mortality rate of the 1755 outbreak was overall significantly lower than that of 1713, its impact on the social composition of Khoikhoi society cannot be overlooked. Many Khoikhoi communities were displaced and never returned to their original places of abode. Much to their dismay, the few who returned did so under trying circumstances as many could not return to their former lifestyle. Given the severity of the situation, a majority of these individuals found it extremely difficult to rebuild their herds, but even more difficult to mend their disrupted lives. Moreover, during the third outbreak in 1767, several Khoikhoi settlements in the Swellendam region were destroyed and set alight by colonists who thought they could combat the spread of the virus by destroying the huts of smallpox sufferers.[55] With forced and rapid changes in the rural landscape, several Khoikhoi communities were left impoverished and marginalized as a result. Thus, the innovative and desperate measures implemented to counteract smallpox seem to have only expedited Khoikhoi decline, allowing the VOC authorities to preside over their lot. The mere fact that some Khoikhoi communities sought colonial assistance to restore their fragile, autonomous existence was a clear indication that some communities had already begun a process of social disintegration and colonial absorption into colonial society.

With regard to the epidemics, the colonial public health regulations embarked upon earlier were also made applicable to the Cape Town Khoikhoi. A clause in one of the decrees stated that all Khoikhoi *kraals* located close to Cape Town were to be evacuated and demolished as soon as possible since they were seen as a potential health risk to white society. This is a good example of how the Cape authorities used the notion of 'disease' and 'sanitation' to ostracize and control the few remaining Khoikhoi communities in and around urban Cape Town.[56] The fact that the VOC authorities could so easily exert control over the local Khoikhoi in the name of public health demonstrates the extent to which health, disease and sanitation had become politicized during the early period of colonial rule in the Cape. Historians of nineteenth-century Cape Town, notably Maynard Swanson, later referred to this social practice as the 'sanitation syndrome'.[57] The disintegration of Khoikhoi society in the light of periodic smallpox outbreaks, together with the loss of land and livestock, fractured Khoikhoi way of life to such an extent that survivors were left very little choice, but to seek employment and refuge on white farms.

As the diseased, displaced and dispossessed Khoikhoi adjusted to their new social status as menials on white farms, colonial medicine acquired new perspectives and lookout. Encouraged by the moderate 'success' in keeping the mortality rates much lower,[58] the colonial authorities increased their commitment to health issues. Shortly after the last outbreak, concerted efforts were made to bring medicine and medical supplies within reach of ordinary white people. Aware of the high prices of medicine, a state-subsidized dispensary was founded in Cape Town, where medicine and medical supplies could be purchased at reasonable prices.[59] In line with these developments, plans were also devised to erect a new hospital near Table Mountain by 1773.[60]

The new developments in the field of medicine and pharmacology hardly made any inroads into the existing Khoikhoi medical practices. These changes only affected the settler population living within the confines of urban Cape Town and not those on the Cape frontier. Settlers living in the outlying regions of the colony hardly reaped the benefits of these changes which meant that the *status quo* of self-medication was largely maintained. Although Khoikhoi society as a whole had undergone drastic social changes since colonial conquest, their medical expertise and medicines remained largely unaffected though. For as long as the need for Khoikhoi medicine in the form of known remedies existed, which there certainly was, particularly on the Cape frontier, it secured its place in colonial society. The fusion of communities on the frontier also brought about fusion of medical ideas and the use of medical knowledge. In fact, Khoikhoi medicine quickly became the backbone of a new type of medicine and medical practices used on the Cape frontier as Khoikhoi and colonists combined their ideas of western and indigenous medicine. Thus, despite the rapid decline of Khoikhoi society and the efforts made by some Europeans to undermine the use of indigenous medicine, colonial medicine was never allowed to dominate or displace its indigenous equivalent.

The status of indigenous medicine and its relation to colonial imperatives and western medicine in India reveals a similar trajectory of encounter in India. In trying to understand this dynamism, Poonam Bala, in her essay in this volume, brings out significant aspects of the engagement of the Indian people, local elites and patrons with the medical and political aspects of colonial rule. As far as the Khoikhoi were concerned, living on a farm was not regarded reason enough to abandon their original ideas of medicine. Even Khoikhoi servants clung to their medical beliefs by regarding most plants and animals as potential medicine. One family who lived on a farm in Swellendam, for example 'looked upon the flesh of wild cats, lions and such like beasts of prey, as a medicine'.[61] In addition, many still rated the fat of a hippopotamus boiled and drunk as a cure for various ailments.[62] According to some knowledgeable Khoikhoi hunters, a peculiar vermin found in the bodies of these animals served as a preventive remedy against piles.[63] Even colonists were taught the medicinal value of hippopotami by Khoikhoi servants who often accompanied them on hunting expeditions. One colonist was informed that part of the skull reduced to a powder and taken in small quantity was useful in treating convulsions among children.[64]

Knowledge of herbal medicine, gynaecology and other indigenous methods of therapy were kept alive mostly by Khoikhoi midwives. As many settlers found themselves isolated from urban colonial society, particularly those living on the Cape frontier, they soon became receptive to the significance and use of herbal remedies. Since very few colonists had access to colonial medicine and doctors, the only medicine they knew was that prepared and administered by their Khoikhoi servants. On one remote farm, two Khoikhoi women treated their master's wife – an asthma patient – with indigenous herbs, presumably *buchu*.[65] It is also no secret that most frontier white women gave birth with the help of Khoikhoi midwives, indigenous techniques and medicine.[66] Peter Kolb, who lived at the Cape in the 1720s, also tells of an incident when a white woman struggled to give birth for three days. Only when a Khoikhoi midwife intervened and advised her to take a decoction of tobacco and milk – an old Khoikhoi custom – was the woman in labour eventually relieved from her misery.[67] These are but a few examples of how indigenous medicine and medical practices influenced colonial medical practices especially on the Cape frontier.[68]

The Khoikhoi's contribution to the development of herbal medicine in South Africa was considerable, yet it was denied in contemporary medical historiographies. Edmund Burrows, for example, ignored their contribution when he referred to the medicinal value of *buchu*. Indeed, Burrows should be challenged on his view that it was the trekboers who first discovered the medicinal value of *buchu*.[69] While his view sparks off new debates, there is much to be said about the role of the Khoikhoi who taught white frontier communities the medicinal uses of herbal plants. This also justifies the long and successful tradition of indigenous medical practice in South Africa. Nevertheless, as Steve Phatlane discusses in his chapter in this volume, over the years, although indigenous knowledge has faced marginalization, it has maintained a willing clientele for addressing sexually transmitted diseases, such as AIDS. While it appears that Khoikhoi medicine was still a sought-after commodity on the frontier, the introduction of slaves, especially those from the Indian Sub-Continent was set to arrive at the Cape with their strong religious beliefs and medical traditions.

Slave Remedies

The introduction of slaves from the East Indies to the Cape of Good Hope in the mid-seventeenth century facilitated the influx and exchange of ideas about medicine, healing and medical practices as understood by individuals captured and enslaved from different parts of the world. Individuals brought to the Cape as slaves from India were mainly from Bengal, the coast of Coromandel and the Malabar coast, which stretched from Bombay (Mumbai) to Cochin.[70] The introduction of slaves taken from regions sporting rich medical and healing traditions suggests that those brought as slaves to the Cape invariably possessed some kind of medical knowledge in order to cure basic bodily ailments. The historian, Vink, for instance, asserts that individuals of Indian origin were drafted into the colonial society as masseuses, nurses, midwives and wet-nurses and spared the drudgery of hard labour.[71]

Slaves of African and Asian origin too were rendered invaluable medical help to fellow servants and slaves, and those who possessed some degree of medical knowledge were often seen as 'doctors' or 'healers' by fellow slaves and Khoikhoi servants. The manumitted slave, Johannes Smiesing for instance, recorded in the Tamil language remedies to heal wheezing, fever, vomiting, griping pain and irritation in the stomach, dropsy, inflammation and venereal diseases such as gonorrhoea.[72] In the 1770s, the botanist and medical doctor Anders Sparrman talks about a slave who treated a slave woman bitten by a venomous lizard-like creature. On another occasion, the slave dressed wounds with oranges and lemon cut into halves. According to Sparrman, the slave doctor was extremely secretive about his many curative abilities, and had apparently 'died with the secret'.[73]

Robert Semple, a merchant and traveller who visited the Cape in 1798, described the slaves that came from the Malabar coasts as 'the best of the household slaves', being 'more intelligent, more industrious' which suggests that many slaves from Malabar, presumably, possessed some medical knowledge after centuries of exposure to indigenous methods of healing in their country of birth.[74] Also, by the late 1790s, the Danish medical doctor and surgeon Theodor Folly had written about the existence of Malabar doctors and those from Tranquebar on the Coromandel Coast of India, the medical knowledge they possessed and how treatment was administered to patients.[75] It therefore seems likely that slaves who hailed from India possessed a fair knowledge of medicine and herbal remedies upon their arrival at the Cape and were, thus, more than likely in a position to treat basic bodily ailments.

Apart from individuals of Indian descent who acted as healers in the Cape slave community, the established sea-route and trading network that fortified Cape–Indo contact further facilitated the transmission of Indian medical knowledge to the Cape. One such major influence was accompanied by the importation and use of the so-called snake-stone to treat and cure snakebite. Engelbert Keampfer, a German-born medical doctor in the service of the VOC, reported in the late 1680s, shortly after having visited Malabar and Coromandel coasts in India, of the existence of two popular antidotes against snakebite: the root of the Mungo plant and snake-stone.[76] Use of the snake-stone in order to treat snakebite proved extremely effective and popular in India and the Cape, regions known for various species of poisonous snakes. In 1772, Peter Thunberg reported that during his travels through the interior of the Cape, near Tulbagh, he was shown what he called 'the much celebrated snake-stone'.[77] 'Held in great esteem' by Cape farmers, the snake-stone was imported from Malabar, India and was priced between ten and twelve rix-dollars, which was very expensive at the time. Thunberg described the snake-stone as follows:

> It is round and convex on the one side, of a black colour, with a pale-grey speck in the middle and tubulated, with very minute pores. When put into water, it causes bubbles to rise, which is proof of its being genuine, as is also, that it put into the mouth, it adheres to the palate. When it is applied to any part that has been bitten by a serpent, it sticks to the wound, and extracts the poison; as soon it is saturated, it falls off itself. If it be then put into milk, it is supposed to be purified from the poison it had absorbed, and the milk is said to be turned blue by it.[78]

The Indian influence and knowledge of the snake-stone and its curative abilities had, by the mid-eighteenth century, become part of the medical culture in treating snakebite, especially among the affluent section of the colonial community. Towards the end of the eighteenth century, a certain Pieter du Preez sold a snake-stone for ten rix-dollars, while Governor Van Assenburgh's last will and testament included a snake-stone.[79] While the colonial elite lauded the medicinal value of the Malabar snake-stone, the arrival of colonial doctors ushered in a new phase of colonial medicine in the Cape colony where the black body of the 'other' would be brought under new forms of medical scrutiny.

Colonial Doctors and the Indigenous Body

A significant development of the post-smallpox era was the appearance of European travellers, some of whom were university-educated doctors. Given *carte blanche* by the colonial authorities to visit the Cape and its unexplored landscapes, many viewed it as an ideal opportunity to test their ideas of medicine among the indigenous peoples of the Cape. The medical doctor Anders Sparrman, for example, boasted of how he once had to rescue a Khoikhoi servant 'from the clutches of his master, who had an unlimited confidence in venesection, and had already whetted his knife on purpose to perform it'.[80]

Apart from promoting western medicine between Khoikhoi servants and Cape slaves, it also enabled these travellers to study the black body and its physical features. Prevailing Eurocentric images of the Khoikhoi which were largely fuelled by fallacious travel reports and contemporary European thought that placed the Khoikhoi at the bottom rung of the social ladder,[81] were to have a major impact on the way medicine was practised at the Cape. European doctors were convinced that whites were not only mentally and socially superior to the African peoples, but were physically and biologically different as well. Compared to themselves, they regarded the indigenous Khoikhoi as a different 'race of men', and their diarized characterization of the Khoikhoi's physical features bears testimony to their perceptions of the black body.[82] To prove their point of racial superiority, doctors used the European male as the yardstick by which to compare the physical features of the Khoikhoi to the very bone.[83] This type of intense medical scrutiny to which the Khoikhoi population was often subjected was the forerunner of the popular nineteenth-century anthropometric examinations involving the measurement of body parts and the dissection of the human body of which Georges Cuvier (1769–1832) was a major exponent.[84] Cuvier's dissection of the Khoikhoi woman, Sara Baartman, in 1815/16 remains the most notorious example to date.[85]

Mesmerized by these so-called physical differences, European-trained doctors visiting the Cape interior were immensely interested in studying the indigenous body, to either prove or disprove their theories and personal perceptions of the black body; curiosity was often the key driving force behind examination of the indigenous body. Sparrman made no secret of his intentions and admitted to 'being curious to examine a negro's flesh'.[86] Subsequently, European doctors created opportunities in which their curiosity with the 'negro's flesh' could be satisfied. Sparrman, for example, was keen to administer medicine to as many indigenous patients and slaves as he possibly could. Thus, the 'negro's flesh' became a subject of intense medical study. In an attempt to find scientific proof that biological differences indeed existed between blacks and whites, Sparrman agreed to treat a servant suffering from an ulcer. He had hoped to prove that the symptoms of an ulcer diagnosed among white people were radically different to those of black patients. A few days later, Sparrman was surprised to notice that 'the raw flesh appeared exactly of the same colour with that of a European'.[87] His medical 'experiment' had failed to reveal conclusively that differences existed between white and black bodies with regard to various disorders and its symptoms.[88] Undaunted by the failure to produce sufficient scientific evidence that biological differences existed, Sparrman sought other ways to substantiate his theory of white supremacy. This time he administered bottled medicine to his patients. In 1775, he doctored an entire Khoikhoi family who suffered from putrid fever (typhus) with medicine he had prepared himself.[89] Months later, he again treated a few Khoikhoi labourers who suffered from bilious fever.[90] At the end of his series of 'medical experiments', Sparrman confessed to being 'amazed to find these people's [Khoikhoi] stomachs require such large dosages'.[91] Such utterances clearly confirm that some European doctors simply administered medicine to the Khoikhoi and slaves to satisfy their curiosity about the black body, and were not at all interested in the physical well-being of the patient. It was also a clear indication that European doctors sought 'scientific' proof to confirm their theory of white racial superiority. Apart from doctoring and exposing the Khoikhoi to western medicine, it was also a deliberate attempt on their part to ensure that western medicine became part of Khoikhoi culture and indispensable in their new 'western' way of life.

In a more recent historical scholarship, Mark Harrison and David Arnold have shown that similar patterns emerged in colonial India when British doctors set out during the mid-eighteenth and nineteenth centuries to study the 'Indian body' in the hope of pin-pointing physical and biological differences as well as identifying Indian susceptibility to various diseases and ailments.[92] Despite the fact that post mortems were strongly opposed in Indian culture, Arnold has shown how colonial doctors based in colonial hospitals often contravened these cultural and religious beliefs. In the mid-1820s, James Annesley reportedly compared the 'effects of disease upon the constitutions of the Europeans and natives'.[93] He concluded that European and Indian males appeared vulnerable to different diseases and ailments. Cholera, fevers and ulcers were more likely to kill Indians, whereas dysentery and liver diseases are listed as the chief causes of death among European males.[94] In 1832, William Twining based at Calcutta's General Hospital ran a battery of experiments on Indian and European patients and concluded that biologically, Indians, 'being constitutionally weaker, could not stand such "heroic" measures as Europeans ... and were more likely to succumb to the onslaught of disease'.[95] The conclusion reached by Arnold commenting on an era when biological differences between indigenous and European peoples is indicative of the direction the world had moved towards by the end of the eighteenth century, as it sought to denigrate indigenous peoples even further, using science, technology and medicine to justify their ideas. With reference to colonial India and British occupation, Arnold writes:

> there was an undoubted growth in the British emphasis upon racial difference, and especially the perceived physical characteristics of race, over the course of the nineteenth century. The concept of race, presented as biological fact, became one of the governing ideas of the high imperial ear, and sustained attempts were made in the name of science to give race an anatomical, even mathematical, precision.[96]

Different opinions regarding methods of medical treatment and medicine frequently arose between Khoikhoi healers who lived and worked on farms and colonial doctors visiting the Cape interior. In one case when western medicine failed to yield the desired result, it was left to two Khoikhoi women to revive the patient who was left for dead after a colonial doctor performed an unsuccessful venesection. In 1775, Sparrman volunteered to treat a Khoikhoi labourer who suffered from a bad disorder. When Sparrman noticed the operation proved unsuccessful, he was quick to admit that he left the patient 'in a much weaker condition than what [he] found him'.[97] Hours later, two Khoikhoi women entered the hut where the sick servant laid and applied their method of healing. By jolting and vigorously shaking the head of patient for while, they eventually succeeded in putting the weak circulation and the other vital organs back into motion as the patient commenced breathing. Sparrman, who witnessed the entire procedure stood amazed at how effective this method of reviving an unconscious person was.[98] Despite the arrogance displayed by some colonial doctors about the healing powers which western medicine seemingly possessed, Khoikhoi medicine, at times still proved more effective than its western equivalent.

Since many European doctors regarded the black body as an object of study essentially to prove racial differences, it begs the question whether or not stereotypical racial ideas regarding the black body played any significant role in social relations on farms and Cape society. If this was the case, then what role could disease and illnesses have played in fortifying existing racial divisions between whites and blacks? As a rule, the black diseased servant was never allowed in the house of the master, or near his family for that matter, for fear that diseased individuals may infect the entire household. For example, one Khoikhoi labourer afflicted with a serious disorder was left unattended for days in his quarters, because his master feared that the ailment might contaminate his entire household.[99]

In Cape society, personal opinions about medical racism based upon colour, race, appearance, anatomy and biological make-up were voiced more openly. The Cape, however, was an inherently racist society and hardly needed a catalyst such as an epidemic to prove the noticeable prejudices prevalent at the time. Yet, it seems as though smallpox did present some colonists and government officials with an opportunity to put their racist ideas into practice. In an effort to allay white fears, the Khoikhoi and slave community seen by many colonists as 'biologically inferior' and 'easily-diseased', were somehow singled out as the ones responsible for the disease. It is, thus, clear that the servile population bore the brunt of medical racism, as they were blamed for the rapid dispersion of smallpox.[100]

In the light of the above, it seems rare that masters would allow their sick Khoikhoi servants to consult a doctor. In 1769, however, a doctor was paid six rix-dollars by Betler Wagner to administer medicine to a Khoikhoi woman in his service.[101] Privately-owned slaves who fell ill were often treated by colonial doctors and paid for by their owners. One Cape doctor, named Jan Blaauw treated a slave for syphilis.[102] However, not all servants were as fortunate, as compensation for medical expenses often proved very costly. On the Cape frontier where medicine was scarce and reliable Khoikhoi labour difficult to hold onto, many farmers saw the medication offered to their servants as a means of control. Compelled by his master, one servant ceded his entire earnings – twenty rix-dollars, a horse and eight cows – to repay his medical expenses incurred.[103] Thus, on the Cape frontier, colonial medicine was often seen and used as an agent of social control, sometimes as in this example the cause of debt and subsequent bonded labour, as early as the eighteenth century.

Medicine, and how it was administered between servants and settlers, gradually became a contentious issue. Needless to say, colonial doctors were often caught in the middle of such disputes. As a result, colonial doctors were often torn between being popular among their peers and honouring their profession. Since doctors generally struggled to establish themselves as full-time private practitioners in the interior, doctoring maltreated slaves and Khoikhoi servants became a sensitive issue. For obvious reasons, some colonial practitioners distanced themselves from master–servant disputes and refused to administer medicine to servants and slaves maltreated by their masters. But there were exceptions, as some doctors valued their profession above an acceptable reputation. At least one such instance is recorded in 1791, when a certain doctor, Frans Sommer, treated the wounds of a Khoikhoi servant who had been badly beaten by his master.[104] In cases of extreme master brutality, the Court of Justice sometimes intervened stipulating that slaves and Khoikhoi servants are treated by doctors. In such cases, Cape doctors had little choice but to treat the less fortunate slaves and servants.

Medical examination of a dead body or an autopsy performed to discover the cause of death was probably the only way in which western medical procedures was imposed on deceased indigenous Khoikhoi servant and slaves, irrespective of their religious beliefs. Even though the Khoikhoi may have been opposed to autopsies for religious reasons, the deceased were subjected to this form of medical examination, especially in murder cases. Family members or friends of the deceased had very little chance of contesting an autopsy. For instance, in April 1764, a Khoikhoi woman who worked at a VOC post was found dead in her room. Without consulting her next-of-kin, the corpse was taken to the hospital in Cape Town where an autopsy was immediately performed.[105] Prior to that, another autopsy was performed on a Khoikhoi labourer who had apparently died in his sleep. The post-mortem revealed that the man had died of suffocation.[106] Since autopsies were performed on a fairly regular basis, colonial practitioners undoubtedly improved their meagre anatomical knowledge by 'operating' on the black body. By demanding that autopsies be performed ostensibly under the auspices of the law was also a clear indication of how the Cape authorities created opportunities which allowed white medical practitioners to use the indigenous body to enhance colonial medicine and medical research. By subjecting the servile population to different kinds of intense medical scrutiny, the state became the principal agent to exploit medicine and the profession as a medium of social control. Apart from the few medical and legal liberties the Khoikhoi enjoyed, they generally had very little say over their bodies after death, as autopsies were performed without permission. VOC law superseded cultural and religious beliefs as shown in the case of a slave woman of Indian descent, Diana van Bengalen. Having been beaten to death by a fellow slave, an autopsy was conducted by two VOC surgeons in the Company hospital and later stated in court that they 'opened the head and inspected' the body of Diana in order to ascertain the cause of death. Kerry Ward questions whether or not the deceased was given a proper burial according to her beliefs, as the slave population at the Cape comprised individuals that subscribed to various beliefs and faiths which upon death was not honoured.[107] However, in at least one instance, an autopsy provided 'justice' to a murdered Khoikhoi servant. In one court case, the body of a deceased servant was exhumed after his friend, who witnessed the murder, insisted that an autopsy be performed.[108] The local *Landdrost* (magistrate) agreed and the state physician, Georg Geering[109] who performed the autopsy reported that the person in question had died of multiple blows sustained from a blunt object. Hans Jurgen Kettner, the person responsible for the murder was subsequently executed and his accomplices banished from the Cape.[110] Even victims of sexual violence and assault, especially women, were at liberty to consult a district surgeon, particularly in cases of rape;[111] perpetrators of this crime were often brought to book after a physical examination was performed on the victim.[112]

As mentioned earlier, despite the fact the autopsies were tabooed in traditional Indian society, as the deceased went untouched and were cremated after
death, colonial medical practitioners in positions of power often ignored the
religious sentiments of these practices. Contravention to Indian religious beliefs
were often performed away from the public eye and executed in a domain of
what Arnold called 'institutional observation – the hospitals, jails and above all
the army'.[113] But as Harrison has argued, it was during the age of exploration,
commerce and empire-building that colonial powers such as the Dutch and later
British infiltrated indigenous societies and saw it fit to impose upon colonized
societies their ideas about medical practice on people that have survived for centuries on their own, relying completely on their indigenous medical and healing
practices. A worrying, but true comment by Harrison, that indigenous 'cadav-
ers were plentiful' and available to be examined and experimented on, brought
into existence a new dimension associated with colonialism and colonial conquest.[114] It suggests that colonial doctors with a meaningful support from the
institutionalized colonial systems such as the law and colonial courts, viewed the
indigenous body as their personal human laboratory, which lead to the production of 'scientific knowledge' that fuelled racial stereotyping.

Conclusion

Here it has been suggested that Khoikhoi communities of the interior were
ostensibly in a better position as far as the use of indigenous medicine was concerned than the first few generations of colonists that settled at the Cape. While
the colonial medical practitioners concentrated on pharmaceutically-produced
medicines and their own version of *boeren-middels*, which their forefathers
brought to the Cape, the Khoikhoi performed surgical operations alongside the
routine treatments and methods they had practised for centuries. Only later,
when colonial medicine at the Cape became 'scientific', particularly with the
discovery of vaccination in Europe, and other cures, did it supersede Khoikhoi
medicine. Although the urban population of Cape Town reaped the benefits of
these developments, rural people continued to rely on herbal medicine. It was
on the outskirts of the Cape colonial frontier society where indigenous medicine
blended with its western equivalent had flourished.

With regard to perceptions of medicine, fundamental differences existed
between the Khoikhoi and Cape colonists. In a Khoikhoi society, medical care
was free and regarded as a 'right', whereas in colonial society this was hardly the
case. In Cape colonial society where western medicine was regarded as elitist, the
notion of cure for cash was very much the order of the day.

The changing social and racial relations in colonial society, undoubtedly,
influenced the way in which medicine was perceived by the various social strata

of Cape society. People with different social and ideological backgrounds formulated their own opinion of how western medicine could be used. Regrettably, not all (including doctors) saw medicine as a means to cure or alleviate pain. With regard to western medicine and the indigenous body, European physicians had their own agenda. Their interest in the black body was essentially confined to two aspects. Firstly, to prove that physical and biological differences existed between black and white, and secondly, curious to see how black patients responded to bottled western medicine. On the other hand, Cape-born colonial doctors expressed little interest in studying and medicating the black body. For them, tending to the medical needs and illnesses of their own people was not only financially more rewarding, but served also as an ideal justification for their distance from the indigenous body. Farmers had a totally different view of colonial medicine. In a colonial society where slave labour was expensive and often scarce in the interior, settlers sometimes used medicine as a tool of social control and a means of securing indigenous labour. Despite these diverse views regarding western medicine, most colonists regarded bottled western medicine as a precious commodity which was not to be wasted on the black, diseased body. These perceptions of western medicine among the colonial authorities undoubtedly influenced the way the Khoikhoi viewed western medicine. For the Khoikhoi, colonial medicine was a foreign substance, imported by whites to bewitch and defile their bodies. Furthermore, it had little healing power and was regarded as untrustworthy and to be avoided at all costs. However, since colonial medicine and colonial law seldom functioned independently, Khoikhoi adopted a less hostile approach towards western medicine.

It is evident that medicine touched the lives of thousands of people across the racial and social barrier, and was destined to play an even greater role in the future history of the entire Colony. Although the Cape Colony, towards the end of the eighteenth-century, was not a fully-fledged medicalized society, it was rapidly on its way to becoming one; one in which the state and colonial doctors were to have a greater say over the lives of marginalized communities which still enjoyed limited access to colonial medicine.

Acknowledgements

This project was funded by the National Research Foundation (NRF) and its support is hereby acknowledged. Gratitude is also expressed to the anonymous reviewers and the general editor of the volume, Poonam Bala.

4 DEALING WITH DISEASE: EPIZOOTICS, VETERINARIANS AND PUBLIC HEALTH IN COLONIAL BENGAL, 1850–1920

Samiparna Samanta

In a district like this in which the majority of the people belong to the Hindoo religion, it is impossible to take the only step which would be efficacious in staying the plague, namely, an unsparing use of the axe on the cattle suspected to be tainted with the disease.

Captain John Gregory 1869[1]

Whenever authorities are able to detect diseased/infected animals, they are sent away to kasai-khanas to be slaughtered by butchers. While there are veterinarians appointed to check diseased meat, it is not possible for them to inspect the numerous animals brought to the slaughterhouses every day, twenty-four hours.

Shree Manicklal Mallik, 'Niramish Bhojon' (Vegetarian Diet) (1916)[2]

On 3 February 1864, John Stalkartt reported to the government of Bengal that a 'malignant murrain' had broken out in Calcutta and the neighbouring area which needed to be checked early. Deeply alarmed at the loss of his own Arab cow and four calves, Stalkratt suggested that

the murrain which attacked the cattle at the Great Agricultural Exhibition is spreading, and some Commission should be appointed to devise means to check it early. Bengal has very few cattle, and should it pass into the villages it will be very serious.[3]

From the mid-nineteenth century onwards, widespread outbreak of cattle plague or rinderpest in Bengal, Punjab and Madras, among other regions, caused panic in the colonial establishment.[4] The government responded to such cattle murrains with urgency, which meant that epizootics of the late nineteenth century stimulated the establishment of state veterinary services.[5] In this chapter, I focus on animal disease, especially rinderpest, to show how it became a site of contestation over appropriate medical knowledge, human health, public hygiene and science. The debate was multilayered and too often diverse tensions manifested themselves at different junctures over class, race and science. Debates surfaced in official circles about the nature and cause of the disease as well as around prognosis; even the conclusion they reached was fraught with anxieties surrounding sale and inspection of diseased meat among the Bengali *bhadralok* (upper middle and middle classes of Bengal). At a different level, I intend to show how animals played a crucial role as social actors in understanding public health in colonial India.

This chapter tells two major stories. First, it discusses the trajectory of cattle epizootics in nineteenth-century Bengal and analyses the impact disease control had on larger debates concerning knowledge formation and the politics of class/ race. While there had always remained a close relationship between animals and human disease, until the mid-twentieth century medical knowledge on the boundary between animal and human health remained blurred.[6] Against this backdrop, this chapter also investigates the relationship between cattle plague and slaughterhouse inspection. Diseased animals increasingly flooded markets because Bengali farmers often rejected the 'English method' of slaughter and culling, as it was economically damaging. In addition, it was cheaper to sell diseased animals than seek veterinary attention. The second story focuses on how rinderpest subsequently revived interest in Bengali diet, as doctors began to discover a co-relation between animal disease and human health. The debate over the safety of meat from diseased animals became fiercer over time and quickly kindled *bhadralok* paranoia over animal disease, public health and sanitation.

Disease Strikes

The Politics of Naming

From mid-nineteenth century onwards, correspondence among commissioners of Bengal, Madras, and the veterinary surgeons in those regions indicates the immediate colonial anxiety to combat 'cattle pestilence'.[7] The symptoms of epizootics were not unknown to the Victorian medical practitioners.[8] Yet, despite this familiarity, there were elements of uncertainty about the nature and cause of cattle plague in the colony. British veterinarians often sought information from England about the nature of rinderpest and ways of dealing with it. For instance, in October 1867, K. M. McLeod, the Civil Assistant Surgeon of Jessore, requested the government of Bengal to help him obtain the *Report of the Parliamentary Commission Appointed to Enquire into the Nature of the Cattle Plague in England*. However, considerable differences of opinion persisted among the British veterinary surgeons as also between the British and Bengali veterinary surgeons when it came to the question of contagiousness.[9] In fact, interpretation of the nature of rinderpest depended on an ever-shifting theory of disease propagation. While some British doctors speculated that the disease was transmissible, others linked it to a range of causes – from heredity, poor nutrition and environmental factors to a weak physical condition of the animals.

While reporting the disease, the first issue to trouble the British veterinarian-authors was its nomenclature. Closely tied to the question of naming the disease was the colonial preoccupation with establishing the roots of the disease – was it an indigenous disease or an imported ailment?[10] Official discourse almost inevitably attributed the disease to 'the machination of the *chamars*' (leatherworkers) who were indirectly responsible for spreading the disease 'by burying the animal skins on the locality where the disease broke out'.[11] If the indigenous farmers understood the disease as an import into Bengal led by north-western bullocks, colonial authorities were quick to deny the role of agricultural exhibitions and cattle fairs, and instead linked it to the nineteenth-century miasma theory.[12]

Nevertheless, whatever be the official confusion over its first occurrence, the British officials consistently claimed to have first 'discovered' the disease. Captain Campbell, Deputy Commissioner of Nowgong reported that a disease that claimed 21,625 heads of cattle in 1853 was believed to be 'cholera' by the natives, but he considered it 'a disease of the nature of the Calcutta epizootic'.[13] Likewise, while acknowledging that the farmers were aware of another disease – the *Puschima* (because it was supposed to have travelled from *Puschim* or western India) – colonial authorities were quick to dismiss the validity of indigenous disease wisdom. Instead, Dr C. Palmer in his Report pointed out that there existed throughout India, very extensively, two distinct and very fatal epizootics. One was the eczema epizootic which corresponded to the foot-and-mouth disease of England, and the other was the Calcutta epizootic of 1864 which was identical to 'Rinderpest, which has for so many years past, devastated Central Europe'.[14] British veterinarians in the colony in the mid-nineteenth century were eager to look to Europe as the reference frame that bestowed scientific legitimacy to the knowledge gathered in the tropics. In fact, British veterinarians not only imposed their familiar European disease names and knowledge systems on cattle diseases of Bengal, but they also brought out claims of 'science' and 'sanitation' in the spread of disease across the world. Commenting on the origins of cattle plague in Bengal, one Professor Symonds argued that,

> the Steppes of Russia are the home of this disease, and that it has spread from there by infection, and that by severe sanitary prohibitions its progress might be limited. It is a highly interesting and important fact that this same disease has traveled eastward, as it has been unchecked by any sanitary restrictions, its progress has been, perhaps, more rapid in an eastwardly and unguarded and unprotected direction than it has been westwardly, where science backed by arbitrary and even despotic government aid, has been called in to check its march.[15]

A partial consensus was reached by 1865 that this was indeed a *new* disease – 'rinderpest' – that was 'unrecognized in the neighborhood by either cattle proprietors' or by civil surgeons.[16] Cattle murrains continued unchecked as several bouts broke out all over Bengal in districts like Dinajpore, Moorshedabad, Malda, Rajshahi and Rungpore from 1863 to 1868, often carrying varying local, native names – *gotee, chupkah*, or the *mour* or *lohomy muska*.[17] Based on observations of the symptoms, the British civil surgeons attempted to relate the disease to something identifiable, arguing that the murrains corresponded to the *Puschima* of Lower Bengal and the Rinderpest of Europe.[18] They repeatedly tried to ascertain if the cattle plague ravaging India was of the 'same type' as the one that affected England.[19] The colonial anxiety to construct the animal disease in Bengal as 'rinderpest' is interesting in that even the act of determining animal plague was debatable and not devoid of power dynamics. However, that the indigenous farmers and cattle-owners were familiar with the diseases affecting cattle is evident from the reference to commonly circulated local, indigenous names.[20] J. A. Voelkar, in his *Report on the Improvement of Indian Agriculture* underplayed the farmers' knowledge and nomenclature concerning the animal diseases by portraying it as both superstitious and vague. He commented,

> The Natives believe that cattle epidemics are visitations of the goddess 'Mata' and that they can only get rid of the epidemic by propitiating the goddess. The variety of names by which diseases are known to the Natives in different parts makes it hard to ascertain how far they really recognize the particular ones and the respective symptoms.[21]

The cattle diseases of Bengal, lacking a common vocabulary or 'scientific' language, was easier to be appropriated with a known European nomenclature than adopt the multiple exotic names given by the indigenous farmers.

Controlling Cattle Disease: Colonial Knowledge and British Veterinarians

Once the legitimacy of rinderpest in Bengal was established, all focus was diverted towards its control. The last decade of the nineteenth century saw frantic colonial attempts to produce systematic knowledge about cattle diseases through surveys and reports, and the ultimate need to create a network of veterinary boards, dispensaries and qualified surgeons who could substitute the village 'quacks' by their professional doctors and, thus, save cattle lives. Ensuring that 'English remedies' reached the indigenous agrarian societies, British veterinarians pushed to circulate adequate Bengali translations of J. H. B Hallen's (Inspecting Veterinary Surgeon of Bombay Army) *Manual of the More Deadly Forms of Cattle Disease in India* to different officers under the government.[22] The government even aspired to introduce veterinary education as a curriculum in colleges and create a class of professional veterinarians who could treat animal diseases – the Belgachia Veterinary College being one such institution established in 1896. While local knowledge of the environment, animals and the indigenous communities was highly sought after, colonial authorities strove to apply metropolitan disease control measures to the Indian colony. As in South Africa, many animal diseases prevalent in India were unknown in Europe and given the lack of research facilities available in the colonies at the turn of the twentieth century, India-based scientists often had to investigate mysterious infections from scratch.[23] However, despite the lack of adequate research facilities, treatment of animal disease and ethno-veterinary practices was not unheard of in the heavily agrarian society of India. Cattle diseases and their treatment featured prominently in indigenous healing practices, as also in several nineteenth-century Bengali agricultural tracts and periodicals like *Krishak, Krishak Bandhab, Krishak Gazette*. If the Bengali farmers were conversant with the more common cattle ailments like *Basanta* (cow-pox), *Daad* (ring-worm), *Bhail* (cholera) and their cures, they were not familiar with rinderpest attacks or its cures. H. Farrell, the veterinary surgeon on special duty ordered to visit different provinces of Bengal in 1869, commented on Bengali farmers' resistance towards adopting colonial measures of disease control, which he believed stemmed from an innate backwardness and bigotry that thwarted any western prevention measures. It is interesting to note that in commenting on indigenous reaction to cattle plague, H. Farrell began his report with an assessment of the character of different indigenous communities of Assam like the Ahoms and Domes.[24] The colonial project of controlling cattle plague became a largely hegemonic process of disciplining and regulating indigenous farmers as much as the diseased animals themselves.

Veterinary Medicine, Status and Colonial Claims

During the mid-nineteenth century when rinderpest first drew the attention of British officials, veterinary medicine was largely an unreformed arena. Historians studying British veterinarians have shown that in the nineteenth century, veterinary medicine had a low status and elite veterinarians were struggling to define their professional domain and to escape the tarnish of the farrier's trade.[25] However, as Michael Worboys has shown, veterinarians had an ambivalent attitude towards the medical profession. They acknowledged that they too practised 'medicine' and were engaged in a similar campaign for status. In a similar vein, qualified veterinarians tried to distance themselves from farriers, cow leeches, knowledgeable farmers and 'veterinary quacks'.[26] Also, as William G. Clarence-Smith has pointed out in his study of diseases of equids in Southeast Asia in the nineteenth and twentieth century, many farmers treated their own animals using traditional remedies, or utilized a range of lay healers, as was only too evident during the cattle plague crisis.[27] British veterinarians in India had to assert their area of competency and define themselves as 'scientific' practitioners to boost their position. Tensions persisted not only on questions of respectability in handling animal diseases and dissections, but also on the boundaries between human and animal diseases. For instance, as early as in 1821, Surgeon-Major C. S Willis (Civil Surgeon) petitioned to the Lieutenant-Governor of Bengal that the order issued by Cantonment Magistrate of Barrackpore requiring him to dissect a poisoned cow, was professionally demeaning because the job of removing the viscera of a poisoned cow was not befitting a civil surgeon.[28] The Surgeon-Major was 'indignant' and 'professionally hurt' because he 'was told to do the job of a butcher'.[29] If British civil surgeons were comfortable dissecting human viscera, they considered the vivisection of poisoned cows demeaning, thus threatening their notions of honour as a product of racial, gender and class superiority. In this case, race anxiety and guarding imperial honour seemed to have gained precedence over the claims of science.

The enormity of the plague paranoia meant that it was not limited to the government alone. If the colonial authorities and veterinarians' agenda of reform and sanitation projected the subaltern classes as unclean masses in need of control or sanitary salvation, records on how the farmers sought to tackle the disease as a health problem are rather scanty. Borrowing Projit B. Mukharji's approach explored in *Nationalizing the Body: The Medical Market, Print and Daktari Medicine* (2009), one possible way of recovering the subaltern medical responses from the educated Bengali sources such as the *Krishak Gazette* and *Krishak Bandhab*, is to look at those cures coded as 'folk' remedies. Scholars have shown how with the development of the Bengali medical public sphere from the late nineteenth century, there was a progressive attempt to appropriate the medical knowledge base of the subaltern orders. However, the Bengali middle class was not so much responsive to animal disease in the initial stages of rinderpest attack. In the absence of more detailed information about the contexts in which some indigenous remedies were developed, it would be impossible to reconstruct the logic that informed them.

By the end of the nineteenth century, in a disease-ravaged Bengal, a general sense of helplessness and loss prevailed. The unpopularity of inspection and slaughtering, along with the economic losses borne by farmers, were powerful reminders of the failure to check the outbreak. The *Evening Mail* captured the despair and anguish in 1885 in a very dramatic way. It reported,

> what strikes us most is the facility with which farmers and veterinary surgeons abandon themselves to despair, so far as regards all hope of successful treatment, and resort to the extreme measure of prohibition and destruction. We could do this, of course, if we were merest savages, ready to believe a demon had passed over our cattle and glad to fall back on our yards and plantains; but we are rather better than savages, and we profess to have some power over the diseases of man and beast. It is a humbling confession that is made by our medical authorities when they tell us to kill at once, for there is nothing at all to be done.[30]

Arnold has examined how the early (human) plague years in Bombay were a major crisis point in the history of state medicine in nineteenth-century India, occasioned by people's hostility towards anti-plague measures.[31] Likewise, in the case of rinderpest, helplessness of the colonial government is evident as it faced a dual crisis of control. Despite the quarantine measures in the villages and the city of Calcutta, the epidemic went on unabated, affecting Bengal, Punjab and Madras. If human plague affected major Indian port cities like Bombay, Karachi and Calcutta, rinderpest affected the rural regions more than the cities, excepting the Calcutta epizootic which equally ravaged the city and the countryside of Bengal. From 1865 onwards, textual evidence indicates the official anxieties concerning rinderpest, which might eat into the profitability of empire. By 1869, it was evident in the official circles that there was 'a considerable decrease in cultivation on account of the want of plough bullocks'.[32] Interestingly, although the colonial authorities praised the European planters' 'intelligence' in arresting the spread of disease among their herds, mortality rates indicate a different story. The disease, in fact, equally devastated cattle of both the Europeans and the native farmers. Thus, while the colonial authorities persistently sought to control both animal disease and the subjects by perpetuating racial hierarchies in a colonial society, yet ironically, animals and diseases easily blurred these actual and invented borders.

Doctors and Diet

Cattle Disease and the Bengali bhadralok

Disease historiography has focused on the ways in which 'western' medicine was deployed in the colony and the manner in which the members of the colonized society appropriated it.[33] In South Asia, the works of Ramanna, Ray, Dutta, Bala and others have focused on South Asian practitioners of western medicine.[34] Regarding the way in which western medicine was received by the Bengalis, Projit Bihari Mukharji through his recent study of *daktari* medicine has revealed how the situation in Calcutta, though not unique, clearly presented some specific dilemmas.[35] 'Western'-style education had been introduced in Bengal for the longest period and as a result, by the 1890s the Calcutta elite were, relative to the other presidency towns, perhaps the most deeply indoctrinated in 'western' sciences.[36] The story of Bengali *bhadralok*'s attitude towards cattle plague is, however, largely different from their response towards human plague. Although the effects of cattle plague were severe and fervently debated in the official circles, it did not significantly affect the *bhadralok*. Generally it was the veterinarians, medical specialists and people involved in live animal trade who actually participated in the debate about the spread and containment of cattle plague.[37] Perhaps the estrangement of the *bhadralok* from the realities of agricultural life also removed them from the immediate economic effects of animal disease? In Bengal, the extent to which any section of society was insulated from contact with working animals and livestock is a debatable point. All kinds of beasts were omnipresent in Indian cities, and links between town and country remained close in Bengal. A serious concern and alarm for the Bengali *bhadralok* over cattle health and disease came much later. Their anxiety concerned the extent to which the great livestock diseases – rinderpest, foot-and-mouth and pleuropneumonia – affected human health. Indeed, the main threat was food poisoning from meat. Perusing through a variety of government and nongovernmental archives – Bengali medical periodicals, pamphlets and so on – I will seek to retrieve the language of *bhadralok* anxieties.

Animal Disease and Humans

A close relationship has always existed between animal and human disease, but the increasing domestication of animals in the nineteenth century in different parts of the world created new opportunities for the spread of disease from animals to humans. The growing urban consumption of meat provided an effective conduit for the transfer of epizootic diseases. The threat of animal diseases was, thus, all too familiar to the Victorian and Edwardian public in the nineteenth century and was widely reported in the press. Rabies prompted hysteria, whilst cattle epizootics generated alarm about the safety of meat from infected livestock.[38] Not unlike Victorian England, in nineteenth-century India, the very visibility of epizootic and endemic cattle diseases led to increasing fear about the threat to human health from diseased meat. In July 1889, medical doctors were 'directed to observe and report to what extent cattle disease was contemporous with human disease, or affected the health of the people'.[39] Along similar lines, the Magistrate of Cuttack demanded 'for submission by the police of two separate reports respectively, through the Civil Surgeon and the Veterinary Assistant, of cattle disease amongst human beings and amongst cattle'.[40] As early as in 1869, the Inspectors-General of Hospitals were requested to instruct the Medical Officers in Assam to report the extent to which cattle disease prevailing in that province was 'calculated to affect the health of the people'.[41] Authorities panicked over the sale of diseased animals, which might find its way into the city markets. Hence the appearance of epizootic cattle diseases in nineteenth-century India called for investigations into diseases of animals, which, in turn, impinged on the *bhadralok* sensibility as discussed in the following sections.

Meat: To Eat or Not to Eat?

Animal disease impacted upon the culture and politics of diet, nutrition and sanitary science. Nevertheless, it intrigued the Bengali *bhadralok* more than ever.[42] Recently, Jayanta Sengupta and Srirupa Prasad have argued how the 'rice-eating Bengalis' countered the challenge of emasculation from the 1880s onwards through medical journals that emphasized the Bengali need for consuming animal protein.[43] Diet and nutrition featured regularly in medical journals like *Chikitsa Sammilani, Bhishak Darpan* and *Swasthya* between 1885 and 1935. The most persistent refrain in these journals, shared by Bengali doctors, was that the Bengali diet was far too rich in carbohydrates but markedly deficient in protein, the 'muscle-forming element'. In order to make good the deficiency in protein, doctors prescribed protein foods of animal origin.[44]

If the *bhadralok* discourse on meat eating in the mid-nineteenth century stemmed from a desire to counter charges of emasculation, the discourse had shifted by the beginning of the following century, which saw an increasing emphasis on vegetarianism. A compelling argument in favour of vegetarianism in India has always been the ethical one. Such perceptions have a long history in the country; hence, the propaganda for privileging vegetarianism should not surprise us.[45] What is compelling, however, is the sharp shift in the Bengali discourse from emphasis on meat eating to vegetarianism within a short time span. Writings advocating meat eating had almost disappeared by the turn of the twentieth century. Vegetarianism was the new mantra – it was the remedy – a curative, prophylactic or reliever of all diseases. By perusing some of the Bengali articles on vegetarianism published in *Swasthya Samachar, Chikitsa Sammilani* and *Bhisak Darpan,* one can argue that the language of the discourse was new – animal disease, human health and nutrition science now came together to determine the Bengali *bhadralok*'s attitude towards meat consumption during this period.[46]

From the early twentieth century onwards, meat was suddenly held responsible for diseases such as tuberculosis. Concerns about diseased and adulterated food projected vegetarianism as the only alternative for maintaining public health. Manifold scientific-hygienic claims were expressed in books, tracts, pamphlets and lectures. In 1916, the writer in *Bangabashi* expressed his anxieties over the fact that Calcutta was flooded with British-styled eateries. He raised serious alarm, 'no one knows what meat they serve, or how fresh it is. They just season it well with onions and chilies, and serve it hot to cover up the staleness'.[47] In 1916, Manicklal Mallick wrote an insightful piece in *Swasthyo-Samachar* where he asserted that in addition to the question of whether the human body was meant for meat consumption, there was also the need for the inspection of meat.[48] Slaughterhouse inspection thus came to assume a significant space in the *bhadralok* fears concerning their meat diet. The defence of vegetarianism came to be identified as a rational, scientific logic that had to be promoted among fellow Bengalis. Manicklal Mallick sought to substantiate his argument by citing examples of 'medical tests' performed by the London Vegetarian Society. The *bhadrolok* anxieties about adulteration, their attack of the meat shops, meat diet and leaning towards vegetarianism raise the crucial question: Why did the discourse on diet suddenly shift towards meat inspection? The answer is evidently clear – rinderpest meant that diseased meat entered the discourse.

Historians have tried to examine how the Bengali middle-class debate on nutrition was a multilayered one.[49] Utsa Ray has shown how an important aspect of the debate was concerned with the question of adulteration and purity, which often had a double meaning.[50] If Ray examines the ritual purity aspect of food, one can study the scientific language of it. In South Asian historiography, very little attention has been directed at the history of slaughterhouse meat inspection, quality of meat purchased and how that came to be tied with *bhadralok* identities, and their claims of science. What made the debate even more intriguing was that from the late nineteenth century onwards, even the ethical reasons for or against meat eating were more often explained away in 'scientific' terms when Bengali doctors attempted to discover a co-relation between public health and meat eating.

The Language of 'Science'

The classic example of the new trend was Ramendra Shundor Tribedi, a science teacher at Ripon College (later its principal) in Calcutta who used 'science' to justify his defence of a meat diet as he established the claim that science did not debar humans from eating meat.[51] Citing Herbert Spencer, Tribedi argued that the natural inclination of humans was towards meat. However, in response to the question of whether or not meat eating was cruel, Tribedi contended that if cruelty was irreligious (*Adharma*), then the person eating meat committed blasphemy (or was *adharmi*). No one better epitomized the Bengali ambivalence towards diet than Ramendra Shundor Tribedi. He became the perfect example of the dichotomy as he was caught between espousals of a meat diet and religious-based anxieties over the ethics of meat eating. His ambivalence came out repeatedly in his attempts to draw from western utilitarianism and Hindu *ahimsa*. He recalled with pride that *Ahimsa* (non-injury to living beings) originated in India and 'not in Christian lands of Europe'. Deeply aware of the built-in ambivalence in Vedic and Brahiminical tradition of animal sacrifices, Ramendra Shundor Tribedi eventually sought refuge in the claims of science. He concluded by hoping that one day, humans with the aid of science (*bigyan*), would be strong enough not to be *cruel* to consume meat any more.

What is the 'science' that Ramendra Shundor Tribedi talks about? Is it a science that grows in a colonial milieu? Indeed this very question – What is colonial about colonial medicine? – has engaged scholars for over a decade.[52] One can demonstrate how the Bengali *bhadralok* came to terms with modern science and imagined it in their own cultural contexts and how the Bengali middle class mediated the language of science in their understanding of meat inspection and food adulteration.[53] The Bengali *bhadralok* defended their knowledge systems and at the same time appropriated new knowledge. It is this interesting moment of borrowing that I attempt to highlight. As Mukherji rightly points out, 'western medicine's links with *repressive* dimensions of (colonial and more recently postcolonial) power have been explored in depth, while its *productive* role in constituting new subjects and subject-positions have been relatively unexplored.'[54] In my study of animal disease and the resultant Bengali *bhadralok* paranoia over meat, human health and science, I demonstrate that while there was asymmetrical flow of knowledge, there were also moments when the *bhadralok* translated western notions of science and health into their own mental worlds. The *bhadralok* were, thus, not passive recipients of this incoming western knowledge.[55]

India and South Africa

Rinderpest vs East Coast Fever

Historians like Keir Waddington, in his study on bovine tuberculosis affecting nineteenth-century Britain, has demonstrated that the experiences of rinderpest had led British veterinarians to investigate the extent to which cattle diseases were contagious.[56] The devastating effects of rinderpest, which plunged the British cattle industry into crisis, served to shock veterinarians into adopting a contagious model that forced a re-evaluation of disease theory. Worboys has also highlighted the role of rinderpest in giving birth to a new 'germ theory'. According to Worboys, attempts to control the cattle plague in Britain provided the veterinary profession with a new public role and raised its status.[57] He has also examined how scientists of tropical animal diseases tended to pursue their studies primarily in the colonies where the infections arose.[58] Military veterinarians were, as some historians like P. F. Cranefield and K. Brown have shown in their study of cattle diseases affecting Rhodesia and South Africa, pioneers of these studies.[59] To consolidate and expand knowledge and research into animal vaccines in the colonies, research institutes mushroomed in South America, the United States and India from the late nineteenth century.

The history of animal disease in colonial India thus has close parallels with nineteenth- and twentieth-century South Africa. In colonial India, where outbreak of *Puschima* called forth the intervention of eminent German virologist, Robert Koch, in the 1902 outbreak of East Coast fever in Southern Rhodesia and the Transvaal compelled several southern African authorities to request Koch to investigate. Recent studies indicate that scientists working in other African colonies no longer automatically looked to Europe for their expertise.[60]

Both India and South Africa gradually turned into what Roy MacLeod has described as the 'moving metropolis' of knowledge generation. Furthermore, the colonies themselves played a significant role in the expansion of an imperial, and increasingly global, scientific culture.[61] Thus, in many respects both rinderpest in colonial India and East Coast fever in South Africa could be considered the turning point for Indian and South African veterinary science, respectively. However, one major point of divergence is the importance that white veterinarians attached to local knowledge in the colonial tropics in India and South Africa. Brown has demonstrated how despite the growing understanding of the role played by germs in causing epizootics, ecology was a key factor in the veterinarian's perception of South African disease environment.[62] In colonial India however, despite efforts to train locals through the creation of the All-India Veterinary School in 1877, racial hierarchies often undermined the efficacy of colonial veterinary services, with Europeans generally monopolizing top positions.

Conclusion: Of Modernity and Non-Human Actors in Disease Ecology

The discourse surrounding animal disease, diet and nutrition was ever shifting and carried within it multiple strands. The Bengali middle class actively imbibed western ideas in the nineteenth century and was not a mere local voice, and in this sense we notice an interesting hybridization. On one hand, they tried to hold on to the Indian knowledge as enshrined in the *Vedas* and *Upanishads*, and on the other hand, they drew heavily on the London Vegetarian Society or Georges Cuvier as they gave voice to the dichotomy.[63] In the end, however, as evident from the foregoing discussion, this scientific discourse overtook Bengali minds. The examples the *bhadralok* cited in the early twentieth century, defined by their demands for slaughterhouse regulation and meat inspection, were no longer borrowed from the *Vedas* and *Puranas* but from European empirical science and rationality. The discourse too was no longer confined to disease control; it ultimately entered public health debates. Colonialism succeeded in controlling not merely the physical space (through quarantines), but also in colonizing the minds of the Bengali *bhadralok* who were not passive recipients but remained engaged in an active dialogue. While acknowledging that colonialism in India was a hegemonic force, a study of colonial knowledge formation has to analyse the nuances within the colonial discourse. That in turn would help us locate the different motives of the different parties in appropriating the overall knowledge creation. This chapter has attempted to dismantle the polarized understanding of the role of colonialism by trying to demonstrate the simultaneous existence of hegemony and appropriation. If colonial animal disease control sought to subvert indigenous healing practices, there were also interesting moments of encounter when the Bengali middle class internalized western notions of disease, diet and sanitation. Identities were forged, challenged and assimilated in response to the multiple colonial impulses.

In conclusion, this chapter has shown that unlike past scholarship that studied microbes as universal agents of empire, we need to examine more critically the role of such non-human actors in disease ecology. This chapter has not intended to focus on the growth of veterinary services in India and its 'professionalization' after the 1920s, which is outside the scope of this work. Rather, here I have attempted to show how animals – diseased, slaughtered or eaten – came to define and exhibit colonial tensions and class hierarchies, and thus reflect the complexities within the empire in India. The actions of non-human actors such as rats, lice or fleas are connected to, not independent of, histories of knowledge production through which such objects gain new meaning and power in the world.[64] 'Can the mosquito speak?' asks Timothy Mitchell in *Rule of Experts* (2002).[65] In a similar vein, historian John R. McNeill examined the relationship between disease and power in the Greater Caribbean, claiming how 'revolutionary mosquitoes' played a crucial role in the struggles for empire and revolution.[66] In fact, in recent years, historians have attempted to 'centre' animals in history, thereby invoking debates as to this project of transforming non-human animals into *central* actors in the historical narrative can make histories less anthropocentric.[67] Acknowledging the methodological difficulty of writing histories from an animal's point of view,[68] scholars have, however, tried to both denaturalize the human/animal binary and yet include animals as another social actor (along with social classes, women, etc.) in histories they write. Borrowing from such works, the above discussion demonstrated that in colonial India, diseased animals were transformed into a powerful force that mobilized the expertise of veterinary surgeons, sanitary officers, *bhadralok* and the vast resources of the colonial government. It has also unravelled the impervious worlds of humans and animals by examining the interplay of human and non-human actors – British veterinary surgeons, Bengali doctors, farmers, cows, goats and pigs – in controlling animal disease and in regulating slaughterhouses for human health. Additionally, this chapter has demonstrated that knowledge produced in the colony was a product of a network of material, social and scientific relations between and among human and non-human actors. In cutting across the categories of human and non-human, animal disease offers up a new vista for revisiting issues of colonialism and public health.

5 MAHATMA GANDHI UNDER THE PLAGUE SPOTLIGHT

Howard Phillips

Explaining why he devoted three chapters of his autobiography to what he labelled 'The Black Plague' – the pneumonic plague epidemic that struck Johannesburg in March–April 1904, killing eight-two people – Mahatma Gandhi wrote, 'the whole incident, apart from its pathos is of such absorbing interest and, for me, of such religious value' that it merited that amount of attention.[1] But, as historians of epidemics, ever since Thucydides, have recognized, epidemics are of interest for reasons beyond these, in particular for the immediate and long-term marks they leave on affected societies, as well as the light they shed on prevailing social attitudes which can sharpen and become more manifest in response to the threat to life posed by a terrifying, runaway outbreak of a lethal disease. As one historian of the Black Death memorably put it, an epidemic is a 'stimulus ... which exposed the nerve system of ... society'.[2]

In this way, attitudes and outlooks which otherwise might not be apparent can be seen – the Romans might have said '*In pestilentia veritas*' ('there is truth in a plague'). In the case of a high-profile individual like Gandhi, views of his surfaced under the duress of the epidemic which show a different side to him, one not wholly in keeping with the popular image of the caste-blind, class-blind, colour-blind, unprejudiced, egalitarian, universalist *mahatma* cherished by his acolytes and many of his biographers. Typical of the latter is the starry-eyed image of Gandhi as an 'Ambassador of God for Mankind in the 21st Century' (to use the subtitle of one volume on his ideas), and the belief that, in everything he did, he was guided by the principle that 'All Men Are Brothers', as the title of an edited collection of his writings puts it.[3]

Accordingly, this chapter will use the powerful lens of the frightening pneumonic plague epidemic in Johannesburg in 1904 to probe Gandhi's attitude to others at that time and also to trace the significant and long-lasting consequences of this outbreak, not only in his own life, but also in the history of Johannesburg. However, in doing so, it is important to bear in mind that in 1904 Gandhi's social, political and personal ideas were entering a phase of rapid transformation. Consequently, it would be just as misleading to conclude that the views he expressed then remained unchanged for the rest of his life, as it would be to view his every thought and deed from 1893 with hindsight, through *mahatma*-tinted spectacles. Indeed, in some ways it may even be the case that his later outlook stemmed in part from his passionate rejection of his earlier opinions. As he himself admitted years later,

> My aim is not to be consistent with my previous statements on a given question, but to be consistent with truth as it may present itself to me at a given moment. The result has been that I have grown from truth to truth.[4]

On four previous occasions before 1904, Gandhi encountered and learnt about bubonic plague or its even deadlier offshoot, pneumonic plague, in which the causative pathogen, *Yersinia pestis*, is spread from person-to-person by coughing or sneezing; in the case of bubonic plague, the pathogen is transmitted to a person by the bite of a rat-flea. Not that Gandhi knew how pneumonic plague was spread. Indeed, like many doctors at the time,[5] he believed that its origin was miasmatic and that it arose from the disease-impregnated soil. For him, therefore, it was a product of dirty and insanitary conditions and constituted a 'messenger which ... comes as a warning against darkness, filth and overcrowding'.[6]

In September 1896, in Rajkot in his home state of Kathiawar, he had served on a committee charged with keeping the disease from spreading there from Bombay. This had heightened his awareness of the need for hygiene and clean latrines as first steps towards disease prevention and control. Later in that year, he had personally discovered that bubonic plague could be used as a means of political control too, when two ships on which he and eight-hundred other Indians were sailing to Durban were quarantined before anyone could land there, supposedly because bubonic plague had been present at their port of departure, Bombay. In fact, 'this quarantine order had more than health reasons behind it',[7] he recalled, being imposed by the authorities under pressure from a European Protection Committee determined to keep Indians out. All through the twenty-three days of quarantine the Committee peppered the passengers with messages warning them to return to India for their own good, but Gandhi and his fellow passengers ignored these calls. However, when he did disembark, he was beaten up by a gang of local whites.

Gandhi's third encounter with plague came when he was doing voluntary work at a small charitable hospital in Durban in 1898–9. Several times he had to attend to patients suspected of having the disease, which meant that he got to know what symptoms to look for if an outbreak threatened.

Thus, by the fourth time he came into indirect contact with plague – when it threatened Durban early in 1901 – he was very well aware of its nature and potency, both epidemiologically and politically. Recognizing that, 'whenever there is an outbreak of epidemics, the executive, as a general rule, get impatient, take excessive measures and behave to such as may have incurred their displeasure with a heavy hand,'[8] he pressed Indians in the city to clean up their homes, especially their sanitary facilities. By the time Gandhi left for India in October 1901, no outbreak had occurred, though it is unlikely that his clean-up campaign was responsible for this.

When he returned to South Africa from India the following year, it was not in Durban that he settled, but in Johannesburg. In February 1903, he opened a legal practice there and was soon winning a name for himself among the local Indian community as a feisty and capable lawyer. Contributing significantly to this reputation, it appears, was his success in securing fair compensation for the Indian property-owners of the so-called 'Coolie Location', a central city site originally set aside for Indians by Kruger's South African Republic in 1893. By 1903, however, it was an overcrowded, multi-racial slum standing in the way of city development. Citing its gravely insanitary state, the post-war, British-dominated Johannesburg Municipality had begun to expropriate properties there in that year. It was to contest the meagre sums it had offered in compensation for these take-overs that Gandhi had been engaged by the unhappy standholders, most of whom were low-caste hawkers, traders, artisans and workers. According to him, his representations to an arbitration tribunal on their behalf were successful in sixty-nine of the seventy cases brought. He thus soon became a popular and admired figure in Coolie Location, even being called *bhai* (or brother) by the residents. In the light of this, it is not surprising that when pneumonic plague broke out there in March 1904, he was one of the first to know.

Hitherto, the few accounts of this epidemic which do exist have drawn almost exclusively on Gandhi's own version of events, either orally or in his autobiography,[9] and so echo it closely. However, as some biographers have only recently realized, what Gandhi says in his autobiography should not to be accepted uncritically, for when he wrote the chapters which comprise it during his time in jail in 1923–4 for 'sedition' against British rule, he had a very real contemporary political purpose for doing so, namely, to use the chapters, at least in part, to show his path to leadership of the Indian national movement which was then beginning to splinter. It was necessary, his associates urged him, to explain to the Indian public the long pedigree of his nationalist campaign. Accordingly, as a modern commentator on his *Autobiography* puts it, this work emphasizes 'the public exploits of the authorial hero'[10] who cared about all Indians, championing their interests with single-minded zeal, integrity, altruism and reliability. In Gandhi's own words, 'Service of the poor has been my heart's desire, and it has always thrown me amongst the poor and enabled me to identify myself with them.'[11]

In *An Autobiography* he, therefore, presents himself as the 'central figure in organising and mobilising the Indians, leading a previously divided, inert and demoralized community in a heroic struggle with the white authorities'.[12] Yet, if one looks beyond Gandhi's *Autobiography*, to his own letters in 1904 and to contemporary accounts by others, some elements at odds with the usual depictions of his thoughts and deeds emerge in his responses to the fearful epidemic.

While Gandhi portrays himself in his *Autobiography* as the first person to whom the outbreak of the plague in Coolie Location was reported, a young Indian doctor with patients there, Dr William Godfrey, recalled that, for over a week before Gandhi was alerted, the rising death toll had been causing panic there, prompting numerous families to flee. 'The exodus became considerable', he told a reporter, 'several hundreds leaving full of fright'.[13] Moreover, by the time that a note was sent to Gandhi asking him to 'come immediately and take prompt measures',[14] Dr Godfrey had already seen thirteen cases, several of whom were 'lying like so many beasts, all half-dying except one, who was dead'.[15] It was only after seeing this calamity unfolding that he recommended that Gandhi be sent for. By the time Gandhi arrived on his bicycle, Godfrey had, according to his account, already consulted with the community which agreed to let him open an emergency hospital in a vacant house. However, Gandhi's account excludes any reference to the community taking an initiative and instead attributes action to a friend of his and himself, describing how he 'wrote to the Town Clerk to inform him of the circumstances in which we had taken possession of the house ... The Town Clerk expressed his gratitude to me for having taken charge of the vacant house and the patients'.[16]

Once he reached Coolie Location, Gandhi certainly did give a lead by taking administrative and humanitarian steps to address the crisis. He persuaded four of his office clerks to assist Godfrey and him in nursing the gravely ill patients in the emergency hospital, but when it became clear that these facilities were wholly inadequate, he asked the Town Clerk for a bigger building to serve as a hospital. This request was granted, which, his autobiography makes quite clear, was his doing. He implied that he alone had 'awakened ... [the municipality] to a sense of their duty'.[17]

Having resolved the question of securing adequate hospital accommodation, he then took it upon himself to visit the location daily to reassure the panicky residents and get them to accept the municipality's orders. 'The people were in a terrible fright', he relates, 'but my constant presence was a consolation to them'.[18] He also makes clear that he spoke out in the press on behalf of the Indian community, berating the Johannesburg Municipality strongly for its negligence over sanitary matters, which in effect made it 'responsible for the outbreak of the plague itself'.[19] What his *Autobiography* is politic in omitting is the fact that, in the said letter to the press, he also pointed a finger at 'the poorer of my countrymen [who] do not observe the laws of sanitation, except under supervision'.[20] Nor was this the only time during the plague epidemic that he was to express a judgemental view of his poorer countrymen's standards of cleanliness, an issue about which he appears to have been especially sensitive, presumably because of his prior encounters with a threat of the disease.

In his sensitivity to unhygienic conditions, Gandhi's vision was much the same as that of Johannesburg's forceful medical officer of health, Dr Charles Porter, whose grudging respect he earned despite their disagreement as to who was to blame for these conditions and how best they could be resolved. At Gandhi's request a month before the plague broke out, Porter had accompanied him on a tour of Coolie Location to witness for himself the deteriorating sanitary situation there and to hear his warning that, 'if the present state of things is continued, the outbreak of some epidemic disease is merely a question of time'.[21] What he saw spurred Porter to intensify his efforts to clear Coolie Location and to take very seriously Gandhi's suspicions a fortnight later that mounting deaths there might be due to plague. These he had investigated, but the conclusion was indeterminate and he dismissed them as 'unofficial and ... from a layman'.[22] Once the epidemic did break out, Gandhi did not fail to point out to his fellow-Indians that he had warned Porter that a severe outbreak of some disease was imminent.[23]

The prickliness of the co-operation between the two men notwithstanding, Porter recognized Gandhi's role in combating the epidemic. In its aftermath, he acknowledged that 'It is due to Mr M. K. Gandhi ... that the M.O.H. has, on various occasions, received ready and valuable help from him in dealing with his poorer countrymen'.[24]

The basis for Gandhi giving this help was clearly their shared antipathy to insanitary conditions and, as indicated above, his contemporary writings (unlike his autobiography) did not spare the criticism of the unhygienic habits of his 'poorer countrymen', the dire consequences of which the epidemic had made manifest in a way he described as 'ghastly'.[25] From his relatively high-caste, London-trained pedestal, Gandhi castigated them. 'It is ... sad to have to confess that the Indian community cannot be held free from blame', he declared,

> The Nemesis that has overtaken it more than any other community is, we fear, more or less deserved. They ought to have protested against neglected sanitation and overcrowding ... The fact that there have been 47 cases among the Indians is positive proof of the low degree of sanitation observed in quarters inhabited by the poorer of our countrymen ... [T]he punishment that the community has received would be too small, if it does not learn a permanent lesson, and emerge from the ordeal well able to take care of the sanitary laws[26]

It is evident that he felt that the Indian community needed some direction and advice, and someone to take charge of their upliftment and sanitary education. Fortunately, Mohandas K. Gandhi was on hand.

'I used all the influence I could command with the Indians to make them submit to the requirements of the Municipality', he wrote in his *Autobiography*. 'I do not remember anyone having resisted my advice'.[27] He had 'an impression that, if I had withheld my cooperation, the task would have been more difficult for the Municipality, and that it would not have hesitated to use armed force and do its worst'.[28]

What he did not say in his *Autobiography* is that to persuade his 'poorer countrymen' to toe the municipality's line, he preached that 'This is not the time for Indians to assert their rights, but to realize their responsibility by suffering'. They should comply as a way of countering negative images held of them by the colonial powers-that-be so as to convince them that they were reputable citizens who merited full civil and economic rights. He went on to add:

> The plague first broke out among them [the Indian community]. The majority of cases are Indians. The popular inference is that the Indian is the cause of the evil. Whether right or wrong, it has got to be recognised. And the community is doing well in living it down by patient suffering.[29]

Not being a resident of Coolie Location himself – he was then living in a room behind his legal practice in Rissik Street[30] – Gandhi cycled over there every day to persuade the residents to accept the municipality's directive that the location be tightly cordoned off by police and a strict quarantine enforced. Although he himself felt that the cordon was 'merely a fiction kept up to satisfy – not the requirements of sanitation – but [white] public sentiment',[31] he believed that it had to be respected so as to establish Indians' civic bona fides and to prove that they were responsible citizens, even in the face of widespread fear and panic in the city. Unfortunately, no evidence survives from the inhabitants themselves to indicate whether they, confined behind the cordon, agreed with him or not. For himself, he was gratified that 'The authorities are perfectly satisfied with the behaviour of the Indians'.[32]

If Gandhi's *Autobiography* does not make clear that he was ambivalent in his support for the cordon, it does not even hint at his support for the next step in the municipality's bid to check the epidemic, viz. the wholesale clearance of Coolie Location, the removal of all of its inhabitants to an isolation camp at Klipspruit twelve miles west of the city and the razing of all the buildings in the location. His silence may be because, by 1923–4 when he wrote, the miasmatic idea on which such a step was premised had been overtaken by germ theory, making such action appear brutal, punitive and gratuitous. Or maybe he was once again being politic.

As early as 21 March, the day after pneumonic plague was officially diagnosed as the cause of thirty deaths in the Coolie Location in three days, Gandhi told the *Star* that 'The only thing now to be done is to burn the whole of the buildings ... and move the people to a temporary camp, and feed them'.[33] Ten days later he spoke of how 'the buildings [being] reduced to ashes', was something which should have occurred months before.[34] Such ideas, it should be noted, were not all that outlandish in the biomedical world of 1904, where modified miasmatic beliefs still retained credibility, even as the theories of Pasteur and Koch were winning dominance. The so-called 'fire cure' had recently been used in Honolulu and San Francisco against bubonic plague,[35] while in Johannesburg Dr Godfrey was just one of the local practitioners to urge, 'fire the whole place down with coal tar'.[36]

Gandhi therefore encouraged the inhabitants of Coolie Location to abandon their homes and to be transported to Klipspruit under armed escort without a murmur, presumably in line with his strategy of 'patient suffering' (in both senses of the phrase). The picture that his contemporary reports present of this compulsory relocation is that, almost incredibly, the residents followed his instructions in the most complaisant manner, thanks to their trust in him and his assurances that it was just a temporary move.[37] '[T]hey quietly moved away to Klipspruit with the quickest dispatch, and without giving the authorities the slightest trouble', he reported.[38] Patronizingly, he commended them on their 'docility' and 'willingness to comply with lawful orders'.[39] His role in thus facilitating this forced removal understandably has no place in the version of events presented in his *Autobiography*. Rather, he focusses there on how, when residents learnt of their fate and did not know what to do with the savings which they had buried under their floorboards, they requested him to look after their money and bank it for them. 'Streams of money poured into my office', he recalled. 'I could not possibly charge any fees for my labours in such a crisis'. He eventually banked nearly £60,000 on their behalf. The larger depositors he advised to put their money in fixed deposit. 'The result was some of them became accustomed to invest their money in banks'. So ends this story of noble altruism in a time of crisis.[40]

Also not part of Gandhi's *Autobiography*'s account are his doubts at the time about the actual – as opposed to the symbolic – value of burning down Coolie Location. Akin to his ambivalence about cordoning the location off in the first place, he wondered if setting it ablaze was any more than

> essentially a theatrical display calculated to fire the imagination of the [white] people ... [N]o amount of argument and cold reasoning by Dr Porter would have eased the public mind as has this burning down of the Location and the isolation of the people residing in it.[41]

Yet, despite these reservations, his principle of 'patient suffering' made him endorse the measure as part of his strategy to promote Indians' reputation in the corridors of power. However, by 1923–4, when he wrote his autobiography, such a strategy had long had its day in India and so probably was not mentioned lest it show the Mahatma in a poor light. Instead, his autobiography tells of how, at Klipspruit, those who had been removed there from Coolie Location were

buoyed up by his visits and soon overcame their sense of displacement and loss.
'Within twenty-four hours', he wrote,

> they forgot all their misery and began to live merrily. Whenever I went there I found
> them enjoying themselves with song and mirth. Three weeks' stay in the open air
> evidently improved their health.

Would that their happy singing and joking had left some independent, corrobo-
rating evidence in the historical record.[42] Certainly, Gandhi's upbeat portrayal of
Indians adapting easily to living in tents in the veld as winter set in on the High-
veld is not corroborated by what he himself wrote in 1904. Describing the camp
as 'not a place for relaxed slumber, rather it is a wilderness' where dysentery had
become 'a common complaint',[43] he lamented that the Indians were 'being treated
practically as prisoner[s]'.[44] They were subjected to 'extremely irritating' regulations which 'uncomfortably controlled their movements in and out of the camp'.[45]
Leaving its premises required a day permit which expired at 8.30 p.m. – failure to
return by then would incur a hefty fine 'or, in default of payment, imprisonment
for three months for the first offence'. This 'more or less ... prison life'[46] contrasts
very sharply with the picture portrayed in Gandhi's *Autobiography*.

There is also a great disparity between the silence of his *Autobiography* about
another community caught up in the forced removals from Coolie Location
and the amount Gandhi said about them at the time. Sharpened by fear and
the threat posed by the epidemic, his candid opinions about the 1420 Africans
who lived as tenants and sub-tenants in Coolie Location in 1904 reveal a racially
prejudiced outlook little different from that common among whites then.

He felt that Africans living cheek-by-jowl with Indians there was 'very unfair
to the Indian population, and it is an undue tax on even the proverbial patience
of my countrymen'.[47] 'Why, of all places in Johannesburg', he chided Dr Porter,

> the Indian Location should be chosen for dumping down all the Kaffirs of the town
> passes my comprehension ... [T]he Town Council must withdraw the Kaffirs from
> the Location.

About this mixing of the Kaffirs with Indians, I must confess, I feel most strongly.[48]

To him, Africans' culture, lifestyle and outlook differed too deeply from
Indians' for them to share space or facilities. Unlike the stereotype in his mind
of 'the African', the Indian was at least 'amenable to sanitary control ... [and] has
no war-dances, nor does he drink Kaffirbeer'.[49] That he believed that such separation should extend even to hospital accommodation, the epidemic brought out
all too clearly. He complained in 1905 that at the plague hospital in Durban,

> no distinction is made between Indians and Kaffirs, all being herded together indis-
> criminately. Anyone with even the slightest knowledge of Indian habits and prejudices

will at once see how great a factor this negligence [of separation] is in impending [*sic*] the good work initiated by the authorities.[50]

Given this antipathy by Gandhi to Indians and Africans being side-by-side, it is very likely that it was his insistence on this fact which helped to convince the authorities that two separate isolation camps should be set up a mile apart at Klipspruit, one for Africans and one for Indians. Indeed, he probably went further along the separation path by arguing that the Indians' camp should itself be divided into separate sub-camps for Hindus and Muslims and even for different castes.[51]

Of the African camp there is no mention in his autobiography and barely a word in his writings at the time.[52] So ethnocentric was his focus, one would hardly be aware that 1420 African fellow-evictees were encamped a mile away.

In the light of this narrow ethnic lens, it is not surprising that Gandhi did not even remark upon the fact that, while, in the months after the epidemic, Indians at Klipspruit were allowed to return to Johannesburg if they could find approved accommodation there,[53] no such permission was granted to the Africans nearby. Indeed, the Johannesburg Municipality decided that Klipspruit should become the designated place of residence for all of the city's Africans not living on their employers' premises in the city; this it began to implement, initially by forcibly removing Africans still living in the so-called 'Kaffir Location' near the city centre out to Klipspruit in 1906. In an operation reminiscent of what had happened in 1904, Porter reported that he acted as their 'shepherd'.[54] Of this, of Africans' opposition and their public petition against this, Gandhi's letters and press articles say nothing, except in passing to 'wonder how the Kaffirs will manage to live at such a distance'.[55] By then he was more concerned about thwarting the Johannesburg Municipality's fresh scheme to develop a new location (or 'bazaar' as they called it in a fit of orientalism) for Indians back at their original Klipspruit site so that it could eventually move all the city's Indians there.

This plan it was forced to abandon, however, when the town council was alerted to the fact that it would face a legal challenge if it tried to force Indians to dwell in a particular place except during an emergency like the 1904 epidemic, and that the Transvaal government was unlikely to overturn this provision lest doing this alienated the government of India and so incur a veto from Westminster.[56]

Klipspruit thus became a site designated for African settlement solely, a role which it went on to fulfil on an ever-expanding scale in Johannesburg's history. Around it, other townships were built over the next decades to accommodate the thousands of Africans flocking to the city. By 1959 twenty-five such townships were in existence, housing close to half-a-million people. In 1963 the city's Department of Non-European Affairs decided to try to foster a common identity for them by conferring a blanket name on all the townships, Soweto. At the heart of Soweto lay the original Klipspruit Location (itself renamed Pimville in 1934) which Gandhi had been so keen to keep quite separate from its Indian equivalent a mile away in 1904. Symbolically, this sums up the deep racial divisions within the ranks of those labelled 'non-white' since the start of modern white rule in South Africa. In the eyes of some historians, Gandhi's racial, class and caste prejudices only furthered this division, as his stance during the epidemic of 1904 makes very clear. He 'facilitated the implementation of the divisive segregationist policies which helped ease the task of white minority rule in South Africa', judged Maureen Swan sharply.[57] From the laundered, heroic account in his autobiography, one would never guess at this.

Looking back at the events of 1904 twenty years later when he penned his autobiography, Gandhi concluded that, for him, its significance lay in how it 'enhanced my influence with the poor Indians and increased my business and my responsibility';[58] how it allowed him to gather a group of volunteers to nurse the sick with faith and an almost religious zeal and how it brought him into contact with a man who became one of his staunchest friends, Henry Polak.

Yet, as this chapter demonstrates, the pneumonic plague epidemic of 1904 is significant in another way too for understanding Mohandas Gandhi, because of the sharp light it sheds on his as-yet superior and paternalist attitude to lower-caste Indians and his outright disdain for those supremely 'other' Johannesburgers, its Africans. To his eye, they were, at bottom, 'persons belonging to uncivilised races',[59] with nothing in common with Indians.

The epidemic also offers a clear example of how Gandhi reshaped his experiences in his *Autobiography* to serve his political and personal interests in 1923–4 by showing his long lineage as a noble and popular leader who identified with all Indians at all times. As historians well know, *when* something is written is as significant as *what* is written. In the words of one scholar of Gandhi's writings, his *Autobiography* 'exemplifies Gandhi's extraordinary talent for self-creation ... [It is] a work of studied thought and artifice'.[60]

But then, perhaps the Mahatama knew this all along. After all, *An Autobiography*'s subtitle is *The Story of My Experiments with Truth*. In its text he freely admits to the reader, 'I am not writing the autobiography to please critics. Writing it is itself one of my experiments with truth.'[61]

6 PLAGUE HITS THE COLONIES: INDIA AND SOUTH AFRICA AT THE TURN OF THE TWENTIETH CENTURY

Natasha Sarkar

Between 1894 and 1909, there had been 243 cases of plague on 139 vessels sailing across various ports of the world.[1] The origins of this third modern pandemic can be traced to the late eighteenth century when plague outbreaks had become frequent in the north-east of Burma and the infection made inroads into the neighbouring Yunnan province of China, firmly establishing itself in the west of Yunnan in the first half of the nineteenth century.[2] It is possible that the infection would have continued to smoulder in west Yunnan without spreading further, but the equilibrium was upset by the movement of troops that were sent in to suppress a Muslim rebellion in 1855. The movement of refugees in large numbers provided suitable means for the spread of disease. Progressing gradually, plague reached Yunnan-fu (now Kunming), the provincial capital, in 1866 but it took an additional twenty-eight years to reach Canton and Hong Kong in 1894. That year, the world confronted a situation unlike that of the pandemic during Justinian I's (c. AD 482–565) time. The introduction of steamships and railways had replaced caravans and small sailing-craft, making transmission of disease much faster.[3] Macao and Foochow (Fu Chou) were infected in 1895 while Singapore and Bombay succumbed in 1896. By 1900, Buenos Aires, Rio de Janeiro, San Francisco, Oporto, Alexandria and Honolulu had all experienced the plague.[4] The pandemic provides us with an opportunity to study urban social history at the turn of the last century in colonial India and South Africa. Colonial medical encounters in urban port cities reveal much about societal attitudes, objectives and priorities, and these perspectives are explored throughout this chapter. The 'idea' of plague as perceived by the colonial authorities dictated the need to implement certain kinds of anti-plague measures. After all, plague aetiology was firmly established only after 1905, much after widespread speculation during the initial years of the pandemic. The infected ports within India and South Africa were also marked by cultural differences that presented diverse responses to anti-plague measures, but a similarity between the colonies was reflected in the typical features of urbanization during the period; a transformation through industrialization, global trade expansion and immigration.[5] Bombay city was the microcosm of urban India, and the British Indian empire was founded on its capitalist system. The late nineteenth century, as we know it, was a period of rapid growth during which trade, transport and communication progressed beyond recognition. Modern urban Bombay drew the wealthy, intellectuals, skilled and unskilled labourers. Unfortunately, increasing foreign, coastal and inland trade brought in not only the Parsis, Muslims, Banias and others on industrial ventures, but also the deadly plague. The expansion of railways and coastal transport carried the plague into towns and villages throughout India. Along with Bombay, Punjab grossed the largest numbers in plague mortality rates but in the instance of the latter, plague was largely a rural phenomenon, offering insights into areas virtually outside the purview of western biomedicine. In South Africa, and in particular, Cape Town, provided a unique situation for the Boer War made it a prime target for the rapid spread of the plague pathogen, given the bustling wartime commerce and movement of refugees. Cape Town had also been transformed into a dynamic port, benefitting greatly from the mineral revolution. It, therefore, attracted hordes of migrant labourers.[6] This chapter provides perspectives on understanding the human experience since urbanization came with its accompanying problems of overcrowded tenement dwellers, insanitation and tensions marked by the complex interactions among colonial authorities and the general public as they confronted alarming incidences of plague. While each region tried to make sense of the extraordinary in terms of the ordinary, what remained central to most experiences was fear, not of the disease *per se*, but of plague regulations. The suddenness and force with which these measures were implemented were unique to this pandemic and threatened to disturb prevalent social and cultural practices and beliefs. The resulting outcome was inevitable in episodes of resistance to segregation, hospitalization and vaccination.

The Outbreak

Bubonic plague officially made inroads into Bombay in September 1896 despite several accounts of its presence in July and August. Waldemar Haffkine, an eminent microbiologist, proposed that the infection was introduced by sea since it commenced near the docks. His alternate theory was that of traders having introduced it from northern India since the southern slopes of the Himalayas had been endemic to the disease.[7] A good many competent authorities, such as R. H. Vincent, the Police Commissioner of Bombay, held similar notions of pilgrims having spread the disease from certain villages in the Kumaon Hills of Uttarakhand, north of India. In early 1896, a stream of pilgrims and devotees moved from the north to the sacred shrines of Nasik while also frequenting the temple of Walkeshwar at Malabar Hill, south of Bombay.[8] Bombay's Police Commissioner, Vincent echoed Haffkine's opinion that the plague had been imported into Bombay from Kumaon by *sadhus* (holy men) who came down from the Himalayas from May through to August 1896, taking up their quarters in Mandvi, also towards the south.[9]

A connection with the Gulf had been suggested, the region being in close proximity to Bombay rather than China. Additionally, communication and trade between the Gulf and Bombay were more frequent than with China, with a large number of country boats plying between Bunder Abbas, other Gulf ports and Bombay. If plague came from there, it was considered possible that it was brought in one of these.[10] There had, indeed, been a brisk commercial intercourse between Bombay and Busrah, the export-centre for Turkish Arabia for centuries, and yet there is no evidence or any existing record that would support assumptions of the disease ever having found its way down the Persian Gulf from the Turkish Arabian littoral.[11] It is also known that a man who contracted plague in Hong Kong, and travelled to Bombay via the *S. S. Bormida* in March 1899, fanned suspicion that the disease travelled from there. The possibility of similar cases having occurred in 1896 was taken seriously. Also, very early in the epidemic, mortality among rats was known to have preceded those of humans in the neighbourhood of a certain warehouse in Mandvi. The building was found to contain goods that had been imported from Hong Kong. The plague was epidemic in Hong Kong shortly before Bombay was infected.[12] A general consensus lay with this 'Hong Kong' theory. That the disease mainly prevailed among the *Lohanas*[13] in Mandvi, and that these Lohanas were mostly employed on board the steamers coming into the port from China offered corroborative evidence. Some of them were even employed as servants to the *Banias*,[14] possibly infecting them.[15] The areas to be affected first were close to the docks and it was logical to assume that plague entered Bombay through its port. The Hong Kong epidemic of 1894 was common knowledge and ships leaving the Fragrant Harbour were quarantined in Singapore. The Indian port of Calcutta was at greatest risk but when the outbreak in Hong Kong was declared under control, the quarantine was lifted. In 1896, when plague recurred in Hong Kong, the government of India did not receive any information as a result of which quarantine could not be reimposed. Thus, ships from Hong Kong enjoyed pratique in India.[16] Widespread official opinion favoured this notion of how Bombay might have been infected.

As a major port of western India with well-connected railways, Bombay was to become a great gateway for the plague bacillus. After the initial slow progress of the disease from Mandvi, the epidemic phase began in December with the sudden appearance of new foci of rat and human plague across the city. The population was panic-stricken, and vast numbers fled until half the inhabitants had departed into the interiors, carrying the infection along with them. Members of the floating population and the merchant community departed in large numbers. The floating population, having nothing to detain them, realized their pay and left. It was from among this class that the early deaths from plague occurred. They left Bombay by sea, some taking with them sick companions, others carrying the incubating disease on their person, ready to break out on their arrival. The plague spread mainly along the main lines of communication, across villages in several districts, and soon appeared in other provinces. Several fugitives from the Bombay Presidency were not long in carrying infection to other parts of India.[17] Punjab was infected in October 1897, followed by Bengal and Madras in 1898. The spread had been slow but certain, and only large tracts of water had delayed it. Year after year, the number of newly infected villages and towns increased.[18] However, the east and south of India never really became strongholds of the plague.

By 1900, plague had reached South Africa during the Anglo-Boer War (1899–1902). Burdened by wartime commerce and teeming with refugees and migrant African labourers from the interiors, the seaports of Cape Town, Port Elizabeth, East London and Durban were exposed to infection.[19] The dreaded disease found southern Africa's ports, harbours and railway stations bursting at the seams with wartime commerce, and with an influx of refugees from the interior and large numbers of migrant labourers.[20] In the latter half of 1898, an outbreak occurred in Tamatave, Madagascar, and a steamer from that port, the *Gironde* which was reported on arrival at Lourenco Marques to have cases of plague on board, was refused pratique by the Portuguese authorities and sent back to Madagascar. About the end of November, suspicious mortality levels among rats occurred in a certain quarter of Lourenco Marques but no bacteriological examinations appear to have been made and the matter was never cleared up.[21] In early 1899, four cases of bubonic plague in male Indians were believed to have occurred at Lourenco Marques. This rumour (which was later proved to be false), created a sensation in South Africa, and hasty measures were adopted, chiefly against the Indians. Indeed, prohibition of Indian immigration was suggested.[22] On 5 March 1900, the steamer *Kilburn* arrived in Table Bay with a cargo of forage from Rosario, South America, with three cases of plague among the crew, and on 1 February 1901, unusual numbers of rat deaths at the South Arm, Cape Town docks, was reported. This part of the port was under the control of military authorities since the outbreak of the Anglo-Boer War in September 1899, and contained large stacks of grain and forage imported from Rosario, Buenos Aires, Rio de Janeiro and other South American ports, several of which were plague infected. A severe epizootic and human epidemic followed and continued until the end of 1901.[23]

Durban was infected in early 1900 when the Diot family arrived at Durban from Mauritius. The family stated that three to four days before the onset of the illness of their son, he had opened a trunk that had been brought from Mauritius. It was believed that infection had probably occurred from an infected flea conveyed via clothing in the trunk. On 12 April 1901, several plague-infected carcasses were discovered in the harbour area of Port Elizabeth, near a large stack of forage imported from Buenos Aires some months before. Steps were taken to localize the outbreak by the erection of rat-proof fencing, but it was soon discovered that infection had spread to certain stores and to a large Military Remount Camp at the northern end of the town. The epizootic quickly spread and human cases followed in its wake. In the latter half of 1902 and the first eight months of 1903, an epidemic claiming 201 cases with 145 deaths occurred in Durban, yet again, but this time, with an extension to Pietermaritzburg. The infection was probably introduced by the *S. S. Kassala*, with its cargo of forage from Argentine ports. In March 1904, an explosive and virulent outbreak of plague occurred in the Coolie Location in Johannesburg, the last case occurring only in January 1905. The original source of infection remained untraceable, but the infection was probably introduced by rail, in grain, forage or crated goods, from either the infected coastal towns of Durban, East London or Port Elizabeth.

'Filth' Disease

The biological revolution of the late nineteenth century marked a defining moment in plague research.[24] Plague now came to be understood as a four-factor disease which required the coincidental occurrence of four distinct factors in order for the infection to be transmissible to humans: an etiologic agent (*Yersinia pestis*), a reservoir (rodents), an arthropod vector (fleas) and a human host.[25] In 1894, Alexandre Yersin, a French bacteriologist, isolated the bacillus from excised buboes and named it *Pasteurella pestis* which was later to be named after him as *Yersinia pestis*.[26] Unfortunately, this knowledge gained little acceptability for plague prevention.[27] Insanitation came to be considered a prerequisite for the disease, and plague came to be regarded as *the* filth disease. Early attempts to understand plague aetiology seemed to be conditioned as much as by the then prevailing levels of scientific knowledge as by the anxiety to justify colonial rule in terms of certain stereotypes. The tendency to attribute the prevalence of disease to poor and unhealthy living conditions was rather pronounced in both India and South Africa. While attributing the outbreak of epidemics to the prevalent insanitary conditions, certain racial stereotypes were evident in the general attitude of the administrators. A correlation was drawn between plague occurrence and filth – a factor that was thought to decrease levels of general health and diminish natural immunity.

The sanitary state of Bombay in the late nineteenth century, when plague hit the region, was deplorable. Dingy, filthy and ill-ventilated structures were quickly associated with the plague. Large numbers were crowded into such houses, for people were in the habit of living close to their workplace which resulted in certain areas becoming densely populated. Kumbharwada, Chakala, Kamathipura, Umarkhadi, Kharatalao and Bhuleshwar were areas that had a population of more than 500 persons per acre.[28] Factory workers lived in extremely insanitary houses, with most of those comprising of simply a room with no ventilation. Some factory owners provided housing to their workers but these were just as bad and over-crowded.[29] However, while it might have been common to associate insanitation with the dwellings of the poor, the houses of the middle class were no different. The Jain merchants of Mandvi were noted for personal hygiene but they neglected public sanitation.[30] The Hindu traders – Banias, Bhatias and Lohanas – lived like the Jains, in crowded houses in bazaar areas where they had their shops and businesses. For instance, in Mandvi, a building on Clive Road, housed 600 people in 133 rooms. These traders had storehouses and go-downs on the ground floors of their buildings.[31] Besides living in overcrowded houses, Indian traders indulged in practices which, it was believed, invited disease. They collected rags and rubbish which were dumped in the *verandah* (porch or balcony), serving as fertile ground for rats and other insects on which to thrive. Since a majority of these traders were strict followers of non-violence, they refused to kill rats. Incidentally, the Jains and the rest of the merchant community suffered the most during the plague years.[32] The ordinary laws of sanitation were neglected. Burning grounds, animal stables, markets, slaughter-houses and factories were sources of ill health. Vehement criticism was levelled against the Municipal Corporation for neglecting its duties, for want of constructive schemes for improving sanitation.[33]

At the turn of the nineteenth century, the conditions prevalent in Cape Town were not very different from those in Bombay. As was typical of colonial societies, the whites lived in favoured surroundings while the slums were home to the Coloured, Malay, Asiatic and African communities. Since the onset of the Boer War, hordes of black rural migrants entered the city. Of its 64,500 inhabitants in 1900, 30,500 were whites, including roughly 7,000 poverty-stricken refugees. Of the rest, some 7,000 were Africans.[34] Medical officers and the Plague Administration focused their efforts on the Africans with whom they associated insanitary conditions. All attention was directed at searching and cleaning out 'Kafir haunts' within the city.[35] For almost a year prior to the onset of the epidemic, proposals had been under consideration for an African reserve or residential 'location' beyond the suburban borders of Cape Town. In September 1900, Prime Minister Sir Gordon Sprigg had appointed a commission to make recommendations for such action. The commission was chaired by Walter E. Stanford, Superintendent of Native Affairs, and comprised Dr John Gregory, Captain J. A. Jenner, Chief of Police, and Dr Barnard Fuller. They had found 'frightful' living conditions, slumlords and support from the African clergy for a government location outside the city.[36] Suddenly this idea of a special location became a priority in February 1901. It was considered logical to proceed from isolating plague victims to creating a permanent location for them. The Cape government rushed to set up a native location at a sewage farm called Uitvlugt, and this was carried out under the regulations of the Public Health Act. There existed no other legislation that might affect municipalities by providing the authority to remove Africans by force if deemed necessary.[37] In March 1901, approximately 6,000 to 7,000 Africans were moved to Uitvlugt. The location had twenty-four huts surrounded by hastily constructed wooden and iron barracks, a twenty-bed hospital and other outbuildings. Several officials viewed this relocation as a major success which would make way for future practice.[38]

In the nineteenth century, the economy of Port Elizabeth centred around trade and commerce.[39] A rise in the population was a response to South Africa's rapid industrialization and capitalist growth prompted by mineral discoveries in the 1860s and 1880s. Natural disasters in the 1890s and the higher wages paid during the Boer War added to the number of Africans entering the labour market. Between the 1860s and 1890s, government legislation was directed towards gaining control of the growing number of blacks coming under colonial jurisdiction. Several laws were passed to facilitate control and to promote cheap labour, limiting competition in the political and economic arena in order to assure white supremacy. These included the Locations Acts in 1878 and 1884, which affected natives in rural areas.[40] It is within this broader context as well as at the local level that we must view Port Elizabeth Council's attempt to remove Africans from the town centre. The black population lived in several areas but primarily at the municipal locations of Strangers' and Cooper's Kloof as well as at Gubbs, a location on privately owned land. The Council was anxious to close the municipal locations because they were situated in the centre of the town blocking expansion of business. As the value of the land rose significantly, civic officials decided that the site should be used more profitably.[41] The Council initiated the Native Strangers' Location Bill (1883) which aimed to close Strangers' location, the oldest African settlement, and to force its residents to move into the 'new' Reservoir location on the outskirts of town. Although there was already a history of some informal separation between the various racial groups, the law was significant because it restricted African land ownership and capital accumulation. However, when the Bill was proposed, government officials invoked 'sanitation' as their reason for removing Africans. Here, as in other places, they argued that the social and insanitary conditions of the 'uncivilized natives' represented a health hazard which endangered both whites and blacks. Not surprisingly, the Stranger's Location Bill won widespread support from the white community, merchants and employers included.[42] Thus, while there existed political pressure for residential segregation, there was also a demand for segregation on sanitary grounds. In a sense, colonial rule and 'racial medicine' were rooted in late nine-teenth-century South Africa.[43]

In Natal, during 1860 to 1913, the majority of Indian immigrants, and in par-ticular the indentured labourers, lived in stringent poverty, while many became hawkers, peddlers and others took to trading. Since immigration restrictions prevented their free movement, they remained confined to Natal.[44] It was here, in South Africa, that Gandhi exhorted the Indian community to protest against neglected sanitation and overcrowding in Durban and also in Johannesburg.[45] That the Town Council allowed for such a state of affairs to continue was consid-ered to be deplorable.[46] The utter incapability of the Johannesburg Town Council to implement sanitary measures was considered as having caused the plague out-break in the city. An important statement of the Health Committee that they did everything they could and that it was not possible for them to fix a new site in place of the insanitary area, was viewed by the *Indian Opinion* as the failure of the Council in protecting the health and lives of the community at large. After all, plague had broken out five months after the Council had taken possession of the insanitary area. Beyond the removal of the inhabitants of the Indian Location to a temporary camp at Klipspruit, there was no sign of an improvement in terms of the selection of a permanent site.[47] It was due to such exceptional circumstances that the Indians held the Council responsible for the epidemic.

What South Africa and India had in common was the absolute neglect of those parts of town inhabited by non-Europeans. In Natal, the conditions in the Eastern and Western Vleis, where the Indians were huddled, were no dif-ferent from that of a bazaar, location or compound under the direct control of the Corporation itself. The Corporation had done nothing to remedy the state of affairs.[48] While one could expect an individual to observe personal cleanli-ness and hygiene, part of the responsibility for domiciliary sanitation certainly lay with the governing body of a locality. While filth was considered to be syn-onymous with plague, a particularly interesting episode suggested that it held but little significance. In the House of Correction, Byculla (Bombay), where cleanliness had been brought to near perfection, a plague outbreak exceeded in severity to that in any of the filthy *chawls* (multi-storied one room tenements) around. There were 345 prisoners confined in this jail when plague broke out on 23 January 1897, attacking thirty-three prisoners, of whom seventeen died.[49] It is significant too that out of 1,579 patients treated at Bombay's Arthur Road and Parel hospitals, there were only sixteen sweepers, and the *halalkhores* (toilet cleaners) who removed the night soil from houses and were considered to be among the most unhygienic of the population were, notably, free from plague.[50]

Concealing Victims

Concealing plague cases by either hiding victims or sending them to a relative's place in the hope of escaping segregation was common. Such actions were hazardous because, first, the patient did not recover due to lack of medical aid, and second, plague spread to newer areas. The Parsis of the Fort area in Bombay were known to have concealed cases. When they knew that house search teams were to arrive, they quickly moved the sick to Marine Street, Girgaum or Breach Candy.[51] Konkani Muslims also hid victims because of their dislike of hospitals.[52] The practice was indeed most common among Muslims, higher-caste Hindus and Parsis.[53] It was rare among Christians or middle- and lower-class Hindus.[54] In the village of Sandhowal, Punjab, graves had been discovered of those who had been secretly buried after succumbing to plague.[55] Several villagers even buried corpses in their houses.[56] And in this regard, South Africa was no exception. Plague cases and deaths went unreported and surreptitious burials were attempted. Gandhi was not in favour of concealing plague cases and deeply regretted that some Indians in Durban were unaware of the serious consequences of such acts. In one such instance, an Indian employed by the Durban Corporation was sentenced to pay a fine of twenty pounds or in default – to three months' hard labour for concealing a plague case. The accused had moved his daughter to an empty house for he did not want European doctors to take her away from him. While this act seemed natural, Gandhi hailed the sentence as exemplary and appealed to the Indians to cooperate with the authorities.[57] The *Indian Opinion* offered a probable explanation for the concealment of cases, suggesting that at plague hospitals no distinction was made between Indians and Africans; that there was an 'indiscriminate herding' of people of all races. Little regard for religious customs and traditional Indian beliefs resulted in the avoidance of hospitals.[58] Opposition to segregation in India would rest upon similar grounds because the caste system restricted the intermingling of people from different denominations. The Jains and Banias were the first to record their complaints against segregation, refusing to send patients to plague hospitals.[59] From fear of 'pollution', Banias even threatened to close down shops as a protest against segregation.[60]

Tracks of Infection

Land quarantine during the plague years included railway inspection with the railway staff keeping watch over the state of health of travellers with the objective of detaining those who showed symptoms of plague. Surveillance was to last for ten days. In Bombay, instances of female passengers being examined on railway platforms drew strong opposition from the native press. The Gurakhi was vociferous in this regard:

> That a female should be publicly asked by a male stranger to remove the end of her sari from the upper half of her body is most insulting and likely to result in loss of life. Native females, whether Hindu, Parsi or Muhammadan, are very particular about their modesty and value it more than their lives.[61]

Tension among the colonial ranks of authority was evident in railway inspection – a measure which was pushed for by the Bombay government, but the Municipal Commissioner P. C. H. Snow questioned its usefulness: 'no medical man, however skilled, would be able to detect a person with bubonic poison incubating in their system. I, therefore, cannot anticipate any practical results of this scheme.'[62] The native press also raised several issues of racial discrimination since Europeans were treated favourably over natives, with the authorities adopting a liberal stance towards the first and second class passengers who were mostly Europeans.[63] Among the natives, some consideration was shown to the aristocracy and the educated middle class. In Punjab, Europeans travelling to Simla were examined within their compartments and those infected were allowed to proceed in the same compartment, while fellow passengers were transferred to a special carriage. On arrival at Simla, the infected Europeans were isolated either in their houses or at the Ripon Hospital. The reason given for not detaining European passengers was that suitable accommodation was not available.[64] In South Africa, complaints arose about how even authorized British Indians were required to furnish medical certificates in order to travel from Natal to Transvaal. But even those with certificates were being subjected to medical inspection at Volksrust. Medical officers gave them letters addressed to the Magistrate which stated that they were to be placed under medical surveillance for ten days. The harassment continued in spite of the removal of regulations and the cancellation of the Plague Notice of the Transvaal government.[65] In the Transvaal, plague had served as a peg on which to hang many a disability on British Indians. On the pretext of plague precautions, the issue of permits to British Indian refugees from all the colonies in South Africa had been stopped. The most plausible explanation for this was that plague-infested rats had been found in some localities in Johannesburg; though not, incidentally, in Indian quarters but in poor European ones.[66]

Affecting the Economy

Soon after plague engulfed Bombay, merchants, traders and labourers (especially mill workers) realized their pay and left the city. They left by rail and steamers, rushing to friends and relatives in the interiors of the province.[67] This general exodus from Bombay drastically affected the city. Most merchants had large stocks of unsold goods lying in their go-downs. A merchant lamented that no sale meant severe losses.[68] In the years preceding the plague, Bombay had exported large quantities of dry fish to Mauritius, Colombo and Rangoon, but with the onset of plague, the fish trade practically ceased to exist. Nearly four hundred men were engaged daily in weighing the fish before export but as plague mortality increased, these men migrated, leaving only one or two men at the scales. About half of the fishermen of Sewri died of plague while the rest fled.[69] In Punjab, shopkeepers in Hoshiarpur suffered following the closure of their shops during evacuation to plague camps.[70] In a similar manner, Delhi's local as well as external trade was paralysed and suffered a setback with the shutting down of wholesale markets.[71] The lime industry suffered as limekilns were located in infected villages and prospective customers were not allowed to enter these villages.[72] At Phillour, timber merchants suffered as the railways stopped trains from plying between Phillour and Ladhowal in 1898.[73] Employers in Cape Town experienced similar labour shortage. A solution was offered in setting up the location as a labour bureau permitting Africans to work for employers through a pass system. The underlying motive was, of course, social control by reorganizing society so as to make black labour easily accessible to white employers while restricting other opportunities for employment. The Native Labour Locations Act of 1899 had even made it possible to house and control workers in private locations.[74] In South Africa at Pietersburg, Krugersdorp and Potchefstroom, measures were undertaken to expel the Indians and not merely to prevent the introduction of plague. On the pretext of plague precautions, Indian trade was nearly ruined and inconveniences were thrust upon the Indians.[75] In the Transvaal region, business among the Indians suffered seriously. Several hawkers were dependent on purchasing their goods from Natal but since they could not afford to obtain the necessary permit, they were practically shut out. In the early years of the plague, the Maritzburg Town Council is known to have issued circulars addressed to Indian shopkeepers, informing them of reducing their stock in the eventuality of removal to a Location. Steamship companies entirely refused to take Indian passengers to other South African ports.[76] There was a total ban on the import of rice and other food-grains from India. Gandhi was convinced that the agitation and panic had their source not entirely for fear of plague but because of an anti-Indian prejudice due to 'trade jealousy'.[77]

Prophylactic with Complexities

Colonial medicine was representative of direct intervention and interaction with the social, cultural and material lives of indigenous populations. This engagement was useful in fashioning the distinct character of colonial medicine in the colonies and also the extent of native reception and assimilation. A plague vaccine was unheard of until Waldemar Haffkine had prepared one on 10 January 1897, and after having successfully inoculated himself, he gave public demonstrations and inoculated many distinguished citizens in Bombay. Among the Muslims, the custom of *purdah*[78] had the force of a religious ordinance but even among other communities, women objected to exposing their arms and wrists to strange men.[79] In Punjab, the upper-caste Hindus resisted vaccination on the plea that it contained substances that went against their religion. The Khatris[80] of Rahon sent a petition to the Deputy Commissioner claiming that the prophylactic serum contained animal matter forbidden by their faith.[81] Where plague inoculations did take place, they were carried out by male medical officers who inoculated women and men, an act that was considered unthinkable.[82] But in any case, compared to their men-folk, women could benefit much less from inoculation. In a village in Banga circle, only 28 per cent of the women and in another village in Hoshiarpur district, 38 per cent could avail of vaccination.[83] This was as much due to ignorance as to the general disregard for women's health. The upper classes threw in the question of honour and custom. In time, only women observing purdah were inoculated in their homes. They covered their arms with muslin and extended them through a small hole in the curtain for inoculation by the assistant surgeon.[84] Interestingly, no serious difficulty was experienced with the Sikhs. It was as much due to the presence of a large number of them in the British Indian Army as to the relative absence of the considerations of the caste system and the purdah among them.[85] No doubt, an element of negligence cannot be discounted. The *Tribune* made frequent references to the most glaring example of negligence, the 'Mulkowal mishap', when in October 1902, nineteen people who were inoculated in Mulkowal, Punjab succumbed due to tetanus contamination.[86] This incident had negative implications for the future of Haffkine's vaccine in the years ahead.

Gandhi was a great experimental scientist. His study and experiments on health convinced him that Ayurveda and Naturopathy were based on sounder principles when compared with Allopathy. Quite naturally, he was not enthusiastic about promoting vaccination in South Africa. He was convinced that vaccination did not extirpate the causes of plague and that unless the insanitary environs (to him, the real cause) were transformed, no real benefit would accrue. Gandhi promoted improved sanitary habits and nature cure.[87] As late as 1913, while writing about health, Gandhi was yet to be convinced about the efficacy of vaccination, but he did suggest elaborate preventives and cures that had their basis in Ayurveda and Naturopathy. Evacuation was, of course, recommended over inoculation.[88] Even after the association between rats and humans in the transmission of plague had been established and was greatly acknowledged, public health initiatives after 1905 centred on educating the masses about the principles of sanitation. With increasing experience of the disease, it cannot be said that the people generally made any endeavour to save themselves in spite of the educational measures that had been undertaken to instruct them in the methods of dealing with the disease. Again, the reach of western biomedicine in providing medical care fell short of the majority of the population.[89] A great number of people resorted to Ayurveda either for preference or for low cost of treatment. While not all Ayurvedic drugs were non-toxic, they were natural absorbents in the body with little or no side-effects. Additionally, the range of indigenous drugs were all tropical and of a bewildering variety.[90]

The vaids[91] acknowledged that Haffkine's serum diminished the incidence of plague attacks on the inoculated population, but the protection it afforded against attacks was not considered absolute. It was believed that plague generally attacked those constitutions that were more congenial to it. Indigestion, over-feeding, fasting, irregular diet, uncleanliness, constipation and general indisposition were the chief predisposing causes.[92] Migration from an infected locality to an uninfected one, personal cleanliness and sanitation, and disinfection and whitewashing of houses were among the preventive measures advocated by Ayurveda.

Conclusion

While the plague bacillus had been discovered earlier in 1894, the mechanism of plague infection was unknown. The authorities were convinced that plague was contagious and that infection was spread through food, air and clothing. The disinfection of contaminated places and the segregation of the uninfected from those infected were based on this misplaced conception of the disease being an air-borne infection. Bubonic plague, therefore, continued to spread in the absence of special measures to destroy rats or to eliminate all possibility of contact between humans and rat fleas. Disinfection did not permanently disrupt the chain of infection and might have even assisted in its spread to other locations. Quarantining plague victims immediately upon infection might have prevented pneumonic plague but it was practically ineffective against bubonic plague. The excessive use of search parties and their overbearing attitude neither mitigated plague nor pacified the people. Early twentieth-century discoveries and the eventual acceptance of the mechanism of plague transmission were, of course, significant in controlling further spread of the disease. The notion of plague contagion was abandoned in favour of fumigation (which replaced disinfection), now targeting fleas. Sanitary policies aimed at making go-downs and houses impenetrable to rats. These measures, no doubt, resulted in a sharp decline in plague mortality after World War I.

If segregation represented the then existing state of scientific knowledge in dealing with communicable diseases, inoculation was new and on trial. Bitter controversy continues even today between advocates of compulsory vaccination and its opponents. The plague epidemic has been a lesson in this respect, making a case for compulsion to be used sparingly. Today, opponents of compulsory immunization continue to invoke religious freedom. The fear of complications that might occur continues to make others indifferent to vaccination. Health education is indispensable today as it was at the height of the plague years. India and South Africa's tryst with plague has brought to the forefront questions of social responsibility and individual freedom. Shared fears and apprehensions had the ability to unite people but latent social tensions were magnified, revealing much about the way societies are structured and the manner of their functioning.

7 THE BLIND MEN AND THE ELEPHANT: IMPERIAL MEDICINE, MEDIEVAL HISTORIANS AND THE ROLE OF RATES IN THE HISTORIOGRAPHY OF PLAGUE

Katherine Royer

Testifying before the Indian Plague Commission in 1898, witnesses described the victims of plague: their anxious expressions, suffused eyes, parched tongues and suppurating buboes.[1] The colonial officials also described hoards of dying rats: falling from ceilings, staggering out of holes and nibbling on the corpses of plague victims. G. Bainbridge, Surgeon-General for the Government of Bombay, reported to the Commission that it was well known to all with experience with plague that 'the illness of human beings with plague follows very closely with the death of rats in or about the dwellings'.[2] His was one of many voices describing the association of rat mortality with the onset of the epidemic in a neighbourhood. Lt-Colonel S. J. Thomson reported that for over fifty years the Government of India had required the evacuation of homes in the foothill villages of the Himalayas, where plague was endemic, at the first sign of significant rat mortality.[3] The Indians themselves had long made the observation that dying rats heralded the onset of the disease and colonial physicians were aware that Hindu texts for a thousand years had advised the evacuation of houses at the sight of dead rats.[4] Yet, when the Indian Plague Commission issued its final report they concluded that Paul-Louis Simond's theory, that a rat epizootic was a precondition for an epidemic of human plague, was inconclusive and that human agency was the most important factor in the spread of the disease.[5] So with rats dying all around them, why did the Indian Plague Commission fail to assign them a primary role in the transmission of the disease? The answer to that question is part of a story that links rats, historians, plague scientists and two separate plague pandemics to tell the tale of the influence of the Plague Research Commission, which issued its report early in the twentieth century, on the historiography of this disease for the next hundred years.[6] However, this is also a story about the seductive power of a one-size-fits-all explanation for a complex biological phenomenon and a reminder of Thomas Kuhn's argument about the impact of dominant scientific paradigms on 'normal science'.[7]

If it's Plague ... there Must be Rats

At the beginning of the epidemic in nineteenth-century India, the rat was not assigned a central role in the transmission of the disease by the Indian Plague Commission, yet seventy years later, John F. D. Shrewsbury, writing on the Black Death in England, stated that 'the historian seeking to identify a particular pestilence as an epidemic of plague must produce convincing evidence that the house-haunting rat was established in the afflicted society at the relevant time'.[8] In other words, if the disease was plague, there must have been rats. Thus once the role of the black rat in the transmission of the Indian epidemic had been established by the Plague Research Commission, historians insisted that if the disease that killed so many in Europe in the fourteenth century was plague, the rat must have played the central role. For example, in her introduction to a collection of primary sources on the Black Death, Rosemary Horrox stated that 'plague can be transmitted to humans only by the agency of fleas from infected rodents'.[9] Ironically, not a single one of the medieval sources in her collection mentions rats dying during the epidemic.[10] Paul Slack also acknowledged that although it was true that references to rats in connection with the Great Mortality were absent from contemporary accounts, he claimed rats must certainly have been there.[11]

Because this particular rodent came to be seen as so essential to the propagation of *any* plague pandemic, when plague revisionists in the last third of the twentieth century began to compare the epidemiology of rat-borne plague in nineteenth-century India with that of the Black Death, they came to the conclusion that the Great Mortality could not have been caused by plague because the patterns of the two epidemics were too dissimilar.[12] Thus, the Black Death and the third pandemic became inextricably intertwined by the belief that if the two epidemics were caused by the same disease, they should behave in the exactly the same manner, even as the responsible bacillus, *Yersinia pestis*, crossed continents as well as time.[13]

Thus the rat is at the centre of a story which links an epidemic in nineteenth-century India with the Black Death in fourteenth-century Europe because after the Plague Research Commission declared that the black rat was essential to the transmission of epidemic plague, the belief that a rat epizootic was an essential precursor to human epidemics came to dominate the scientific, as well as historical literature. Dead black rats were thought to be essential to the transmission of the disease because the rat flea, *Xenopsylla cheopis*, was believed to be the principal vector that transmitted the plague bacillus from its host, *Rattus rattus*, to its human victims. Importantly, this flea abandons the rat only after it has died from the disease, so a rat epizootic was deemed to be essential to epidemic plague.

However, plague is a disease that involves multiple vectors, hosts and victims and can be transmitted in a variety of ways.[14] The black rat is only one of many potential carriers; nevertheless, it has been assigned the central role in the transmission of *all* plague pandemics.[15] This belief is a testament to the influence of the work of the Plague Research Commission on generations of scientists and historians. This Commission, which was the third of the British directed plague research efforts, investigated the third pandemic which, although global in scope, had its greatest impact in late nineteenth- and early twentieth-century Asia. Its conclusions were then applied to earlier plague pandemics by both plague scientists and historians alike. So assumptions were made about the Black Death in Europe based on research done in an entirely different climate and in different social conditions. The Plague Research Commission's full embrace of the germ theory of disease and its enthusiasm for a unitary explanation for the transmission of epidemic plague led generations of plague scientists and historians to discount observations made about the disease in both nineteenth-century India and medieval Europe. Along the way, a more nuanced appreciation of this complex disease by some colonial scientists fell by the wayside, especially for many in the historical community. For this reason when it comes to plague, too often historians have acted like the blind men in the parable of the Indian blind men and the elephant, each drawing conclusions about an entire animal based on feeling only one part of a beast with thick legs, a small tail and a very large trunk.

Plague in India, Contingent Contagionism and the Reluctance to Assign the Rat a Central Role in the Transmission of the Disease

The road from the rejection of the rat as central to the transmission of epidemic plague by the Indian Plague Commission to the acceptance of the rat as essential to all plague pandemics began in June of 1897 when Ogata suggested that rat fleas possibly acted as vectors that transmitted the disease from rats to man.[16] In 1898, Paul-Louis Simond offered what would come to be the accepted hypothesis for the transmission of the disease.[17] Yet despite this research, the Indian Plague Commission argued that although rats played a role in the first outbreak of the disease in infected areas, once plague was established human agency was a more important factor in its spread than the activity of rats. Like the Indian Plague Commission, most of the international scientific community did not initially embrace a dominant role for rats in the transmission of plague and as late as 1921, the seventh edition of *Manson's Tropical Diseases* listed multiple animals, including dogs and oxen, as carriers of the disease.[18]

Important to this story is the fact that the onset of the third pandemic in India in 1896 was not the colonial medical establishment's first experience with plague. The Government of India had received over twenty-four reports of outbreaks of plague between 1812 and 1894, of which many, but importantly not all, described significant rat mortality associated with the disease.[19] Significantly, some of these earlier epidemics had been in the plains and not just in the foothills where the disease was known to be endemic. Thus, W. J. Simpson's *Treatise on Plague*, published in 1905, discussed plague in the Levant and Asia and Ernest H. Hankin's article in the *Journal of Hygiene*, published in the same year as Simpson's work, examined the previous outbreaks in India.[20] Although associated rat mortality was well known, neither author fully embraced Simonds hypothesis. Simpson called it 'fascinating' but felt he needed to see more evidence.[21] His scepticism may have been, as L. Fabian Hirst reports, because he and William Hunter had not been able to infect rats with the plague using infected rat fleas.[22] Hankin noted that rats were described during the second pandemic in Constantinople, but not in Europe, and reported that some of the epidemics in the foothills of India were not accompanied by rat mortality.[23] Like Simpson, he also did not reject the rat as a vector, but rather believed it was not *always* the vector largely because of the history of the disease in India. In particular, Hankin noted that rat mortality was seen in only eight out of forty outbreaks of the disease in Garwhal. In fact, it was the behaviour of plague in Garhwal that Hankin cited when he proclaimed that 'rats are not a necessary factor in the spread of the disease'.[24] He also presented evidence that monkeys had played a role in spreading the epidemic in Kankhal, as well as remarked upon the failure of Tidswell and Kolle to transmit plague to healthy rats by means of infected fleas.[25] Additionally, Hankin pointed out that Simond himself only succeeded in transmitting the disease in two out of four experiments.[26] The Indian Plague Commission and Hankin and Simpson were not alone in their reluctance to give the rat primacy of place in the transmission of plague. The German Plague Commission thought lice might be the vector and Yersin believed many different animals, including pigs and oxen, were involved in the transmission of the disease.[27] So multiple scientists involved in investigating the epidemic believed that rats and their fleas were just one of several carriers of the disease.

Simpson and Hankin, along with other colonial scientists, did acknowledge the evidence of significant rat mortality in the Indian epidemic, but there already existed an epistemological framework within which the imperial medical establishment could place this information. The rats described falling from the ceilings in India were simply considered fellow victims, who did not themselves play a role in transmitting the disease to humans. As David Arnold has argued, this position allowed the British medical establishment, domestic as well as colonial, to slip the evidence of rat mortality into an existing paradigm that associated rats with filth and filth as the incubator of disease.[28] Michael Worboys has demonstrated that British medicine in the second half of the nineteenth century, both at home and abroad, embraced a plurality of germ theories of disease incorporating them within the dominant metaphor of 'seed and soil': bacteria were a seed that would only grow in the right soil.[29] Simpson said as much when he attributed the varying behaviour of different plague epidemics to 'a great growing seed' sometimes being planted in 'barren ground'.[30] He argued that epidemic plague was influenced by many different factors, citing the fact that its virulence, history, symptoms and mortality varied from place to place and from epidemic to epidemic. For example, Simpson noted the differences in mortality between the epidemics in Hong Kong, India and Chile.[31] Thus, the seed did not always find fertile soil. Therefore, in his opinion the unsanitary conditions within which rats thrived were what constituted the fertile ground for a plague epidemic and so it was the filth in India, not the rat, that facilitated the spread of the pandemic. Of course, Simpson had been an enthusiastic supporter of sanitary reform even before plague hit India. In 1894 he had published 'The Need of a Sanitary Service for India' in the *Transactions of the First Indian Medical Congress* and in his introduction to the *Treatise on Plague* he argued forcefully for an aggressive sanitary establishment in the empire and blamed the deficiencies of the Sanitary Service in India for the spread of the epidemic.[32]

Hankin was also an advocate of contingent contagionism, but as a microbiologist he was more inclined to focus on possible biological vectors. So he, in contrast to Simpson, argued that plague was not a disease associated with filth; yet he did posit that it may be a 'miasmatic-contagious' disease.[33] Although Hankin did not fully believe that rats were essential to the transmission of the disease, he did claim that perhaps in some localities fleas were a factor because of the history of the epidemic in Agra, which abated when the weather turned hot.[34] In an addendum to 'On the Epidemiology of Plague' written after the original paper had gone to press, Hankin commented on Glenn Liston's recent observation that guinea pigs had died of plague at the Bombay Zoological Gardens after being bitten by rat fleas.[35] This, for Hankin, offered definitive evidence that rat fleas would attack other mammals after the rat had died. So Hankin gave serious consideration to the role of fleas in the transmission of the disease, even though he did not believe rats were an essential feature of all plague outbreaks.

Therefore, the influence of contingent contagionism, enthusiasm for sanitary reform and the experience with plague in India throughout the nineteenth century, where significant rat mortality was not reported in every outbreak, led to the reluctance of colonial scientists to give the rat an essential role in the propagation of the third pandemic. Additionally, many other possible hosts and vectors were given serious consideration by much of the international scientific community. So for this first generation of plague researchers, rats were simply a subplot to a larger story that involved multiple potential vectors, a dark, fetid and unhealthy India and a disease with a long and varied history in the subcontinent.

The Plague Research Commission and the Road to the Acceptance of the Rat as Essential to Epidemic Plague

When the epidemic hit Australia in 1900, the hypothesis that rats were simply fellow travellers in the unsanitary environments of China and India where plague seemed to flourish came under increasing scrutiny. The epidemic in Sydney, in contrast to India, was less virulent and the majority of victims were Europeans; whereas the European population in India had largely been spared.[36] This made it more problematic to blame the disease on dirt. It was this pattern of behaviour of plague in Australia that convinced J. Ashburton Thompson, Chief Medical Officer for the Government of New South Wales, that the disease was not transmitted directly by human agency, as claimed by the Indian Plague Commission, but was rather a disease associated predominantly with an epizootic among rats.[37] This led Thompson to concur with Simond's hypothesis, although he acknowledged that the mode of diffusion of plague did exhibit 'slight variation in detail under different conditions which obtain in other countries'.[38] Nonetheless, he argued that it 'must hold good in all essentials'.[39] Significantly, in his opinion there was one overriding reason why those 'essentials' had been identified in Australia and not in India. In his 1906 article in the *Journal of Hygiene*, Thompson pointed out that the population impacted by plague in Australia was 'not merely wholly white, of English extraction, and speech, and fully civilized, but intelligent, instructed and orderly, accustomed to direction and amenable to it'.[40] Because of the nature of this population, Thompson believed that the epidemiological observations made in Australia should be privileged over those from India and China, where language and cultural differences prevented scientists from collecting accurate data.[41] Thus, he argued that the research done during the epidemic in Australia constituted 'normal observations' and, in his opinion, the results of the investigations there, which he believed confirmed that plague was primarily a disease of the rat and a suctorial parasite, should be considered the 'normal results'.[42] Thus, the protean history of the disease in India was brushed aside as plague scientists came to privilege the experience with the disease in Australia over its more varied behaviour in the subcontinent.[43]

By this time, there was also the fact that sanitary cordons, inoculation with Haffkine's vaccine and a programme of aggressive rodent eradication appeared to have had some success in controlling the epidemic. Many believed that these efforts had brought plague under control and in Brisbane in 1904 a programme of rodent eradication begun in January appeared to have brought the epidemic to an end by September.[44] Needless to say, the Australian experience of consistency in the association of plague and rat mortality, coupled with the apparent success of a programme of rodent eradication in stemming the tide of the epidemic, raised the profile of the rat among plague scientists.

It was in this environment that the Plague Research Commission began its work in 1905. The work of this commission played an important role in elucidating the role of the rat and its fleas in the transmission of plague and for the rest of the century its conclusions would cast a long shadow over how plague was understood. The Plague Research Commission was established at the direction of the Secretary of State and its advisory committee was comprised of representatives of the Office of the Secretary of State, the Royal Society and the Lister Institute; thus, much like the Indian Plague Commission, it was dominated by members of the metropolitan medical establishment.[45] More importantly, it did not undertake a broad inquiry directed at investigating multiple potential vectors or means of transmission.[46] The Commission began its research having already accepted the premise that epidemic plague was essentially a rat-borne disease and explicitly stated that its research would be directed at elucidating the exact mechanism by which the disease was transmitted among rats and from rat to man.[47] Not surprisingly, the Commission's final conclusions were definitive as to the primacy of rats and their fleas in the initiation and maintenance of epidemic plague. However, despite the fact that he was a strong supporter of the conclusions of the Plague Research Commission, L. Fabian Hirst did note that it failed to fully investigate the human flea, *Pulex irritans*, as a possible vector after it found few of these fleas infected with *Yersinia pestis* in afflicted Bombay households.[48]

This certainty regarding the essential nature of the rat flea to the transmission of epidemic plague was not universally accepted. The French scientists George Blanc and Marcel Baltazard argued that in North African epidemics the human flea, as well as lice, played an important role in the spread of the disease.[49] Their conclusions, however, were dismissed by most British scientists because of questions regarding their methodology and the evidence from Arthur William Bacot and Charles James Martin that a flea needed to be blocked to be infective.[50] Blocking was considered such an essential condition for the transmission of plague that the human flea was discounted as a significant vector in major epidemics because it was believed that it could not ingest enough bacilli when feeding on humans to block and so could not efficiently transmit *Yersinia pestis* to a human population.[51] Although Hirst believed that human fleas might have played an auxiliary role in the Black Death, he did not think they could sustain an epidemic on their own, so he supported the Plague Research Commission's conclusion that epidemic plague was essentially a rat-borne disease.[52]

Hirst played an important role in ushering the Plague Research Commission into the pantheon of the Whig history of medicine with his book, *The Conquest of Plague* (1953), in which he contrasted the work of the Commission to that of earlier colonial scientists, whom he described as incapable of 'freeing their minds from the current misconception and influence of old established orthodox ideas'.[53] Robert Pollitzer would argue that along with Yersin and Simond, the Plague Research Commission laid the foundation for modern plague science.[54]

This narrative endured throughout most of the twentieth century, in part because it fit comfortably into the scholarship on colonial science.[55] Much of this history explored the claims to specialized knowledge by physicians practising in the tropics in the late eighteenth and early nineteenth centuries and argued that their authority was undermined by the cholera debates of the second half of the nineteenth century.[56] The resistance of the Anglo-Indian medical establishment to contagionism during these debates had so sullied the reputation of Anglo-Indian medicine that its claims to specialized knowledge of diseases in the tropics was undermined. So embedded in this history of imperial medicine and science is the story of the rise of the germ theory of disease and how plague science, like that of cholera, led to the triumph of one medical epistemological system over another.[57] Therefore, the view from the microscopes and culture plates of the Plague Research Commission came to be privileged over the observations of the men on the ground in India as bench science was given primacy of place in the history of plague science. And with the certainty expressed in that Commission's final report regarding the essential nature of a rat epizootic to epidemic plague, 'no rats, no plague' became the mantra of the second generation of plague researchers for whom this dictum applied, no matter where or when a pandemic took place.[58]

The Second Generation of Plague Scientists and the Historiography of the Black Death

This second generation of plague scientists, which included Hirst, Pollitzer and Wu Lien-Teh, were all strong adherents to the position that major pandemics were due to rat-borne plague, even as they described outbreaks of disease which did not involve rats, such as the Manchurian epidemics in 1910 and 1920 in which marmots were the source of the infection.[59] While they acknowledged that plague could be transmitted by vectors other than the rat flea and appreciated the complexity of the disease, they remained committed to the position that all human plague pandemics were essentially a rat-borne disease.[60] Along the way, the fact that the disease had not expressed uniformly in India became lost in the enthusiasm for the work of the Plague Research Commission by this generation, who then retrospectively applied the Commission's conclusions to the Black Death.[61]

Yet, there remained the problem that there were no descriptions of rat mortality during the second pandemic. In *The Conquest of Plague*, L. Fabian Hirst acknowledged this, but he justified his 'no rats, no plague' position on the argument that conditions in medieval Europe would surely have been conducive to rats and that the behaviour of the Great Mortality fit the pattern of rat-borne plague because of its recurrent nature and eventual location in urban centres.[62]

Like Hirst, Pollitzer also believed that the rat was the primary agent responsible for the Black Death.[63] So a rat epizootic was considered an essential precondition for a human epidemic in both the second and third pandemics, even if there were no descriptions of significant rat mortality in fourteenth-century Europe. Everyone kept coming back to the same argument: that if it was epidemic plague, there must have been rats. So once the rat-borne plague hypothesis had gained acceptance for the third pandemic, more than a few plague scientists were willing to look past the fact that descriptions of dead rats were missing from medieval accounts of the Black Death. And significantly, medieval historians followed suit.

The Revisionists and the History of the Black Death

Ironically, it was the belief in the universal role of the rat in the transmission of pandemic plague, regardless of the climate or the century, that led a group of historians, zoologists and epidemiologists beginning in the 1970s to question whether the fourteenth-century epidemic was indeed plague, even though they never questioned the role of rats in the transmission of the disease.[64] In fact, it was the epidemiology of rat-borne plague in late nineteenth-century India that led them to argue that the second pandemic was either not caused by plague or it was not the only disease responsible for the Great Mortality. Interestingly, it was not so much the absence of descriptions of rat mortality in the medieval sources that concerned them, although they made note of it, but rather it was the disparate epidemiologic footprint of the two pandemics that formed the basis of their argument.

One of the earliest volleys in this battle came from a microbiologist, John F. D. Shrewsbury, in 1970. He argued that because the epidemiology of the second pandemic did not fit that of rat-borne plague, plague alone could not have been responsible for the mortality seen during the Black Death, suggesting that perhaps typhus was an additional factor in the fourteenth-century demographic collapse.[65] The zoologists Graham Twigg and Christopher Duncan, historical demographer Susan Scott, the epidemiologists working with George Christakos and historian Samuel Cohn, Jr, were far more willing than Shrewsbury to reject the assumption that the Black Death was caused by plague. Among the many arguments presented by this group was the fact that fourteenth-century Europe did not have the conditions necessary to support a large population of *Rattus rattus*, that the animal moved too slowly to have spread the disease as fast as the Black Death travelled, and the incubation period, pattern of spread and mortality of the Black Death were very different from that of the third pandemic, which moved slowly and was less lethal. This led some of them to posit that the second pandemic was caused by diseases other than plague, such as viral hemorrhagic fever or anthrax.[66] However, although all of the revisionists predicated their arguments one way or the other on the disparities between the transmission patterns of the second and third pandemics, they all accepted the hypothesis that bubonic plague is essentially a rat borne disease. So the influence of the Plague Research Commission continued to dominate the work of revisionists and non-revisionists alike.

The Palaeogeneticists and Plague Science in the Twenty-First Century

Of course, the ground shifted under the revisionists in the autumn of 2010 with the publication of Barbara Bramanti's work on DNA extracted from plague pits throughout Europe which confirmed that *Yersinia pestis* was involved in the second pandemic in Europe.[67] This work was followed by further confirmation by Verena Schuenemann and colleagues in 2012.[68] Schuenemann's research also indicated that the plasmid identified in the East Smithfield plague pits, pPCP1, was not significantly different from the pPCP1 found in the modern plague bacillus. Since this plasmid is one of three believed to be responsible for the evolution of *Yersinia pestis* into a lethal organism from its less virulent precursors *Yersinia pseudotuberculosis* and *Yersinia enterocolitica*, Schuenemann's work offered no immediate genetic explanation for the difference in mortality between the second and third pandemics. And since the Plague Research Commission issued its report, plague science has identified over 200 different species of animals that can serve as hosts for the disease and research has demonstrated multiple mechanisms through which it can be transmitted, many of which do not even involve the black rat or its fleas, such as ingestion of contaminated undercooked meat or the handling of infected animal tissue.[69] In 2008, a multidisciplinary group of scientists acknowledged in their summary of the conclusions drawn from a meeting of plague scientists that humans can be infected with plague through handling of infected animals, including rodents, cats and camels, that cats can develop *Yersinia pestis* and transmit pneumonic plague directly to humans, and the fleas, as well as the bacillus, can live for some time outside the mammalian hosts, and thus, can play a role in human to human transmission.[70] Additionally, the basic premise of the Plague Research Commission regarding the essential nature of the rat flea to the transmission of the disease has been challenged. *Pulex irritans* is believed to be the vector responsible for a more recent outbreak of the disease in Tanzania and Hirst's argument against the human flea as a vector in major epidemics has also been challenged by research that has demonstrated that fleas do not need to be blocked to be infective.[71] And another group of scientists have argued that the human body louse, *Pediculus humanus*, can transmit plague.[72] They posit that in colder climates lice may have played a role in transmission of the disease, which makes a bit more interesting Shrewsbury's observation that the Black Death had the epidemiologic footprint of another louse borne disease

– typhus. Yet, the protean nature of plague demonstrated in this research had been ignored by many in the historical community, who like Ole Benedictow, remained largely committed to an explanation for the transmission of the disease based on the conclusions of the Plague Research Commission.[73]

Plague Reconsidered

Yet, the early plague scientists acknowledged the protean nature of a disease which can present in multiple forms, bubonic, pneumonic, tonsillar and septicemic, each of which have different rates of mortality. Like more recent plague scientists, they also believed that *Yersinia pestis* could be transmitted directly through skin lesions or by eating infected material.[74] They also appreciated that plague is a disease which can be transmitted through a complicated chain of events which frequently, but not always, involve a variety of mammalian species and insect vectors and that each of these hosts and vectors, as well as the bacillus itself, are influenced in different ways by their physical environment. Yet the fact that plague has been transmitted by different host/vector combinations in different locations from marmots in Manchuria to ground squirrels in California and human fleas in Tanzania, has rarely been considered a possibility for the fourteenth-century epidemic by Anglophone historians. Instead, the predominant assumption has been that if plague was a rat-borne disease in the third pandemic, it must have been one in the second.[75] However, both Simpson and Hankin recognized that plague is like an elephant; a creature with a variety of features. They noted that not only was rat mortality not associated with every outbreak, but that the pattern of the disease in India changed with the location. Simpson reported that the 1853 epidemic began in fulminate form in the foothills and then its virulence declined as it moved into the plains.[76] At other times and in other locations an epidemic would build strength as time went on, as it did in Pali in the 1830s.[77] Simpson also observed that in 1853 plague killed 25 per cent of the population in the foothills of the Himalayas, a mortality level similar to that seen during the Black Death, but then the virulence declined as the disease moved to a lower altitude.[78] For these reasons Simpson was not wedded to the idea that plague must behave uniformly in every circumstance and instead posited that different plague epidemics may involve a variety of incubation periods, as well as presentations, depending on the vector, victim and physical environment.[79] Hankin also noted that occasionally in India an epidemic would flare immediately and at other times it took longer to establish as the disease moved through populations of animal hosts before it broke out in epidemic form in humans.[80] He also pointed out that sometimes there was evidence of rat mortality months before the first human case was reported, but at other times the disease struck a location and then only several months later were dead rats observed.[81]

Yet this nuanced view of this complex disease was overlooked in a century-long embrace of the conclusions of the Plague Research Commission by many historians who also failed to take into account that none of the Commission's research was done in conditions similar to those found in fourteenth-century Europe. As L. Fabian Hirst revealingly remarked in his dismissal of *Pulex irritans* as a dominant vector in pandemic plague – such a contention must be rejected because of the 'practical experience in *Asia*'.[82] However, fourteenth-century Europe was not nineteenth-century India.[83] Nevertheless, the trunk of the elephant proved to be so fascinating that historians failed to examine the rest of the animal. And despite recent moves towards taking a more regional approach in understanding the history of plague, the desire for a unitary explanation that can be applied to all plague pandemics lives on.[84] Some of the DNA hunters of the twenty-first century have been just as seduced by their own paradigm of genetic determinism as were the germ theorists of the early twentieth century. They believe that the answer to the mystery of the disparity in plague virulence between the second and third pandemics will be revealed by further sequencing of the entire chromosome of *Yersinia pestis*.[85] This may prove to be true; but this contention assumes that the most essential component of a virulent epidemic like the Black Death was the genetic makeup of the responsible biovar. So the history of plague is a story about the tendency of modern science, as well as historians, to grasp tightly to the dominant paradigm, whether it is the germ theory of disease at the turn of the twentieth century or the genetic determinism of the twenty-first, as they seek one size fits all explanations for biological phenomena that are often quite complex and protean in nature.

8 PHYSICIANS, FORCEPS AND CHILDBIRTH: TECHNOLOGICAL INTERVENTION IN REPRODUCTIVE HEALTH IN COLONIAL BENGAL

Arabinda Samanta

Introduction

This chapter seeks to engage in two important issues: first, it explores the historical trajectory which made scientific and technological intervention in reproductive health and childbirth in colonial Bengal a pressing imperial/medical imperative, and second, it will attempt to explicate the cultural implications of this intervention in an era of enforced transition from pre-modern to 'modern' under the British rule. On both these counts, it will examine the role of colonialism and the nature of 'enforced modernity', and look at how the colonial interventions, consequent upon considerations of medical market, constricted the adoption of a modern technology in childbirth that was devised through painstaking indigenous initiatives.

In recent writings on reproductive health, a sharp historical focus on the use of surgical instruments and its socio-cultural and technological implications for a tradition-bound society like India is curiously lacking.[1] All the major scholarly interventions made so far in this direction have been confined only to casual references to surgical instruments and their impact on the colonized. Postcolonial feminist histories also are curiously silent on how colonial contentions over issues like marriage and reproduction produced bodies as accessible sites to modern science. Even in nineteenth-century Britain, when the medical profession was characterized by tradition and prejudices about women were slow to recognize the real needs of women, the development of obstetrics and gynecology was not a smooth one. The medical world in India was experiencing the same predicament. The same holds true of caesarian section which slowly made its way into the Indian medical vocabulary at the beginning of the twentieth century, but was slow to gain recognition and social acceptance in the cultural milieu of 'modern' Bengal.

In fact, a few further questions are in order: First, how was the 'body' of the colonized women imagined during colonial encounters with reproductive health? How were changing scientific notions informed by the production of a 'normative' woman? Second, when did forceps, an important surgical instrument designed to aid in delivery, trudge its way into the Indian medical world and how exactly did it make a dent on the socio-cultural taboos that characterized the contemporary Bengali society? What was the implication of the use of such techniques for the Bengali society where the cultural stereotypes and colonial intervention often worked in tandem to impede free acceptance of any innovation? Given the fact that childbirth was traditionally perceived as a natural process that warranted little or no technical intervention and was looked upon as an exclusively female domain, impact of the introduction of forceps, vis-à-vis colonial modernity, merits fresh interrogation.

Managing Birth Pangs

It has been a standard argument in recent historical scholarship, shared equally by Indian and western historians, that the British colonial authority in India had little interest in Indian birth practices and that they took the initiative in promoting medical care for Indian mothers only when the missionary women in India made it an issue. Miss Beilby, as the current narrative goes, came to Lucknow as a medical missionary in 1875. While she was there, the Maharaja of Punna, a Native State in Bundelkhand, asked her to come and attend his wife. The Maharani recovered and told Miss Beilby: 'I want you to tell the Queen ... what the women of India suffer when they are sick'. Retuning to England Miss Beilby had an audience with Queen Victoria, who reportedly said, 'We had no idea it was as bad as this. Something must be done for the poor creatures. We wish it generally known that we sympathize with every effort to relieve the suffering of the women of India'.[2] When Lady Dufferin was leaving for India, in 1883, the Queen instructed her to initiate some plan for providing medical aid to the women of India. The Countess of Dufferin Fund that started in 1885 is generally treated as the starting point for a history of western medical care for Indian women. The Indian initiative in this whole story, particularly by the men folk, is relegated to the background. The story of indigenous initiative needs to be told afresh in proper historical perspective. For we have ample evidence to believe that much before the medical missionaries as also the British high officials intervened crucially in the domain of reproductive health and childbirth, indigenous initiative was not at all lacking. And here the role of some male physicians such as Dr Madhusudan Gupta and Dr Kedarnath Das merits fresh attention.

The management of childbirth in India emerged as a crucial agenda in colonial and nationalist discourses in the late nineteenth and early twentieth centuries, as it did in other colonial settings around the globe.[3] Writings on medicine and health became an important genre of vernacular publishing with a wide nonmedical readership by the late colonial period, with journals and textbooks exalting medicine and reproductive health as a primary sign of modernization in Bengal.[4] In fact, the professionalization of obstetrics was considered by the colonists and nationalists alike as an antidote to the problem of high maternal deaths and infant mortality. Hence, debates in the late nineteenth and early twentieth centuries revolved around the question as to how and to what extent childbirth could be brought within the emerging western medical establishment in India.[5]

The medicalization of childbirth in colonial India consisted of two related projects. The first project endeavoured to provide a new setting for childbirth, seeking to reform or even modify the *zenana*, or the women's quarters, on the basis of sanitary principles, as well as to integrate the lying-in hospital into a hierarchy of resort for the birthing woman. The second project entailed replacing childbirth attendants. In particular, this latter project sought to marginalize the role of the indigenous *dai* and to replace her by a trained midwife or a qualified physician.[6] But the British rulers as such were not particularly interested in the health of their colonial subjects. It was the western educated Indians who took the lead and, gradually, the whole-scale acceptance of western-style birthing practices, regarded as scientific and rational, became an integral part of a progressive Indian society. These ideas readily found expression in the magazines and journals of the time, which contained articles on 'scientific' birth practices and congratulatory notes to medical graduates. New medical institutions for women appeared: lying-in hospitals and institutions, especially designed for female doctors and nurses. Concerned with the traditional process of birthing and the resultant high mortality rates, women's organizations also took up the issues of pre- and post-natal care.[7]

Concern in the Print World

The agenda of women's health drew interested attention of the medical fraternity in nineteenth-century Europe which subsequently led to a proliferation in literature on the subject; books written specifically on the subject, such as Dr Fleetwood Churchill's *On the Diseases of Women* (1874), were noteworthy in this respect. In addition, male doctors began to contribute regularly to women's magazines. Women's hospitals multiplied to provide special care for women at the same time utilizing them as a fertile field for experimentation on their health problems. It was from these centres, through the mediation of a few pioneering individuals, such as James Young Simpson and Robert Lawson Tait, that the path-breaking theories of technological developments and surgical procedures were elaborated.[8] Pregnancy, for the first time, addressed though its profound complexities, was just beginning to be perceived. The profound impact it had on the intimate relationship between mother and child came to be realized in a more explicit fashion. The growing concern over motherhood was reflected in a spurt of burgeoning literature that began to flood the market; examples include Dr Alfred Bull's *Hints to Mothers for the Management of Health during the period of Pregnancy and Lying-in-Room* which first appeared in 1833 and quickly went through fourteen editions in 1877. Mention may also be made of Dr Conquest's *Letters to a Mother on the Management of herself and her Children in Health and Disease: Embracing the Subjects of Pregnancy, Children, Nursing, Food, Exercise, Bathing, Chloroform* etc. and Dr Albutt's *The Wife's Handbook: How a Woman should Order herself during Pregnancy in the Lying-in Room, and After Delivery with Hints on the Management of the Baby and Other Matters of Importance Necessary to be Known by a Married Woman*. In addition to the hundreds of manuals published, there were also periodicals produced expressly for mothers and their particular problems, such as the *British Mother's Magazine* and the *Mother's Friend*, both of which existed from 1848 to 1895.[9]

The impact of these works continued well into nineteenth-century Bengal, when male physicians started writing books on midwifery carrying prescriptions and advice for expectant mothers.[10] The agenda of social reform in the nineteenth century, led by the Bengali male intelligentsia, was informed by an attempt to improving the lot of women, but much of their endeavour was also directed towards an urge for reshaping the norms and functions of middle-class family as a site for the moral and cultural restructuring of the nation. The large number of pedagogical texts written in this period produced a normative discourse on family which framed new rules and laid down guidelines for an ideal housewife for proper home management, scientific nurturing of children, regulation of dietary habits, and creation of hygienic environment and so on.[11] The modernization project of the nineteenth century also looked upon the family as a site where nationalist restructuring was to be carried out and the women's question was addressed within the restrictive parameters of domesticity. The Indian middle class internalized some of the imperialist critique of Indian/ Hindu domestic life, yet at the same time modified some of the prevalent ideas about bourgeois domesticity, privacy and individuality to suit their own needs. Comparisons between the 'Indian' and 'European' home were made by Bengali authors, the latter being described as the epitome of perfection while the former seemed to suffer from a grievous lack of order, discipline and cleanliness. The Bengali *bhadramahila* was expected to master the technique of becoming a *sugrihini* or good housewife by acquiring elementary knowledge of all sorts of medical remedies for treating at least common ailments to save the family a lot of expense in doctor's fees.[12]

A new genre in popular Bengali print culture emerged in the second half of the nineteenth century. These normative texts, or advice manuals, were a cultural production of the middle class which came to project its women by carefully distancing them from other social classes. Informed by a changing notion of domesticity, the 'Manual' (these instructive texts generally go by this name) writers, ranging from the ardent nationalists to the aspiring lower class, charted out the role of an ideal Bengali housewife. The new concept of womanhood was a fine blending of the self-sacrificing Hindu wife and the Victorian helpmate. These texts were written mostly by middle-class men of different religious persuasions and their target audience was the new Bengali *bhadramahila* whose roles and obligations they projected in these manuals.[13]

Male Physicians in the Doman of Women

Against this backdrop of historical trajectory of reproductive health and childcare we intend to look at the work of two major physicians, Madhusudan Gupta and Kedarnath Das. Madhusudan Gupta (1800–56) hailed from a *vaidya* family of Baidyabati, a village in the Hooghly district of Bengal. He joined the newly created Ayurvedic classes in Sanskrit College, Calcutta, in 1826 and was promoted to the post of a teacher in the Calcutta Medical College (CMC) in view of his great interest and enthusiasm. Indian students at the time were not interested in joining the CMC, particularly because they hailed from aristocratic families with evident disdain for surgery, for it involved touching the dead body, a taboo in Indian society. Nevertheless, Madhusudan Gupta had made a significant contribution to the CMC during his time. A Sanskrit scholar and an Ayurvedic doctor, Madhusudan Gupta proclaimed that he would dissect the dead body and thus became the first man in India to dissect a cadaver in 1836, a feat highly disapproved by tradition and the orthodox Hindu society. The momentous event was celebrated in a rather militaristic fashion by firing a fifty-round gun salute from Calcutta Fort William.[14]

Contrary to what most other doctors would call it a sacrilege, Madhusudan Gupta undertook a project of determining the average age of menstruation among the Hindu girls. One really wonders how, though not a gynaecologist himself, he was able to extract such private information from respectable and conservative Hindu families. Such questions, asked by a male doctor to a girl could have been construed as a direct affront to the family's cultural insularity. There is no evidence of how he took on this onerous task, what methodology he adopted, nor how he avoided public outrage. We do, however, know that he conducted a survey among 127 Hindu girls to ascertain the age of their first menstrual experience. He observed that menstruation had started among eighty-one girls at an average age of twelve, but as many as eighty girls had had their first sexual experience at an average age of nine. Twenty-eight girls had even given birth by the age of fourteen. He thus concluded that in India, most of the girls had had their first menstrual experience at an average age of twelve, an age pre-scribed by Manu, the ancient law-giver, as the appropriate age of marriage. This revelation distressed him so much that he devoted his career to the concern for mothers' health and childbirth.

Madhusudan Gupta argued that much before the introduction of western medicine in British India, Ayurvedic practices had been firmly established. But childbirth in India was considered a matter exclusively within the family domain, outside the purview of the medical gaze. And since the cutting of the umbilical cord was considered dirty, an elderly *dai* or midwife from the *dom* caste (low caste, 'untouchable') was supposed to do the job. He was aware of the consequences of illiteracy and superstition in reproductive health. His evidence to the Fever Commission is revealing when he observed that the arrangement for the lying-in-room (*aturghar*) was anything but hygienic. The lying-in-rooms resembled 'the abode of death' or 'prison houses'. Its floor was very often damp and ill-ventilated with only one door and no windows. The inside temperature was often no less than 90 degrees since a fireplace was always kept alight. Living in such a lying-in-room often led to death – three or four out of twenty mothers would die in these rooms. While purity was attached to the process of concep-tion of an offspring, birth was conceived to be highly polluting.

The Bengali normative texts or the advice manuals, in fact, did not propagate the cause of hospitals, although they had begun to cater to women's health by the middle of the nineteenth century. Till the turn of the nineteenth century, hospitals were not regarded as entirely suitable places for 'respectable' women.[15] The new medical wisdom laid down that a mother should not remain in the *suti-kagriha* for longer than one week, but it is not known how many families would have dared to defy traditional taboos in this regard. A woman was to take care with her diet; traditionally approved foods such as pepper, lime, hot ghee, fish, meat, roti *luchi*, *parota*, were considered harmful; a medically recommended diet included milk, arrowroot, barley, sago, boiled rice, among others. In extreme cases, brandy could be taken for relieving pain. About the same time, although women's health during childbirth had not yet remarkably improved, there was some recognition of the importance of post-natal care.[16]

Very few women from respectable and influential families used to go to the Medical College Hospital in Calcutta for delivery of a child, presumably because all the attending doctors were male. In view of this, Madhusudan Gupta sug-gested that prospective mothers would be encouraged to visit a hospital if the government arranged for provision of Hindu *dais* and female attendants. The traditional *dais* would also be trained there in modern scientific delivery practices. This, he believed, would dispel any myths and superstitions pertaining to childbirth with a gradual introduction and acceptance of western medical practices by the indigenous population.

Madhusudan Gupta empathized with the pains and sufferings of motherhood, and sought to remove them through modern scientific medical birth practices. He sought to introduce some sort of a cultural regeneration in reproductive health of Bengali women. Much against the social taboo, he was the first physician in India and, perhaps, in Asia to dissect a human body for medical education. This iconoclastic zeal inspired him to rethink various issues concerning the health of the mother especially at a time (early nineteenth-century Bengal) when women's issues were considered a social taboo. On 25 May 1869, the *Amritabazar Patrika* newspaper included in its pages:

> there are very few in Bengal who think about the emancipation of women. This has become customary to laugh at the women's question. One is very often ridiculed if he sympathized with the pitiable plight of the Bengali women. He is in fact held in public contempt as being henpecked.[17]

Madhusudan Gupta was well aware of the repercussions and the public ridicule he would face in his supportive endeavours for the betterment of women. Nevertheless, this did not deter him from pursuing his goals. He wanted to have an adequate number of well qualified female Hindu midwives on moderate fees who might accomplish the job. If a hospital with a lying-in-ward were established with proper Hindu midwives and attendants, a great number of married women of higher castes would be encouraged to avail themselves of it, and many a life would be saved as a result. Employment would be generated for a good number of midwives in such a hospital. And these women, employed and instructed by European teachers of midwifery, would readily find employment at a moderate charge among Hindu women of all castes and rank at their houses and many of their lives and those of their children would be saved.[18]

At the risk of public disdain, Madhusudan Gupta appealed to the Government of Bengal to look into the health of Bengali mothers. Almost fifty years after his appeal when the government brought in generous funds for the cause of women, its recognition went to Missionary intervention and the Queen's benevolence, instead of its mastermind, Madhusudan Gupta and his efforts. It is true that women missionaries from Great Britain and America who came to India in the late 1860s, tried to break the rigid boundaries of the seclusion of the *zenana* or the 'uncolonized space' and to wage battle against ignorance about health and hygiene. Dr Clara Swain, Dr William Elmslie, Miss Fanny Butler and several others took the initiative in providing western medical care to train midwives and nurses by establishing private clinics. But this kind of missionary medical establishments created 'family discord and strife, and it was difficult for the *pardanashin* or the lady in veiled seclusion to avail of the benefits of western treatment. Several years later, the Queen asked the Countess of Dufferin to study the matter and decide what could be done. The Countess Dufferin Fund that was instituted in 1885 became the first programme with official support to focus on medical care for Indian women. But in this highly publicized official story, the Indian initiative, particularly the one taken by Madhusudan Gupta, occupies an insignificant place. Madhusudan Gupta had tried hard to break loose the cultural taboos pertaining to childbirth and sought to introduce western scientific method in reproductive health. His negotiation with modernity underpinning science and rationality, although cautious, helped create a cultural space in which later reformers aspired to intervene.

The Physician and his Forceps

A mother's death during or as a result of labour is, perhaps, the oldest tragic saga in a reproductive narrative the world over. In India, one man who endeavoured to prevent it was Dr Kedarnath Das, India's greatest obstetric guru, for he was the first Indian to call attention to the need of western methods for stemming its dreadful maternal and infantile mortality; and this he did in the public forum and in books and journals for over forty years. The principal and professor of midwifery and gynaecology of Carmichael Medical College, Calcutta, Dr Kedarnath Das was perhaps the greatest obstetrician India has ever produced.[19] He wanted to ameliorate the conditions of the women of Bengal. Having devoted his life for the progress of science and midwifery in Bengal, he laid the foundation but did not live to see his dream of a fully functional maternity hospital in Calcutta become a reality. His publications were numerous and indicative of the vastness of his clinical experiences and outlook. His first book, *A Handbook of Obstetrics*, was published in 1914 and was followed in 1920 by *A Textbook of Midwifery* which is still regarded as one of the greatest midwifery classics of all times. Equally significant was his *Obstetric Forceps: Its History and Evolution*, published in 1929.[20] The book describes as many as 878 types of forceps along with a picture of each one. It took him more than twelve years to compile, and will remain an enduring monument to his knowledge and patience. He toured Europe and America collecting materials for this last book, and was made an Honorary Fellow of the American Gynecological Society, and the American Association of Obstetricians, Gynecologists, and Abdominal Surgeons. He was also a Foundation Fellow of the British College of Obstetricians and Gynecologists. He received many accolades from different British medical institutions in recognition of his exemplary service to medicine in India; his knighthood in

June 1933 was a deserved tribute to an Indian who for forty years had striven to reduce maternal and infantile mortality in the country of his birth.

Born in 1867, Dr Kedarnath Das was engrossed in research on female diseases. He stood First in the M.B. Examination in 1892 from Medical College, Calcutta, securing the highest grade in gynaecology, a record which stands unbroken even today. He spent his initial years of medical training at the Campbell Medical School which he joined in 1899, and later in 1919, he joined the famous Carmichael Medical College (present R. G. Kar Medical College). His enviable skill in surgical operation tended to strengthen the sagging confidence of conservative Hindu women who wished not to die in labour at the hands of an inexperienced gynaecologist. Professor Green-Armitez, the renowned gynaecologist of Calcutta Medical College, often referred to him as 'my guru'.

While concerned about women's issues, Dr Kedarnath Das came to the realization that a comprehensive treatise in English on the gradual evolution of obstetric forceps was a desideratum. According to him, such a work should have contained not only the history and evolution with detailed descriptions of the instrument but also its indicators, use and abuse, methods of application, dangers both to the mother and the child, its value as compared with any other feasible operation, its medico-legal aspect and statistics. Ambitious as he was, Dr Das started collecting materials for such a work in 1917. All the monographs and journals available in Calcutta were consulted and the references verified as far as possible. The labour involved in collecting materials for the book and arranging them had been enormous, as practically every reference had to be verified. His lack of knowledge of the different languages from which the compilations had to be made, namely, French, German, Polish, Russian and Japanese, added to the difficulties which he sought to overcome through consultation with friends who knew these languages. Moreover, his preoccupation with his regular professional duties as well as the arduous work in connection with the Carmichael Medical College and Hospitals, also limited the time he had to be able to work on these issues.[21]

Dr Kedarnath Das was a teacher par excellence and also a keen researcher on reproductive health. For twelve long years he worked on surgical forceps, and finally in 1912, he won acclaim for his success in designing Bengal Forceps. The history of obstetrical forceps goes a long way back. Sanskrit writings from approximately 1500 BC contain evidence of single and paired instruments. Similarly, Egyptian, Greek, Roman and Persian writings and pictures refer to forceps.[22] Perhaps, the earliest mention of instrumental delivery in the Vedic period is 'Ankush'.[23] Amputations were a regular part of surgical practice, and a large and varied number of instruments, more than hundred, were said to have been available to the surgeon: forceps, specula, scissors, saws, needles, syringes and catheters.[24]

Dr Das modified the traditional Simpson Forceps which was much in use in Great Britain[25] at the time and redesigned it to suit the physical and biological requirement of Bengali mothers. This surgical manoeuver was based on his observation that the pelvic area of the Bengali mother is generally seven eighths of that of a British mother, and that an average weight of a Bengali baby is sixth sevenths of that of a British baby. So the insertion of the traditional forceps might cause tear and make wounds in the vaginal canal of a Bengali mother. In order to relieve pain and reduce any damage made, he designed his forceps more delicate in weight and more appropriate to the foetal head and pelvic curve of a Bengali mother. This was, indeed, a very crucial technological intervention in the birthing process in twentieth-century Bengal.

Reproductive Health in Bengal Revisited

The importance of Dr Gupta's and Dr Das's achievements can scarcely be understood if we fail to situate it in the context of contemporary colonial Indian indifference to child birth and maternal health. Beliefs and cultural values embedded in society in different parts of India affect significantly the health seeking behaviour of women. In Bengal, in particular, some unfounded beliefs persist even today that prolonged labour is a punishment for past infidelity and unassisted delivery is a sign of courage. Traditionally, in colonial Bengal, pregnancy was considered to be a natural state of being rather than a condition requiring medical attention and care. Shame during the first birth made newly pregnant girls anxious and inhibited. They were expected to exhibit modest behaviour by remaining calm throughout their crucial carrying months. They were also enjoined not to talk about the pregnancy at all. This birthing environment constrained a lay-health culture and compromised the process of corresponding treatment.[26] These traditional beliefs about childbirth, coupled with misconceptions and fears of medical institutions, led many women to maintain a reliance on home births in India.[27]

At the turn of the nineteenth century, arguably under compulsion of 'enforced modernity', childbirth in Bengal underwent a complete transformation. The process of birth was now transferred from the domain of women and the female *dai* or midwife to the dominant realm of male obstetrics. This male intrusion, however, required both social sanction and medical legitimacy to overcome the associated suspicion. Such legitimacy came in the form of a conjunction between midwifery and anatomical dissection: a scientific practice that had long been considered one of the most important sources of medical knowledge.

To assess the significance of medical intervention in childbirth in Bengal, no matter how limited its impact, we need to revisit the nature of traditional management of birth. After all, birth is never a purely natural event in an animal sense, but proceeds in a cultural setting.[28] Whereas medicine is marked by tell-tale signs of professionalism and specialized knowledge, midwives or *dais* clearly belonged to a pre-modern area of occupation. Without any formal training, the *dais* formed a hereditary, caste-based group. They had neither the anatomical knowledge of the body, nor were they any sort of professional salaried group. A certain community feeling became a strategy for survival in an often uncertain world. But unlike their European counterparts where midwives without formal training were often represented as drunken, dirty and immoral,[29] the *dais* were considered an escapable part of the birthing process. It seems that delivery-at-home or non-medical attendance was somehow more natural.[30] However, 'a further subdivision of culture within complex societies is seen in the various professional sub-cultures that exist, such as medical and nursing. In each case, these people form a group apart with their own concepts, rules and social organization' and, during a process of enculturation, 'they also acquire a very different perspective on life from those who are outside the profession'.[31] Traditionally, the *dais* were an inseparable part of the destiny of a birthing mother in pre-modern/pre-colonial Bengal.

During the beginning of the twentieth century, childbirth gradually started taking place in hospitals because there were few alternatives: under the dispensation of 'enforced modernity' obstetrics had been projected as successful – not in creating safe childbirth but in creating a monopoly market under western therapeutic intervention for its own professional gain; organized medicine had 'medicalized' childbirth, a process that in Bengal and in Bengali tradition rarely took place outside hospitals with little medical intervention.[32] Under colonial dispensation delivering modernity, traditional midwifery, marked by private, unregulated old-style midwives, was transformed into modern midwifery through the adoption of a highly medicalized and state-sponsored birth model.

The situation is comparable with conditions in twentieth-century South Africa. A long-term historical view of medicine in South Africa offers a fascinating picture of subtle shifts in the relationship between western and traditional medicine. The colonial rulers tended to see indigenous medicine as merely superstition with 'witch doctors' practising magic and sorcery.[33] Therefore, in rural hospitals, administered by missionaries, the government sought to train many African nurses who would function as 'culture brokers' between the 'modern' western medical model and the African 'traditional' medicine. The nurse as 'the agent of displacement' was predicated on the assumption that she would eventually distance herself from her own traditional culture. Thus the model of nurse devised by the missionaries was viewed partly as an agent of substitution.[34] Again, in the early nineteenth century, Cape doctors implemented training and licensing for traditional midwives, which indicates that they viewed midwives as junior partners rather than dangerous competitors.[35]

By contrast in Bengal, in order to colonize Indian body, the state replaced the *dais* by trained midwives and physicians. It amounted to a role reversal, perpetrated at the behest of the government: earlier, the traditional *dais* were at the helm of affairs with a holistic and indigenous method of birthing; but later, the *dais*' role was appropriated by the midwives and the physicians who doctored the whole process of birthing driven by western medical technology. Indeed, in the twentieth century, biomedical technologies altered the process of childbirth on virtually every level. What had been a matter of private interest, focusing on family and lineage, became a state priority, a symbol of the new citizen who would participate in the creation of a revitalized state. This transformation of reproduction coalesced with the broader story of the social transformation, marked by an emphasis on science and modernity. The roles of the state and western medical personnel were paramount in affecting these changes, but equally important were the intense social and cultural shifts that occurred simultaneously. The dominant themes of reproduction in twentieth-century India were thus characterized by expanding state involvement, shifting gender roles, escalating consumption patterns accompanying the commercialization of private lives, and the increasing medicalization of the birth process.

Besides the economic potential of gaining control of childbirth practices, obstetricians in India were eager to use new European surgical instruments, such as forceps, and interventions that quickly became their specialty, using them to assist with labours which seemed problematic or were obstructed. This division also included a distinction between a midwife's knowledge, gained through apprenticeship, and the new formal education that came with the proliferation of medical schools across the country. The new scientific knowledge and development of new technologies provided the theory on which the female midwives' definition of normal could be challenged and was used to construct the pathological potential of pregnancy and childbirth. Thus, obstetricians were able to gain control over all births by exploiting this pathological potential and treat childbirth with an 'as if' or 'in case' syndrome that could only view childbirth as 'normal' in retrospect.[36]

As a matter of fact, during childbirth the medical gaze and its accompanying power are directed at the woman in labour, rendering her a patient under an obstetrician's supervision. This surveillance operates as part of a structure of control. For pregnant women, biomedical hegemonic rituals begin well before labour and continue in the hospital as soon as nurses meticulously chart notes for the doctor, and medical students observe and use women as tools of practice. She is fully shut out and isolated from her own real world: community, family care, enshrouding concern for the mother and child. The panoptic layout of the hospital ward works to maintain social control; and though a woman in labour may carry along all her moral and physical strength, upon entering the hospital she is immediately reduced to play to role of patient, marked by a loss of autonomy. This loss of agency may be seen in something as subtle as a change in dress from a woman's own clothing to a hospital gown. Knowledge is crucial to this situation, and the scientific knowledge of childbirth assigns the doctor an overriding primacy over the patient who is at the receiving end. The whole process reaffirms the hierarchical relationship between and separation of the patient and the doctor.[37] This is the process of childbirth acknowledged to be 'scientific' and practised world over.

By contrast, the reality of India's maternal health is that the majority of maternal health-care providers were represented by the widespread indigenous system of *dais*, cord cutters, Unani and Ayurvedic practitioners and a host of other women who cannot be dismissed. By far, the majority of births in the country, even in the early twentieth century, happened at home with indigenous practitioners or 'other' women.[38] The inability of biomedicine to account for a patient's symptoms and desire opened up an interpretive space. Following this, the voices of the patients and the preference of their community reasserted in favour of the *dais* taking charge of the whole affair.[39]

Love's Labour Lost

The Bengal Forceps, even though its maker was hailed as a precursor of technological obstetrics, had few takers in the contemporary medical world. Bengali society could not accept Dr Kedarnath Das's labour of love, and there were two reasons for its lukewarm response: the first socio-cultural and the second medico-psychological or psycho-medical. Culturally, as their historical experiences had proved time and again in the nineteenth and early twentieth century, the Bengalis were generally too slow to accept anything novel and innovative; they were slower still if, with the resources at their disposal, they could negotiate any exigency. But perhaps a more crucial reason for its rejection was psycho-medical, prioritized by colonial imperatives of power/knowledge. The most sustained objection to the use of modified midwifery forceps came from the British medical fraternity itself. Dr William Stephenson, Professor of Midwifery in the University of Aberdeen, for instance, observed as early as in 1888 that 'a medical man cannot, like a dentist, provide and carry about with him a number of forceps ingeniously modified to meet varying conditions'.[40] Dr Stephenson, like many others in the profession, would 'recommend' no forceps other than that of Simpson. Even by the end of the nineteenth century, objection to the early and frequent use of forceps persisted, as evidenced by Dr Japp Sinclair's Address to the Section of Obstetrics and Gynaecology of the British Medical Association in Montreal.[41] These objections always met with vehement opposition and continuing protests from dissenting doctors.[42] But their voices were overpowered and muted by opinions of the largely supported logic of advancing medical science.

By the middle of the twentieth century, obstetrics as a science underwent phenomenal changes with more comprehensive understanding of the process of pregnancy and childbirth. Labour management improved with multiple modalities of ante-partum and post-partum foetal monitoring which equipped the obstetrician with precise knowledge of the foetal condition. Moreover, the development in the field of anaesthesia, antibiotics, blood transfusion, surgical aids and techniques arguably made the once-dreaded operation, caesarean section, very safe. Reproductive health now came to be progressively attached to the notion of beauty, and attempts were made to arrest impaired health and stunted beauty, consequent upon pregnancy and childbirth. This new-found notion of beauty vis-à-vis reproductive health brought in fresh debates about technological intervention in women's health and contraception. As the colonial era drew to a close, the government set up in 1944 the Bhore Committee to report on public health. The Bhore Committee Report, published in 1946, dwelled upon the alarmingly high levels of morbidity and mortality among mothers and children in India. The Committee recommended services for the antenatal supervision of expectant mothers and for skilled assistance at childbirth.[43] It also noticed the accelerating pace of population increase and recommended three possible courses of action: (i) raising the age of marriage for girls; (ii) improvement in the standard of living; and (iii) controlling fertility through self-restraint. The last of these was rejected as neither healthy nor practicable in a majority of cases, and the first seemed fraught with particular difficulty, for the Sarda Act in 1929 had produced a storm of protest even in raising the age of marriage for girls to fourteen years. The Bhore Committee, therefore, rehearsed the arguments for and against contraception and agreed that 'when childbearing is likely to result in injury to mother or infant, there is every justification for the practice of contraception'. There was also unanimity in respect of state control over the manufacture and sale of contraceptives. This was however just an opinion, and the members of the committee could not go beyond arguing that 'in view of objections to it on religious grounds in certain quarters', the state should only proceed 'if there is substantial support from public opinion'.[44]

The role of the press in communicating ideas and opinions on the new developments and popular response cannot be overlooked at this point. In the mid-1930s, the popular press also took up the issue of contraception when it disseminated information on contraceptives through vernacular newspapers.[45] Methods of contraception and technological innovations were advertised to capture popular attention on important and sensitive issues. For instance, *Santannigraha kee dava* was advertised as possessing unique properties of preventing pregnancy, quite akin to the role of a contraceptive. Though the sales of such contraceptives were often promoted through a specific pedagogical approach that linked childbirth and women's impaired beauty, there is no evidence to suggest what impact, if any, such advertisements of contraceptives may have had on the public at large.

Conclusion

I would like to tentatively suggest that technological intervention in reproductive health and childbirth in colonial Bengal was extremely limited. Partly explained in terms of cultural distance, it was largely due to the prevailing economic imperatives of colonialism. Admittedly, the Bengalis were not too keen to accept anything new. They were extremely reluctant to open up domains which they considered their own private space; in particular, the sites that strongly related to *antapur* (the inner apartment of a household, exclusively earmarked for women) were considered sacrosanct and hence could not be shared with colonial rulers. Though they were at the forefront of western education, one also notices a lamentable lack of initiative in social engineering which one might expect to be taken up by members of the educated middle class. Historically speaking, they undertook to reform their society and its religious practices in order to adapt them to western modernity, but at the same time they sought to preserve the core of Hindu tradition.[46] The literati was, in fact, a divided house: conservative, progressive, traditionalist, modernist and traditional modernist. The paradigm used in this debate involved not only science, technology, applied technology and medicine, but also culture and colonialism. The educated Bengalis failed to contribute to the socio-scientific logic that was very crucial to discourses on the modernization of the colonial Bengali society. This brings us to the role of the Raj in introducing modern technology in reproductive health in Bengal. The colonial rulers oscillated in a negotiation between the cultural imagination of a Bengali obstetrician and the profitability of a medical market marked by a competing technology. The government decidedly weighed in favour of the latter. In addition, the colonial government had its own private agenda in matters of public health and women's health. It displaced the *dais* and replaced them with trained midwives through a process of 'enforced modernity'. The forceps devised by an Indian obstetrician were dislodged and put to disuse with the introduction of a medical technology, underpinned by profit and medical market under colonial dispensation. In doing so, the colonial government preferred to speak a language of 'science' and 'modernity' to discount all that went to inform the 'native' discourse of science and culture in a situation where indigenous attempts at legitimization of modernity through its own cultural idioms experienced much obstruction by the colonial trope of 'science'.

9 NOT FIT FOR PUNISHMENT: DIAGNOSING CRIMINAL LUNATICS IN LATE NINETEENTH-CENTURY BRITISH INDIA

Jonathan Saha

Introduction

In an appendix to the 1911 census of the Andaman and Nicobar Islands, Major J. M. Woolley, the Senior Medical Officer, noted an apparent statistical anomaly. Among the population of male convicts transported to the penal colony, the rate of insanity was 11.4 in every thousand. Using the rather scant statistics available to him, the limitations of which he readily acknowledged, he estimated that this was fourteen times higher than the figure for British India as a whole, which he calculated to be 0.8 in a thousand. Indeed, the figure was nearly four times higher than the 'regrettably high' rates of insanity in England and Wales, which he cited as 3.6 per thousand.[1] A year later, in an article published in the *British Journal of Psychiatry*, Woolley highlighted a similar trend regarding the numbers of male suicides in the Andaman Islands' penal colony. It appeared that suicides were over sixteen times more frequent in the Andamans than in Bengal.[2] In both cases his explanations for these exceptionally high figures were the same, shielding the penal system from any share of blame. Emphasizing the leniency of the regime and the general health of convicts on arrival, Woolley argued that there was a pathological link between murder, insanity and suicide. The high rates of insanity and suicide in the penal colony could thus be attributed to the high proportion of transported men convicted of murder, a figure of roughly 90 per cent. The vast cellular jail in which some convicts were initially incarcerated apparently had little impact on the convicts' mental health. This point Woolley spuriously supported by noting that most of the convicts who committed suicide or became insane, did so within their first few years of incarceration, whereas, if the prison itself was a factor, longer-serving convicts would have figured larger in the statistics. He made this argument despite the fact that the construction of the jail had only been completed five years before he wrote his report on insanity

– 127 –

and so there were no convicts who had been in the prison on a long-term basis. For Woolley, the regular cases of suicide and insanity were the result of the psychasthenic and psychopathic tendencies of murderers, particularly, according to his ethnographic enumerations, the Hindu convicts.

Woolley's writings were the product of the colonial government's tendency to reduce social phenomena to statistics.[3] The manner in which he used vague and rough data on the number of 'lunatics' in India and Britain to form sweeping conclusions with claims to scientific truth was commonplace in the production of colonial knowledge.[4] However, notwithstanding this crude Orientalist enumerative impulse, Woolley's two pieces on insanity in the convict population of the Andaman Islands' penal colony reveal the crucial intersection between criminality and madness in British India. This is evident in his claim that there was an inherent link between psychopathy, suicide and murder, as well as the basic statistics that he provided. Of the total asylum population in British India, those defined as 'criminal lunatics' made up roughly 20 per cent, totalling some 1,605 individuals. This figure is significant. In England and Wales, Woolley calculated that there were 1,100 criminal lunatics, almost a third fewer. The overall population of India was vast in comparison, and the number of criminal lunatics constituted a tiny fraction of this, but when situated within his comparable numbers on the non-criminal lunatics (133,000 in England and Wales, 5,579 in British India), it sets into relief the peculiar proportion of criminal lunacy in British India.[5] The question raised by Woolley's work is why were there so many criminal lunatics, not only on the Andaman Islands but also in British India as a whole?

Historians who have researched colonial psychiatry in British India have never claimed that it was a science of much significance.[6] Both Waltraud Ernst and James H. Mills, authors of the two major monographs on the topic, have been careful to note the limited impact that asylums have had on Indian society at large.[7] There was no 'great confinement'.[8] This has not diminished interest in the subject, important studies have been published that focus on different aspects of colonial psychiatry in India: for example, the racial divisions implicit in psychiatric practice and discourse;[9] the everyday routines in the lunatic asylums;[10] and the challenges posed to colonial psychiatry by Indian conceptions of mental health and the rise of psychoanalysis.[11] Despite the fact that very few Indians entered colonial lunatic asylums, these studies indicate that the practice of psychiatry can reveal much about the nature of colonialism in India. Overall, however, the significance of linkages between psychiatry and discourses of criminality and justice has been overlooked.

In her recent book on punishment in colonial India, Taylor Sherman argues that rather than studying colonial coercive institutions in isolation, they should be studied together as a network of interlinked sites and practices: the police, the courts, the prisons and also informal, improvised forms of violence.[12] Our understanding of colonial psychiatry too is furthered when it is situated within the framework of an overarching coercive network. One of the principal purposes of colonial asylums was to enable medical officials to make judgements on the sanity of those standing trial.[13] Colonial psychiatry was also important both in policing and in penal discipline for determining the sanity of criminals and convicts. The role played by colonial psychiatry would be understated if the tiny proportion of the population confined in asylums is taken as the measure because, despite this, it became an intrinsic part of the colonial disciplinary system during the nineteenth century.

Situating psychiatry in this coercive network also nuances our understanding of colonial justice and punishment. The very presence of concerns about knowing the minds of Indian criminals challenges how colonial discipline has been characterized. Anand A. Yang and David Arnold argue that in the Indian penal system, punishment remained fundamentally corporeal.[14] Unlike the modern disciplinary regime emerging in Europe,[15] the British remained ambiguous about reforming the 'soul' of the 'native' criminal. Additionally, instead of discipline being an individuating process, colonized criminals were often targeted, judged and punished in collectives.[16] However, the efforts made to establish the sanity of suspected criminals suggest that the colonial regime was at least cursorily interested in individual 'souls'. Deciding whether a convict or criminal was of sound mind was axiomatic to determining whether they were responsible for their actions and, therefore, whether they deserved punishment. Although colonial punishments may have continued to target the body, knowing the mind of the Indian criminal was a related aspiration.

The role played by psychiatry in colonial discipline is unsurprising. As Arnold has argued, the prison was an important site for the production of colonial medical knowledge and an enclave of western medical practice.[17] This was also true of colonial psychiatry. However, the relationship between criminality and insanity, as categories of colonial knowledge, has attracted little attention. Mills touched on the history of insanity among convicts in his study of the late nineteenth-century 'native-only' lunatic asylums of British India. He argued that prisoners were transferred from the penal system into the medical care of the asylum when they had become disruptive to prison discipline. In this analysis, colonizers instrumentally deployed insanity as a useful classification to 'justify' the removal of difficult individuals.[18] This argument was part of Mills' broader contention that Indian lunatic asylums were used to house 'unproductive' individuals, an argument which resonates with historical studies of asylums in nineteenth-century Britain.[19] Although Mills is correct in noting that the presence of insane prisoners in colonial jails did cause problems and disrupted prison routines, he does not explore the moment of diagnosis itself. As a result, it might be assumed that distinguishing between a criminal and a criminal lunatic was an unproblematic act: simply label a disruptive convict as mad. But, as Arnold has shown, colonial prisons were riddled with resistance and disruption, some of which the authorities acquiesced with.[20] Not all of the disruptive behaviour of convicts and criminals was pathologized as insane. Indeed, distinguishing between insanity and criminality was a contingent and an often contested act.

Historians who have researched mental illness in colonial sub-Saharan Africa have explored the moment of diagnosis taking into account this complexity. Jonathan Sadowsky and Meredith McKittrick have both written micro-historical studies examining an individual case in which a colonized subject became entangled in colonial disciplinary systems and diagnosed as insane.[21] Different actors within the colonial state as well as figures from the colonized society, not to mention the individuals under observation themselves, contributed to and challenged the eventual diagnosis. Similarly, but on a larger scale, Megan Vaughan's and Lynette Jackson's studies of colonial psychiatry reveal the multiple meanings attributed to disruptive, deviant behaviour.[22] It is apparent from these studies that disorderly African conduct was interpreted by colonial states according to a number of overlapping and indiscrete yet competing discourses, of which psychiatry was only one. This was also applicable to British India during the late nineteenth century. When diagnosing insanity, medical officers had to negotiate related discourses of race, gender and, importantly, criminality. It was not always clear to officials whether disruptive acts were the characteristic behaviour of an unruly racial 'Other', signs of criminal activity or the symptoms of mental abnormality. To complicate the matter further, the boundaries between normality, criminality and psychopathy were ill-defined and permeable. In the inherent ambiguities of this process, there was always scope for dispute and disagreement between state officials. In the practice of psychiatry, as in all aspects of their existence, colonial states were not unified and homogenous actors.[23] The differing jurisdictions, interests and imperatives of colonial officials often informed their diagnoses.

In addition, as these Africanist scholars show, the state was not the sole actor involved in the diagnosis of the insane. In British India, the colonized also attempted to characterize individuals as insane, particularly when attempting to militate against colonial punishment for family members or attempting to have family members returned to them for treatment at home.[24] How far these local uses of psychiatric discourse reflected a shared understanding of deviance, and how far they were an example of an instrumental appropriation of a dominant language, is difficult to say. Nevertheless, it appeared that the colonial state and colonized society could concur on the diagnosis of individuals.

A related and almost intractable problem for British medical officers was the chance that criminals and convicts were feigning insanity. As Satadru Sen has argued regarding the Andaman Islands' penal colony, medicine was used to regulate colonial punishment. In this context, establishing the health of a convict was a contest between the patient and the doctor, with the former attempting to deceive the latter into believing that their condition was worse than it was to avoid the full rigours of penal discipline.[25] Determining whether an individual was genuinely mentally ill or merely pretending is a futile task for a historian to undertake retrospectively, but at the time medical officials were often unsure and imagined malingering to be a reality. In a 1908 publication, the long-serving superintendent of a lunatic asylum in the Punjab, G. F. W. Ewens, detailed his strategies for determining whether convicts were acting insane to avoid punishment. His suggestions included checking whether they slept (the acutely insane were, apparently, unable to), and checking whether they were 'overacting' and behaving 'too' insane. But he also suggested introducing harsher treatments, such as forced nasal feeding, to discourage convicts from continuing to feign insanity.[26] Psychiatric treatment and corporeal punishment overlapped,[27] and the relationship between colonial doctor and suspected lunatic was a fraught one based on mistrust.

Separating the insane from the criminal was a complex, incomplete and inchoate process that cannot be adequately explained with reference solely to the colonial state's desire to maintain order. Every diagnosis was to some degree dependent upon a constellation of contingent factors. This entanglement of criminality and insanity in British India may explain why the proportion of criminal lunatics was higher in Woolley's statistics. This chapter examines two examples from British India in the 1870s and 1880s, a time when, as Sally Swartz has demonstrated, metropolitan imperial oversight of psychiatric practice had increased and when uniformity of practice was (theoretically) being implemented.[28] First, it explores cases of lunacy that emerged among convicts under transportation to the Andaman Islands, and second, it discusses the medico-legal disputes regarding criminal lunatics in Lower Burma. These examples demonstrate some of the ways that the diagnostic indeterminacy of insanity caused problems for the colonial regime. By studying these cases, and situating colonial psychiatry in the broader coercive network, the history of a creeping medicalization of state practices is also revealed.

Transporting Lunatics

In March 1874, the Superintendent of Port Blair penal colony on the Andaman Islands, Donald Stewart, called out to a convict named Russool Buksh who, disconcertingly, was singing while performing hard labour. 'Who are you?' asked Stewart. 'Who are *you*?' replied Buksh. It was only due to the Senior Medical Officer's insistence that Buksh's seemingly insubordinate act was the result of him being a 'harmless lunatic' that severe punishment was avoided; although Buksh was latter refused promotion in his convict status due to his notoriety, much to the ire of the medical establishment.[29] As unimportant as this episode

may seem, it resulted in a clash between the medical authority and penal authority, marking a moment in the increasing medical regulation of punishment in
the penal colony, highlighted by Sen.[30] In this medically monitored disciplinary
regime, diagnosis as insane could protect convicts from punishment. Indeed, on
at least one occasion during the 1870s, a convict avoided execution because of a
diagnosis of insanity.[31]

Individuals such as Buksh were perceived as a threat to both the productivity
and order of the penal colony. As a result, so-called 'harmless lunatics' like him
were separated from the rest of the convict population and subjected to a greater
degree of surveillance. Under this observation, they were thought less likely to
disrupt the labour regime or, as Buksh had, undermine the hierarchical social
order. Their symptoms of insanity ranged from singing and 'jabbering about anything and everything', to muteness.[32] Convicts suffering from more acute forms
of insanity, particularly mania, were housed in a special ward at Haddo, a settlement on the Islands. Initially, in the late 1860s, these individuals did not present
too great a problem for the penal colony's government. They were mostly viewed
as 'eccentric' individuals who experienced a temporary bout of 'acute mania'
upon arrival.[33] However, with increasing numbers of convicts being sent to the
islands who upon arrival were deemed unfit by Port Blair's medical officers, the
numbers of lunatics became a concern and were subsequently viewed as a burden. During the 1870s, their presence was portrayed by officials as unproductive
and potentially dangerous. As a result, diagnosis became an area of dispute.

In 1872, Stewart drew the attention of the Government of India to six convicts who had arrived at Port Blair even though they were insane. He used this
case to complain more generally about the numbers of prisoners who were, in
his view, unfit for transportation but who were being sent to the islands nevertheless.[34] The arrival of the *Scotia* in January 1874 which, according to Stewart,
contained an exceptionally and unacceptably high proportion of unfit convicts
– including a 'congenital imbecile' and a convict missing a hand – resulted in an
angry missive from the Superintendent. He pointed out that despite the assurances from the governments sending the convicts that they all left in 'perfect
health of body and mind' the 'gangs of insanes, imbeciles and cripples now in the
settlement' were proof otherwise.[35] Stewart was not a lone voice in this respect.
Sir Henry Wylie Norman, aide-de-camp to Queen Victoria and military member of the Supreme Council in India, noted during a visit to Port Blair in August
1874 that there were a number of 'unmistakable lunatics' whose symptoms were
such that he found it 'difficult to understand how they escaped detection as lunatics [prior] to transportation'.[36]

Determining which part of the colonial bureaucracy was responsible for
ensuring that convicts were fit for transportation for a long time remained an
unresolved and disputed matter. Although all convicts were transported directly

from Alipore Jail in Bengal,[37] the Government of India maintained, in response to Stewart's complaints, that it was the duty of the local government of the place in which a convict had been initially incarcerated to make sure that they were fit for transportation. This meant checking that they were 'fit for labour', and younger than forty-five. In addition, it was emphasized that, 'Lunatics and idiotic criminals are on no account to be transported to the Andamans'.[38] Alipore Jail could only remove those convicts who had become ill during transfer from the local jails. Stewart argued that responsibility should instead be placed on the medical staff at Alipore Jail to ensure that convicts were fit enough for transportation. In response to his accusations, the authorities in Bengal questioned the ability of Port Blair's medical staff.[39] This dispute resolved little; it resulted from the insurmountable epistemic problem of convict identity.

Clare Anderson's research on convict transportation in the Indian Empire has demonstrated that the various attempts made in the colonial penal system to fix a criminal's identity to his/her body in the late nineteenth century were, at best, imperfectly implemented. Descriptive rolls, *godna* (tattooing), clothing and photography all failed in making convicts' bodies entirely legible to colonial rulers.[40] The health of convicts proved an even more intangible piece of information to maintain on convicts as they moved through the penal system, in part because it was something inherently liable to change over time. Additionally, convicts could affect their physical condition by harming themselves or each other. Information on mental health was more elusive still. Medical officers at Port Blair noted that insanity could come and go. A predisposition to mental distress could be stimulated by external factors such as 'intoxicating drugs, mental excitement, or excess'.[41] Stewart accepted that 'a criminal may have lost his senses somewhere on the road between the place of his conviction and his destination' and that there was a 'great deal of feigned madness'.[42] An individual's mental state was not a stable piece of information which could be fixed to the body of the convict.

Stewart cited the case of Doorjodhan Sawunt (hereafter, Sawunt), who arrived at Port Blair in 1874, in a successful attempt to prohibit local governments from transporting convicts who had suffered from any previously recorded episode of insanity. However, Sawunt had not previously been diagnosed as a lunatic until he underwent observation on the islands, as we can see by tracing the changing view of his mental status from his conviction to his arrival on the Andamans. During his journey, he was recategorized from an individual who once acted 'without reason' to a lunatic who enjoyed 'lucid intervals'. He was initially sentenced to transportation for murdering a two-year-old child and stealing jewellery. Judged sane at the time of the murder, his nominal roll described him as a cultivator of 'good' character.[43] In the penal colony, in contrast to criminal tribes, murderers from this background were seen as 'decent' killers by the Port Blair establishment.[44] Their eventual objection to him circled around his actions the day after his conviction when he murdered a fellow convict but was acquitted on the grounds of 'momentary unsoundness of mind'.[45] However, importantly, as he was not certified a lunatic and he was still eligible for transportation.

The Superintendent of Alipore Jail re-categorized Sawunt's character from 'good' to 'dangerous', advising the authorities in Port Blair that he required 'careful watching'.[46] What Sawunt had done in custody to warrant this is not stated, but there was no indication that he was viewed by the officials at Alipore as insane. However, once on the Andaman Islands the Senior Medical Officer Dr J. Dougall and the Second Medical Officer Dr J. Reid came to conclusions different to those of the officials at Alipore and diagnosed Sawunt as a lunatic, writing in no uncertain terms, '[We] find that he is a man of weak intellect, and a monomaniac. Judging from his criminal history we consider him to be a man liable to paroxysmal attacks of madness with a homicidal tendency'. Sawunt's 'moment' of madness after his conviction, when set alongside his behaviour under observation, was used to classify him as a lunatic. Stewart wrote to the Government of India, referring to this case, that, 'Lunatics who are subject to lucid intervals are obviously the most dangerous in a community like that of Port Blair, where every labouring man has deadly weapons habitually in his hands'.[47] This time the Government of India acquiesced to Stewart's demands and prohibited the transportation of convicts who at any time exhibited symptoms of insanity.[48]

The diagnosis of Sawunt as a lunatic was informed by the administrative disputes between Port Blair and Alipore Jail. It was a case successfully used by the Port Blair authorities to have further restrictions placed on the types of convicts sent to the penal colony and thus, it was hoped, to minimize the number of unproductive and unruly members of the population. The act of diagnosis, in this case, was inseparable from the politics of the administrative disputes surrounding it. But prohibiting the transportation of criminals with any history of mental disturbance did not stop the arrival of convicts that the Port Blair medical establishment deemed insane and unfit.

Reinforcing this resolution, the Government of India sought to tighten the transportation procedures further and increase the amount of medical observation in order to ensure that lunatics were not transported. European medical officers became a prerequisite for boats transporting convicts so that they could monitor transportees' health during the 'middle passage', which had previously been a blind spot for the colonial medical gaze.[49] The Government of Bengal was now made responsible for the medical examination of convicts on arrival at and on embarkation from Alipore Jail.[50] The threshold for prohibiting the transportation of convicts was raised with the Government of India ordering local governments that, 'prisoners as to whose sanity doubts may be entertained should be detained under observation until the true mental condition is clearly evident'.[51] Following this, a special medical committee was established at Alipore

Jail charged with judging the sanity of convicts sent for transportation.[52] Common to all of these orders was the belief that greater medical observation would reveal objective and lasting truths about convicts' minds.

Between 1873 and the 1880s the intensity of the colonial medical gaze increased and Alipore Jail came to take on a greater burden of responsibility for ensuring that lunatics were not sent to the Andaman Islands. Despite this, Port Blair continued to complain about the numbers of convicts arriving insane.[53] However, these complaints were mirrored in those of the local governments arguing that the Alipore authorities were being too restrictive and returning healthy convicts.[54] In this new distribution of responsibility across the coercive network, in which Alipore Jail acted as a gate keeper, disputes about the diagnosis of insanity continued. The Government of Bengal bemoaned the 'constant fault-finding' and 'impossible' standard expected by the Port Blair authorities, and sought to bolster the authority of the Alipore Jail officials.[55] The Port Blair regime argued for the deportation of all lunatics currently held in the penal colony to asylums in India.[56] These opposing administrative concerns shaped the diagnosis of Khorda Manjhee.

Manjhee was deported back to Alipore Jail as a lunatic after spending nine months under medical observation and treatment in Haddo. On arrival at Port Blair, medical officers initially deemed Manjhee to be 'eccentric' and 'insane', and their opinion of him did not change during his spell under observation.[57] The Alipore Jail committee set up for judging the sanity of convicts disagreed and found him to be of sound mind due to his ability to converse in Bengali, to answer questions rationally and to make twenty hand-sewn bags a day. Although they conceded that because he could not speak Bengali well this might have made him appear 'stupid and slow at understanding' to the Port Blair authorities, they firmly concluded that he showed no symptoms of insanity.[58] A member of the committee who had been present at the original examination of Manjhee put forward his opinion on Manjhee's mental state and why medical officers at Port Blair had misdiagnosed him:

> It is quite possible that the man, being an uneducated, uncivilised Sonthali, was somewhat dense and boorish, and not intellectually up to the standard required of convicts in the Andamans, and evinced a not unnatural dislike to penal labour whilst at the settlement. That he is insane, I deny, but that he may be both clumsy, stupid and cunning I think quite possible.[59]

The Alipore committee's diagnosis was eventually upheld and in 1887, after two years in Bengal under observation, Manjhee was returned to the Andaman Islands having shown 'no signs of insanity'.[60] This diagnosis sought to simultaneously expose what they believed to be the excessively high standards held by the Port Blair medical staff, and to restrict definitions of insanity. Both of these strategies relied on reading Manjhee's behaviour alongside ethnographically derived expectations of behaviour that contrasted the tribal Santal population to Bengalis. According to this colonial discourse it was not necessarily a pathological sign that a Santal man appeared unintelligent and backward, although the same might have been considered symptoms in a Bengali.[61] When diagnosing insanity thus, Port Blair officials did not make enough allowance for varied mental ability across ethnic differences when diagnosing insanity. But by emphasizing that although Manjhee may have been stupid, he was not insane, Alipore officials were also attempting to limit which forms of mental disorder fell under the rubric of insanity and would thus prohibit transportation. Port Blair medical officers routinely cited 'weak intellect' as a symptom of insanity when returning convicts as unfit for transportation. Indeed, just after Manjhee arrived in Alipore another Santal convict was deported from the Andaman Islands for possessing a 'weak intellect'.[62] This was consistent with broader contemporary psychiatric nosology which included dementia praecox, a 'weakening intellect'.[63] By arguing that stupidity did not always mean insanity, the Alipore regime was attempting to limit and determine who would be deemed unfit for transportation.

In the network of institutions involved in transporting convicts to the Andaman Islands' penal colony, the diagnosis of a convict's mental state was not a straightforward act. Given that mental health was an inherently unstable characteristic that could be shaped by the knowing acts of the convicts, it was unsurprising that disputes between different colonial authorities occurred regularly, resulting in convicts being sent back and forth across the Bay of Bengal. The different diagnoses made in Alipore and Port Blair can be accounted for by the differing administrative imperatives incumbent on the medical officials in those branches of the state. Officials in Bengal were more inclined to find convicts sane and fit for transportation, whereas officials at Port Blair, fearing an accumulation of unproductive and unpredictable convicts, found insanity where other colonial officials had not. Yet despite the indeterminacy of psychiatric diagnoses in this context, these disputes led to a gradual medicalization of the penal system during the 1870s. Although no diagnosis was definitive, the decision to punish a criminal through transportation was mediated by psychiatric observations in court, in the local jail, at Alipore Jail, during the 'middle passage' and on arrival at Port Blair. The failure of colonial psychiatry to produce secure diagnoses paradoxically led to greater a medical observation of convicts' minds.

Insanity in Burma

On 30 March 1874, Myat Hnit's wife fled their home and informed the local police of his erratic behaviour. When the police sergeant eventually arrived at the scene, roughly an hour later, he found Myat Hnit brandishing two knives and was unable to prevent his escape into the jungle. It soon emerged that in the time between Myat Hnit's wife's warning and the sergeant's arrival, Myat Hnit had killed one woman and wounded two others. He was apprehended and brought under police custody later that evening when he attempted to return home.[64] This case came to the attention of the Chief Commissioner of Burma, Ashley Eden, because it appeared that the murderous attacks could have been prevented if the police had shown more urgency, since the station was only two miles from the scene. However, the investigation into the case led by the local Deputy Commissioner exonerated the police from blame. According to his enquiries it seemed that Myat Hnit's mental health had been a local concern for some time and that he had been receiving treatment from what were described as 'native practitioners'. Indeed, just moments before his attacks, the Deputy Commissioner reported, 'a native doctor was about to, or had been, treating him for mania, and that he had escaped from the first stage of this treatment'.[65] Given that the police were aware of his history of mental disturbance and were oblivious of the violence that had occurred, it was felt that the sergeant was not in dereliction of his duty.

The above incidence is equally as revealing as it is frustratingly opaque. It demonstrates willingness on behalf of the colonial state to acquiesce with indigenous medical practices for treating mental illness, when during the late-nineteenth century a more antagonistic dichotomy between western bio-medicine and local practices was taking hold in most branches of colonial medicine.[66] The colonial state did allow medically certified lunatics to be released to their families for treatment and care in the home, indeed towards the end of the nineteenth century this was actively encouraged in an attempt to reduce the cost of maintaining a growing number of 'incurable' lunatics in the asylum. But, as in the case of Myat Hnit, violence was the decisive factor for colonial officials when deciding whether indigenous treatments would be allowed without state interference, or whether instead intervention and incarceration were necessary. In 1874 the brother of criminal lunatic Nga Shwe Loon petitioned successfully for his release, 'in order to enable them to try him with some other medicine'.[67] His release was allowed because although Nga Shwe Loon was still deemed insane he had shown no signs of violence. In contrast, the uncles of Pha Htau, also a criminal lunatic, had their petition declined in 1873 because of Pha Htau's violent past.[68] The Burmese population regularly mobilized the judicial category of mental 'unsoundness' through petitions attempting to mitigate colonial punishment and to have family members released from confinement.

Myat Hnit's case reveals the informal space allowed for the indigenous treatment of insanity and is also suggestive of the overlap between local and state understandings of mental disturbance, but it tells us precious little about what indigenous practices consisted of or what meanings mental disturbance had for Myat Hnit and his neighbours. Colonial officials exhibited little interest in

Burmese conceptions of mental health. Translations of Burmese medical texts by contemporary British officials simplistically applied western bio-medical designations to Burmese terminology and obscured their meanings.[69] The writings of even the most sympathetic colonial scholar-officials treated Burmese medical practices, including those for healing mental illness, with condescension and outright hostility.[70] Although British officials were supportive of indigenous medical practitioners to treat non-violent lunatics, or even criminal lunatics, they cared little about the nature or content of Burmese conceptions of mental illness.

Following his arrest, Myat Hnit was sent to court for his trial, where he was acquitted for possessing an 'unsound mind'. This was a breach of how court procedures were supposed to operate in these cases. The Commissioner of the Tenasserim Division, which incorporated Myat Hnit's district, argued correctly that he should have been held under observation in the local jail until he was deemed fit to stand trial or, if there was no recovery, until orders came to commit him to the asylum.[71] Despite the fact that his diagnosis was uncontested by the judge, medical officers, police or witnesses, the procedure through which he was formally diagnosed as insane was disputed. His case was not the only one to cause concern over the decisions made by the lower courts when diagnosing insanity. It also raised questions over the effectiveness of the procedures, or lack of them, through which officials made these diagnoses. Several court cases were a cause for concern for the Chief Commissioner in the 1870s leading to a standardization of how criminals' mental states were to be ascertained.

The procedures for distinguishing between criminals and criminal lunatics were a particularly acute problem in Burma because it had the highest crime rate and prison population of the provinces of British India.[72] A related feature of this overburdened and dysfunctional penal system in colonial Burma was a disproportionate number of criminal lunatics, mostly Burmese men.[73] The increasing numbers of criminal lunatics in late nineteenth-century Burma highlights the importance of studying the interactions between the colonial judicial system and psychiatry. In colonial Burma, tensions between British judges and medical officials attempting to diagnose insanity in criminal cases exposed the lacunae between ethnographic, criminological and psychiatric discourses. As in the case of convicts sentenced to transportation to the Andaman Islands, differentiating between criminals and lunatics was axiomatic to dispensing colonial justice and punishment in Burma, but the problem was that diagnosis was attained through procedures that were both inconsistent and irregular.

In February 1873, the Commissioner of Pegu highlighted to Chief Commissioner Eden two cases of murder in which the accused had been acquitted due to an unsound mind. In one, the accused had killed a man while apparently under the influence of a drug administered to him during tattooing and was consequentially acquitted by the judge, without consulting medical expertise, as temporarily insane.[74] In the second case, the accused attacked his wife and a police sergeant with a knife. The medical officer's evidence was overruled by the judge who acquitted him as insane. His reasons for doing so were revealing: testimonial evidence of a previous bout of insanity and 'the appearance of the man ... his dull dazed look, such as one who has some deep mental worry passing on his brain' were enough to convince the judge.[75] On receiving the details of these cases the Chief Commissioner wrote to the Government Advocate asking his advice on appealing these decisions, as he believed 'that the two men who have committed very grave crimes ... escaped punishment on very insufficient grounds'.[76] In a different case that same year Eden again called the attention of the colonial judiciary 'to the necessity of greater care being paid in disposing of pseudo-lunatic criminals'.[77] His term 'pseudo-lunatic criminals' neatly encapsulates the suspicion around the legal defence of insanity.

These matters culminated in a case in 1876 in which the accused was acquitted of causing grievous hurt with a dangerous weapon because of a fever that rendered him unconscious of having done anything wrong. The Chief Commissioner, noting the lack of medical evidence, wrote bluntly that the 'excuse is worthless'. He went on to summarize the broader problems as he saw them:

> there is throughout this province generally too great a readiness on the part of Magisterial Officers to accept the plea of unsoundness of mind, the result being practically tantamount to an acquittal of the accused person, as it is observed that, should a prisoner happen to be sent to the Lunatic Asylum, he is generally immediately after being admitted declared sane[78]

The government appealed against the case and the decision was overturned. But, as with the diagnosis of convicts in transportation procedures, the difficulties surrounding the diagnosis of criminal lunatics in Burma were insurmountable. Most officials, irrespective of the extent of their medical training, based their judgements on the demeanour of suspected individuals. Insanity had to be visually evident.[79] In a case noted above, the suspect was acquitted by the judge as insane in part because of his 'dull dazed look'.[80] In another, a convicted murderer was referred to a medical officer because the Commissioner had 'observed a silly look about the prisoner'.[81]

However, simply observing the demeanour of a suspected lunatic to reach a diagnosis was a process rife with problems. Officials were aware that a suspect could be feigning insanity.[82] In addition, they found it difficult to clearly distinguish between pathological, criminal and normal Burmese behaviour as they were all inextricably linked in colonial discourses. In police reports the Burmese were commonly described as having a 'marked homicidal tendency'.[83] In the asylum reports it was noted that Burmese lunatics had a tendency towards violent outbursts of 'acute mania'. And colonial ethnographic writings produced gendered stereotypes of Burmese men as usually passive, hen-pecked husbands who expressed their frustrated masculinity through bouts of violence.[84] British officials saw insanity among the Burmese as an exaggeration of their stereotypical flaws and criminal propensities. There was no clear break between insane and normal behaviour.

In the face of these intractable difficulties, tensions between judges, administrators and medical officers were resolved by establishing clearly whose observations carried the ultimate authority, and the medical gaze was made the principal authority. In 1879 the Chief Commissioner ruled that criminal lunatics had to be held either in the asylum or in the prison hospital in Rangoon for medical observations.[85] The asylum was further marked out as a privileged space for diagnosis later in the same year when the Chief Commissioner emphasized that all non-criminal lunatics should also be sent for observation in the Rangoon asylum whenever possible.[86] By the 1880s medical observation became the sole authority by which the suspected insane were diagnosed. This did not resolve the abstract difficulty of distinguishing between the criminal, the lunatic, and the normal Burmese man in the British mind but it made the decision a matter exclusively for medical specialists.

Conclusion: Fixing Minds and Bodies

In his ground-breaking study on state medicine in British India, Arnold argues that the colonial state attempted to use the bodies of the colonized as a site for the construction of its own authority.[87] In enclaves of colonial power, such as the prison and the army, the state used its access to colonized bodies to produce knowledge and practise western medicine. This framework undoubtedly helps to shed light on the diagnosis of insanity in the Indian penal system. However, in order to formulate an extensive account of the indeterminacy and uncertainty of colonial psychiatric diagnoses the existing framework requires modification. Indeed, the colonial desire to know the minds of criminals and convicts caused more problems for the state than it solved. Instead of focussing solely on how medical practices were used instrumentally to reinforce the moral and material authority of the state, we need to also understand how medical authority came to structure state practices.[88] In other words, writing the history of colonial psychiatry only in terms of the function it served for the state can lead to a diminution of the important historical effects it had on the penal system.

Although colonial psychiatry was, as Shruti Kapila puts it, 'an enclave of practices',[89] they were not practices that were exclusively confined to the small and neglected lunatic asylums of British India. Rather, psychiatry was routinely practised across the colonial judicial and penal systems. As discussed in this chapter, examining the colonized convicts' minds was an intrinsic part of judging their criminal responsibility and fitness for punishment. During the 1870s, the procedures for determining the mental states of criminals were ad hoc and irregular. As a result, disputes routinely occurred over the diagnosis of individuals. While the minds of the colonized remained beyond the reach of British officials and were fundamentally unknowable, these disputes were resolved by the 1880s through an increasing reliance on and faith in medical observation to produce definitive statements on convicts' mental states. In both the India-wide procedures for transporting convicts and the particular problems of British Burma, the medical gaze was extended and intensified to monitor criminal minds. Both of these cases corroborate the role psychiatry played in advancing the medicalization of the coercive network.

It should be apparent from these studies that the numbers of people confined in lunatic asylums is a limited measure of the historical impact of colonial psychiatry. A quick glance through the routine matters of British Burma's prison and judicial proceedings, for any year in the late nineteenth century, will show the frequency of reports on the sanity of criminals under observation, numbering as high as several hundred every year. Put simply, psychiatry was important not only for the rather small numbers labelled insane but also for those criminals, the majority of cases, who after observation were found sane. Although it was not a separate, professionalized branch of colonial medicine (medical officers' psychiatric training only involved a brief few weeks' experience of asylum management),[90] psychiatric judgements were an implicit part of colonial discipline. An important Foucauldian observation is to be made here. In colonial justice, penology and medicine we can see two interlinked features of modern disciplinary systems at work. Firstly, they were attempts to reform colonized bodies through healing or punishing. Secondly, they were attempts to know colonized bodies by generating a body of normative information on them. In these processes, colonial psychiatry played an important role in fixing colonized bodies, where we take the verb 'to fix' to mean both 'to mend' and 'to cement'. Psychiatry sought to determine how criminals should be reformed, whether through the penal system or through the asylum, and it sought to render the minds of the colonized into knowable objects. The expanding scope of colonial psychiatric observation revealed in this chapter is best understood as part of this unfolding of disciplinary logic, rather than simply in terms of utility to the state. The state did not only deploy psychiatric practice; psychiatry also shaped state practices.

10 MULTIPLE VOICES AND PLAUSIBLE CLAIMS: HISTORIOGRAPHY AND COLONIAL LUNATIC ASYLUM ARCHIVES

Sally Swartz

The flimsy line between historical fact and fiction – between accurate summary of the contents of an archive and the construction of a gripping tale – is at the centre of the historian's craft. The choice of focus and angle, spotlight and commentary, make the difference between overwhelming detail and pattern, repetition and forward movement. Historians' choices, as they lead their audience through a sequence of 'facts', are weighty matters: the most mundane of detail, such as the price of a cake of soap in 1897, becomes significant in a story about – for example – gender, laundry and household budgets.

This chapter addresses the narrative truths and fictions of colonial asylum histories, and the significant challenges posed by their archival traces. It is partly an exploration of the complexity and ethics of writing about the everyday lives of the insane; it also explores the discursive structures that continue to shape scholarship in this area, and the effects these have on interpretations of the archive.[1]

Patricia Allderidge sketches the shape of the problem in an article about historians' willingness to perpetuate a certain kind of spectacular history in relation to the Bethlem Royal Hospital, without ever consulting primary sources. She notes:

> I have therefore come to the conclusion that, on the whole, historians of psychiatry actually do not want to know about Bethlem as a historical fact because Bethlem as a reach-me-down historical cliché is far more useful ... Bethlem as the ultimate symbol of all that is evil is far too useful a space-filler to be risked in the refining fires of academic research: and it does not really matter too much what it symbolizes, so long as it is sufficiently discreditable to be credible.[2]

As a historian immersed in the Bethlem archive and deeply knowledgeable about its complex, contradictory relationship to the care and custody of lunatics, the rise of madhouse professionals and the general public's insatiable curiosity about all things mad, Allderidge is well placed to remind asylum historians to mind their archives, to do the sure-footed historical thing, and to attend to the facts of the matter. Of course, post-Derrida and the deconstruction of the very idea of 'an archive', this is easier said than done.[3] 'Facts' are hardly self-evident, and the idea of histories as multiple – a conglomeration of more (or less) credible narratives, reflecting events, speech acts, geography, the whimsy of archival policies, lines of power and ideology, the selective memory and access to voice of those writing/recording, and perhaps most significantly of all, the perspective of the historian – is common cause. In this reading, the ground between Bethlem 'fictions' and 'facts' is obscured in the disappearing mirrors of factual fiction and fictional fact, and the motives for why historians peddle them. After all, we will never know what Bethlem was 'really like'. However, the collapse into radical relativism that such lines of argument possibly imply flies in the face of two things: the materiality of the world upon which we do leave traces, no matter how open to multiple interpretations they may be; and the relationship of credibility to intersubjective truths. In her commentary on colonial archives, Ann Stoler returns scholars to the issue of 'what we take to be evidence and what we expect to find'. She warns against a too-easy slide into readings 'against the grain', without immersion in the textures of the archive. She adds that, in order to disrupt the process of finding what we 'know' to be there, we must first be aware of 'what we think we already know. For students of colonialisms, such codes of recognition and systems of expectation are at the very heart of what we still need to learn about colonial policies'.[4]

Histories of psychiatry in French and British African colonies now form a substantial body of knowledge. These histories begin with Franz Fanon's groundbreaking and still unsurpassed narrative reconstruction of colonialism and subjectivity as decisive in its effects on later histories of colonial psychiatric histories as Foucault's 'great confinement' narrative on the northern hemisphere accounts of lunacy management.[5] Histories of colonial psychiatry in Africa include M. Vaughan's influential 'The Madman and the Medicine Men' in *Curing their Ills: Colonial Power and African Illness* (1991); Jock McCulloch's *Colonial Psychiatry and 'The African Mind'* (1995); Jonathan Sadowsky's *Imperial Bedlam: Institutions of Madness in Colonial Southwest Nigeria* (1999); Robert Edgar and Hilary Sapire's *African Apocalypse: The Story of NontethaNkwenkwe, a Twentieth-Century South African Prophet* (2000); Lynette Jackson's *Surfacing Up: Psychiatry and Social Order in Colonial Zimbabwe, 1908–1968* (2005); and Julie Parle's *States of Mind: Searching for Mental health in Natal and Zululand, 1868–1918* (2007).[6] There is also a steady accretion of scholarly articles and chapters in books on colonial asylums in and beyond South Africa.[7] In recent years, 'new imperial histories' have focused attention on similarities and differences between colonial spaces, and their links with each other, as well as with a colonizing centre; this decentring focus draws attention to studies of colonial psychiatry beyond Africa as an essential comparative resource.[8] Here the work of

Waltraud Ernst, James Mills on British India, C. Coleborne on Australasia, Jonathan Saha on Burma and Hans Pols on the former Dutch East Indies, contribute to a rich account of colonial diversity.[9]

Histories of colonial psychiatry in Africa have one unifying theme – the relationship of colonial psychiatry (and psychiatric institutions) to racism and oppression. There is a great deal of evidence at this stage that colonial psychiatry institutionalized racist practices and constructed scientific justifications for neglect of the black insane, an acutely vulnerable group under colonial rule.[10] The aim of this chapter is not to review this literature, but to reflect on the colonial psychiatry–oppression link as a 'reach-me-down' historical cliché. It expands arguments already formulated along these lines, most notably by Shula Marks, but also raised and elegantly explored by both Sadowsky and Parle. Its concerns are historiographical and address the kinds of evidence that would be needed to describe the relationship between colonial psychiatric practices and the inmates of colonial lunatic asylums. The chapter will outline the provenance of the cliché, perhaps more accurately described as a discursive formation about colonial psychiatry and the black insane.[11] This discursive formation works to place narrative constrictions on ways of writing about this complex relationship. A description of the Valkenberg Lunatic Asylum archive is then used as a point of departure in an exploration of an intertextual, intersubjective way of writing for/about the colonial insane. It argues that the construction of a credible historical narrative about lunatic asylums requires a reading of the archive against and along the grain, accounting for both the deep ambivalence of colonial authorities towards those in their care, and for the faint subaltern voices of the incarcerated insane. Here, I attempt to identify questions that can be answered, but for many these answers will always be straws in the wind. I conclude with a challenge to historians of psychiatry about questions that should never be asked.

Not Sufficiently Other

In *Curing their Ills*, a groundbreaking work on African colonial medical history, Vaughan describes the way in which 'normal' African mentality was pathologized in medical writing. She goes on to make the following observation:

> The madman and madwoman emerge in the colonial historical record not as standing for the 'Other' but more often as being insufficiently 'Other'. The madness of colonial subjects is to be feared, for it is indicative of 'deculturation' and the breaking of barriers of difference and silence.[12]

There is ample evidence in colonial archives and published psychiatric papers that colonial doctors assumed, and found illustrations for, the difference between African and European mentality. Africans were typically characterized as childish, impulsive, hypersexual and biologically incapable of suffering more 'refined' forms of mental illness, such as melancholia.[13] Two medical superintendents in Cape Colony, Doctors T. D. Greenlees and J. Conry, both used their experience of the black insane in their asylums as the basis for a description of 'normal' African mentality.[14] They insisted that the black and white insane suffered from different forms of insanity. They also blamed increases in numbers of black insane men and women on increased contact with the pressures and temptations of 'civilization'. At this stage, the traumatic effects of racism, economic oppression, inadequate housing, migrant labour and other civilized offerings were not in view. What *was* in view was the spectre of growing numbers of black men in urban areas, not docile bodies, but disruptors of the peace. There were similar fears about the effects of living in the colonies on European sensibilities.[15] In both cases, 'deculturation' as a potential cause of insanity was at the root of the unease. Their speculations about this, echoed over the following several decades by psychiatrists across the British empire, was never related in any systematic way to asylum case records.

The black *and* white colonial insane therefore broke 'barriers of difference and silence' in a number of ways. The black insane called attention to their capacity for suffering (by being not different enough), refusing to be the stolid workforce that the colonial machine required, and in their madness they commented directly on sex, money, race and politics. On the other hand, the white insane failed to *maintain* their difference (in terms of culture, intelligence, standards of civilized behaviour) from the colonized masses, and they, too, were noisy about it.

Vaughan is careful to state that African mental institutions were too small and poorly resourced to be regarded as a significant means of social control for the rebellious, and the archival record is clear on this point: there was no great confinement in Africa, and colonial psychiatry was never a serious challenge to an ongoing plurality of beliefs about the nature and causes of insanity among indigenous peoples. There is evidence that in both Cape Colony and in Natal, African families used both indigenous healers and western medicine when confronted with the impossibilities of managing an insane family member.[16] As Sadowsky points out, colonial institutions were often 'too shifting and diffident to accomplish hegemonic domination'. Similarly, Parle concludes that on detailed examination, it is 'not so much the power of colonial psychiatry that becomes evident, but its effective limitations'.[17]

The 'insufficiently other' trope does, however, invoke images of rebellion, expressed by Vaughan as 'individuals who had "forgotten" who they were, and had ceased to conform to the notion of the African subject, who most often found themselves behind the walls of the asylum'.[18] The Robert Edgar and Hilary Sapire account of NontethaNkwenkwe's long period of institutionalization as a mental patient in South Africa (1922–35) summons this narrative strand. In a section entitled 'Troublesome persons' they argue that colonial authorities invariably only confined deranged Africans in asylums when they disrupted the regimes and disciplines of work on white farms, in the kitchens, and mines or when they threatened social peace more generally, whether in the street or 'native reserves'. The primary concern in confining mad Africans thus was less with 'curing' or alleviating their mental pain than with removing them as a source of disturbance to society as a whole. [19]

During this period, as elsewhere in Africa, accommodation in mental institutions always fell short of demand for prospective white and black patients. The 'troublesome persons' who were 'confined' were indeed often disruptive, and included black *and* white men and women from all walks of life.[20] This line of the argument is taken up by Jackson in her study of Ingutsheni Asylum in colonial Zimbabwe where she characterizes Vaughan's argument as suggesting that colonial psychiatry, an arm of 'the colonial state's repressive power apparatus' targeted the 'insufficiently other'.[21] She uses case records to argue that 'the mobile African woman elicited suspicion':

> The most common reason for admitting African women to the colonial mental hospital was 'strayness,' meaning that African female admissions were generally those who, for one reason or another, were thought to be in the wrong place.[22]

She notes a 'dramatic increase in the African female population in both the towns and the mental hospital during the 1930s, 1940s, and 1950s'. In the same paragraph, she records the ratio of African male to female asylum inmates as remaining steady at 1:4, and of African women to total asylum population as slightly under 1:6 in the same period. The African female inmate population rose from fifty-two in 1929 to 286 in 1956, which, in the given general population growth and gradual increase in available accommodation for the insane during this period, might constitute a *decrease* over time in numbers of African women in the population being identified as needing institutional care.[23]

Through these accounts – different though they are on the surface – a discursive formation takes root, a system of expectations, *despite* the archive and, in fact, despite the often nuanced analyses in which they are embedded.[24] Drawing its oxygen from words such as 'confined', 'repressive', 'deranged', 'rebellion', it creates a dense intertextual web with an impressive genealogy. The African 'incarceration' summons the ghosts of well-worn arguments from asylum historians to feminists and the anti-psychiatry movement, all characterizing custodial care in mental institutions as political or inhumane, an attempt to discipline unruly bodies or rebellious souls. However, while building on this genealogy, this particular 'law of what can be said'[25] about colonial asylums, rehearses race and oppression as the organizing codification of archive data. Ironically, this discursive formation demands that the black insane *were* other, which is to say *different* from their white counterparts. We must, therefore, return to the 'insufficiently other' trope, but with a new reading. For colonial asylum historians, there is an insufficient otherness indeed, one suppressed in readings of the archive, and which shapes narratives about them. The white insane were insufficiently other – in fact they had 'gone native'.[26] This has led in some instances to a curious myopia about the archive as a whole, and resistance to readings that might confront the layers of similarity and difference, contradictions and ellipses that characterize an along/against the grain description.

The Valkenberg Archive: Material Remains

Valkenberg Asylum opened as a whites-only institution in 1891. Initially, a handful of lunatics were housed in old farm buildings. These were soon replaced with buildings designed by the Scottish architect, Sydney Mitchell, of Sydney Mitchell and Wilson, Edinburgh. Many of these buildings still stand, and some are still in use as accommodation for the mentally ill: they are, therefore, not only a substantial material trace, but a living archive, one that can be explored and imagined and experienced side by side those in care.[27] The locked wards in the older buildings have changed little in over a century of use, apart from occasional refurbishing. Some single rooms originally designed for the seclusion of noisy or violent patients have 'learnt' to be offices or consulting rooms, but the day rooms in which patients wait, dance, talk, undress, quarrel and sing have changed very little either in dimension or function.[28] The faces change more rapidly than they once did.

Until those folders dating back to the period before 1950 were rehoused in the University of Cape Town Library's Manuscripts and Archives Department, the old buildings held a musty registry of all patient folders, organized by number, with recent and very old admissions in a jumble together. Before Valkenberg's racial desegregation in the early nineties, black and white patient folders were housed in separate buildings, one on each side of the Black River. When the patients were brought together, their folders merged into one constantly moving, shuffling, vast set of papers that kept together the living and the dead, men and women, people of all races and cultures, a material trace of a new democracy.

The herding together of old and new folders is testimony to a significant strand of asylum life. No-one knew when – if – patients would return. Sometimes a relapse occurred within six months, but sometimes patients stayed out of the asylum for decades. Some never returned, yet their details were relevant once again with the admission of a relative, a cousin or child perhaps; when a genetic history came into sharp focus. Thus, throughout Valkenberg's history, two institutional 'truths' shaped folder life: the transmissibility of insanity, from parent to child to grandchild, and the improbability of 'curing' it. Families passed through Valkenberg generation after generation, and individuals came and went, some many times over decades. It was quite fitting then, that in the old registry, the folder life should enact this reality, insanity threading together the texts of generations of institutional life.

The folders vary in weight: some are slim and contain nothing more than admission documents, some spill out of their covers, bursting with correspondence, often about money – maintenance fees, estates, *curator bonis* proceedings – but also about cycles of admission and discharge, physical illnesses and their treatment. The notes about the form of insanity and its progress through the years are always brief: there are a few lines of statutory periodical reports and these are sometimes separated by years of silence, with no intervening words. Some records contain a photograph of the patient, which contains a promise of a 'knowing', an intimacy seldom delivered by the surrounding text. The folders say much about doctors, a system of asylum governance, evolving psychiatric knowledge: but the subaltern voice, the subject of it all – the patient – is a black hole in the centre of the archive.[29] The folders are full of text 'about' (around, surrounding) a patient. His or her own account of events, either current or past, tends to be reported only as a symptom of delusions (for example) or disorderly speech. In the case of black patients this is compounded by doctors' lack of access to indigenous languages, and often, their infrequent contact with relatives. In the absence of a clear narrative about the patient's illness, and a way of engaging directly with current symptoms, a diagnosis and observations of behaviour carry the full weight of the patient's 'history'. As Vaughan has remarked, 'hearing the authentic voice of the mad African in written documentation really does involve straining the ears'.[30]

There is a rich set of documents relating to Valkenberg Asylum in the Cape Archives. They include Colonial Office, Public Works Department, Treasury, Medical Officer of Health reports and correspondence, and range from the lengthy and official (debates about asylum location, for example, and drafts of lunacy legislation with commentary) to the intensely banal (sewerage pipes and recovering the cost of hay for an asylum superintendent's horse). The boredom and delight of archival searches, the chase for missing puzzle pieces and orderly disorder are familiar ground and need not be repeated here.[31] There is much to be learned about asylum administration, doctors' attitudes to their patients, relationships with each other, and the trials and behaviour of lunatic asylum staff. Again, the archive has little to say about the patients themselves, except to record movement into, or out of, the asylum, and to note occasional accidents, pleas for release and, in one source, a number of urgent requests (from an inmate) to send troops, hammocks and stimulants to Valkenberg so that the Princess of Wales's sons might be freed from imprisonment.[32]

A further archive resides in the university library, in scientific journals read and annotated by asylum doctors, some of them containing articles written by the doctors on the colonial situation. This is the primary source of information about doctors' emerging curiosity about, and attitudes to, perceived differences between the white and black insane.[33]

The Valkenberg archive also includes discussions of, and blueprints for, building plans designed to accommodate lunatics. These are a rich source of information about proposed management of bodies within the asylum. A close reading of the plans and the surrounding correspondence allows the possibility of imagining daily routines, staff concerns and patient experience. This includes the separation of patients by gender and race in separate buildings; separation of day and night spaces, and of patients in good bodily health from those with physical illness; structural provision for the confinement of violent or disruptive patients in single cells and for constant staff surveillance of all patients at all times; the policing of sexuality; provision of accommodation for staff on the grounds of the asylum; and a variety of support buildings – administrative offices, workshops, barns, sheds, kitchens and laundries.[34]

Then there are the buildings themselves. Although many Valkenberg buildings have 'learnt' several functions since their construction, their original function has left material traces: heavy doors and barred windows, observation hatches, high-ceilinged large spaces once used as dormitories and day rooms, clearly designed to accommodate thrity or more bodies at any one time, and the many banisters that were polished by patients as a part of their regimen of occupational activity. The wood-panelled dining room (now used as a boardroom) is testimony to the fine quality of materials used in the original construction. The imposing façade of the Administration building, with its tower, large entrance and tiled lobby must surely have carried the stamp of security and authority for those bringing in their insane relatives. Money had been spent on this substantial edifice. It was not homely, however: it spoke of governance and docile bodies within, and imperial influence; safety perhaps, but also invasiveness. The main buildings of Valkenberg still cast a long shadow.

The other side of the imposing public façade of the Valkenberg buildings can be found scattered over the extensive grounds, and includes utilitarian blocks once used to accommodate various groups of acutely ill, intellectually challenged or chronically institutionalized patients, nurses' homes, hydrotherapy or occupational therapy buildings. Over the Black River, where once the black patients were accommodated separately from their white counterparts, is a similar scattering, now housing a community of small business enterprises (one that includes a pot-bellied pig). The buildings conform to a single (standard issue government) style on both sides of the Black River and, therefore, they speak of *uniformity* in the creation of docile bodies, regardless of their race. Their echoing dormitories, barred windows, narrow staircases, minimal provision in terms of domestic comfort – kitchen space, bathrooms, toilets, gardens, views – are evidence more of a herding together for surveillance and incarceration, than rest, tranquillity or release from stress.

Reading the buildings of Valkenberg is an interdisciplinary task and unsettles the security of text-based history. Even its scope is unsettling: it spans a large tract of land, two rivers, the Liesbeeck and the Black, a flourishing reed-bed home to a paradise of birds, and many buildings, some almost derelict, some relatively new. Within this jumbled expansiveness, there are small and confined spaces – cells, toilets, pantries within which the horizons are very confined. A project that takes the physical Valkenberg as its centre has a rich scholarly literature as a guide, crossing the disciplines of architecture, archaeology, human geography, social anthropology and cultural studies.[35]

Intertextuality and 'Both/And' Narratives

The material traces of the buildings are shells without surrounding text. What makes plans – even a walk through the buildings themselves – 'readable' as evidence is their location within a web of case notes, reports and official correspondence. The boundaries of this web are wide, and may expand to include documents about other local asylums, asylums in other colonies, provision for lunatics in asylums at 'home' and the history of the Empire itself. The use of different kinds of source material, produced by a range of speakers talking from contrasting class, gender, employment and positions of accountability, is likely to highlight contradiction or tension, and creates the possibility of resisting narrative 'smoothing'. A superb explication of this as a narrative strategy can be found in Stoler's account of one violent event at Dutch Indies colony in 1876.[36] Her telling draws on a single thirty-page handwritten letter, which she embeds in multiple texts, producing a narrative replete with contradiction. She rejects, however, the notion of 'a multistranded set of equally plausible claims',[37] opting instead for:

> a different kind of coherence, not one that elevates this text to master narrative, nor one in which only subaltern voices have truths to tell. Rather I have sought to recoup the inconsistencies of these narratives, to explore how subaltern inflections entered these stories retold in disquieted European voices, tangled by multiple meanings that could not easily be read.[38]

There are many examples in the Valkenberg archive of the kinds of narrative tensions to which Stoler refers. Under Dr Dodds, the superintendent and the colony's first Inspector of Asylums, provision for lunatics was transformed from grossly unsanitary, poorly regulated 'dumping grounds' into modern, efficient institutions; moreover, legislation was put in place to protect those identified as lunatics.[39] The legislative measures were taken directly from British law, and were marked by careful attention to 'humane care'. Many documents in the archive record Dodds as implementing the legislation meticulously, and also bolstering it with rules and regulations for the running of asylums that aimed to prevent abuse.[40] There is a complaint from Dodds about patients being brought to the asylum by police in uniform, because of the distress caused to inmates: 'In the weak state of their minds, the sight of the police escort troubles them; they think they have committed some crime, and I have seen it difficult to disabuse them of the ideas aroused'.[41]

The above commentary positions Dodds as vigilant about standards of humane care for all patients. However, the narrative does get murkier. In the 1913 *Select Committee on the Treatment of Lunatics*, Dodds's testimony was unreservedly in favour of maintaining strict segregation between the races. Moreover, his remarks reflect his belief in the intrinsic superiority of the white race. When asked about the 'native' insane, he said,

> Personally I do not know very much about natives. Only a comparatively small num-
> ber of natives are insane, in relation to population. You cannot expect in a race like
> the natives that you can have anything like the same amount, or proportion of insane
> as among civilized people.[42]

So how does the archivist make a credible narrative around the substantial figure of Dr Dodds? It is an ambivalent, contradictory both/and narrative. He was concerned for the humane care of all the colony's insane and there can be no doubt that the colony's asylums steadily improved and were possibly the most advanced to be found in sub-Saharan Africa during his term of office. On the other hand, he certainly regarded the black insane as different to and separable from the white insane, and ultimately less deserving of the best quality care. He was infuriated by what he seemed to see as careless attention to black patients, and yet allowed a form of provision that issued in significantly deleterious consequences. The narrative must reflect both sides.

Discourse analysis, postmodernist deconstructive, subaltern and psycho-analytic methodologies have in different ways drawn attention to the archival reading of absence to detect resistance, unrecorded voices, 'truths' beyond the hegemonic, those structures that are imagined beyond regimes of expectation. Part of the construction of both/and narratives that read along and against the grain must consider absences. Here the challenge resides in the 'speaking for' the subaltern, and two examples will illustrate this problem.

The Valkenberg archive contains a set of letters written by patients to the colonial government – requesting release, or complaining of abuse, or reporting on various financial matters – some even warning of secret conspiracies against the government. Surrounding documents show that every letter was read and responded too, and in many instances, the superintendent was asked for his comments. All of this was required by law, and seems to have been meticulously implemented.

A similar set of letters from black patients is absent. There is an issue of literacy here: some black inmates of colonial asylums did not read or write. However, it must be presumed that some did, and of those, might some have been moved to write to the Colonial Office: Were they offered pen and paper? Did they write, and were the letters not sent? Embedded in this is a narrative thread that would need to be pursued through another archival source, one perhaps less empty of evidence one way or the other. There is an archive specific to the questions of colonial education and it includes material about the perceived threat of literate black subjects. The issue of absence is then reconfigured as one of presence, but displacement, resistance and repression, not lack.[43]

A different kind of absence is constituted in the lack of voice. Apart from occasional direct or indirect quotations of their speech in doctors' notes (almost always used as illustration of delusional thinking or cheek), these letters are one major archival source for patients' voices. Delusions amplify social, political, economic and religious concerns and desires, especially when they affect matters of personal identity. It is not uncommon, therefore, to find examples of patients who believed themselves to be of royal birth, wealthy landowners, Christ or, in the case of tortured melancholic men and women, even Satan. There are some patients identified in the system as black, but who during their illness had the 'delusion' that they were white; similarly there are cases of white patients who felt anxious enough about how they had been classified racially to feel the need to insist frequently that they were indeed white. For example, Sarah S. was quoted as saying, 'She is really white but for some reason became pale brown. Delusions of being of royal blood, that she is the Queen of England'.[44] Similarly, where 'cheek' is reported, it carries a remarkably clear subaltern voice, speaking as it does in defiance of the manufacture of mad speech through doctors' notes. For example, Phillip D. was described on one of his medical certificates as 'not the respectful boy I know him to be, he refuses to do what I tell him and says he is my "baas"'.[45]

From the symptoms of insanity, a certain amount can be surmised about patients' existential anxieties. The occasional defiance of the racialized social hierarchy affirms the strength of its existence, even under conditions of mental confusion and suffering. Moreover, patients often spoke of their wish to go home, to be freed; they also climbed out of windows and absconded – surely all 'readable' subaltern texts. It is, however, the leap from these suggestive passages to a broader picture of bullying and racist colonial psychiatric practice, or to repeated intolerable misreadings (by doctors) of rationality (or more appealingly, 'divinest sense') as 'nonsense' that the archive cannot sustain.[46]

In reading patient records either with or against the grain, they must be understood as discursively shaped by psychiatry as a discipline, with the purpose of accounting for an illness, with an aetiology, symptoms and a prognosis. Doctors cannot be held accountable for failing to produce biographies or for calling spades delusions. Secondly, alongside the doctors' commentary runs a second stream of observation – this time from relatives, no longer able to shoulder the burden of care. They too amplified symptoms, in order to secure the institutional care they had struggled to achieve, often for years. They colluded with the reduction of patients' life scripts to an illness narrative. Finally, there is a startling uniformity of narrative across all patients, regardless of their race, class or gender, and this in itself is a caution to those seeking the subaltern voice.[47]

Another major source of information about Valkenberg's patients is to be found in a variety of family records: birth and marriage certificates, census findings, court cases and bankruptcies, and police reports and correspondence with resident magistrates and district surgeons. Taken together with official asylum casebook entries a picture gradually emerges – not of a single voice, nor of the experience of insanity or incarceration – but of a life embedded in a family, a community and a colonial context.[48]

Crossing Disciplines

It is critical that asylums be examined as one form of social institution, with connections to many others. It is likely, for example, that asylum life had parallels in some respects with colonial prisons, reformatories and hospitals – a point elegantly made in Jonathan Saha's chapter in this volume.[49] However, lunatic asylums are extremely complex institutions, and are peculiarly suited to excursions into theory beyond the single focus of one discipline. Apart from the role to be played by architects, archaeologists and social anthropologists in relation to the physical remains of lunatic asylums, and anthropologists, psychiatrists and psychologists have been major contributors to work on the symptoms of mental illness and culturally-specific illnesses.[50] The colonial madness/race narrative is produced in its least nuanced form in social historical accounts that engage with psychiatry as a particularly cruel form of 'cultural imperialism', with no benevolent intent or effect.[51] In the period during which Cape colonial asylums were being reformed, psychiatry itself was undergoing a revolution. It was during this time that 'mania' was redefined into dementia praecox and manic-depression; the organic psychoses and their causes came more clearly into view and the neuroses and personality disorders began to be described and identified. It is in the psychiatric, not historical literature, both past and present, that the lived reality of insanity is described in ways that begin to make sense of asylum social conditions – the gangrenous limbs of catatonic patients, the spread of enteritis through patients who played with their faeces, the noise and scuffles, the unstoppable violence.[52] The historiography of any asylum needs to incorporate an account of the practical management, in wards of thirty or more patients, some of whom were making violent attacks on patients and nurses, some who were silent and unmoving but incontinent, some tortured by their delusions. A patient like Harriet H., who 'knew' of 3,000 girls being kept in dungeon brothels between Sea Point and Newlands and 'heard' them being beaten at night, who knew too that her own life was in danger as a result of what she could hear, needed extraordinary care.

The Single Case

Asylum and psychiatric histories are replete with extraordinary stories of individual cases, from James Norris and James Tilly Matthews from the early nineteenth century, through to Sylvia Plath's bio-fiction, *The Bell Jar* (1963).[53] In the colonial asylum scholarly literature, there are case studies that are used to illustrate both the typical and the singular; it is the tension between these *as method* that needs to be addressed. It is a slippery narrative structure: the extraordinary case is citeworthy not only because it is a story worth telling, but rhetorically it becomes emblematic of a wider truth, a 'typical' case. So, for example, the extraordinary story of Nontetha Nkwenkwe, prophet, is told as a unique instance, but comes to represent both colonial oppression of dissent and colonial psychiatry's insensitivity to the expression of visionary experience except as a symptom of psychotic illness. On the other hand, Charles Van Onselen uses the case of Joseph Silver, who seems to have been a petty criminal, thief, pimp and psychopath, as an extraordinary tale of villainy and ingenuity, worthy of an extended narrative. The heroic status given to Silver would certainly have satisfied his own grandiosity, but fails to reflect the many others whose lives were similar to his.[54]

The case cited as 'typical' is rhetorically just as slippery. The very act of telling it makes the typical extraordinary, by lifting it out of the archive and examining it minutely. In the process a weighty accumulation of detail 'told' in stories not picked out for description is lost. Illustrations, drawn from case notes, affect credibility equally – if not more – than statistical tables recording diagnoses, death and recovery rates, and lists of symptoms. For example, the Valkenberg archive contains the record of Engela F., a woman whose insanity took the form of racial attacks on her person: hallucinations of 'kaffirs hitting her over the head'; the 'idea that she [was] being "Malay tricked" by her husband and another woman'. The record notes that she was removed from laundry work because she attacked one of the 'native' workers there.[55] This is a case that could be used in a number of ways to illustrate a form of delusional insanity, the colouring of delusional content by a particular social and political context, and even white anxieties about incompletely segregated lives. She had tried to throttle 'an old coloured woman', her neighbour – in itself of interest to the colonial historian – and the record is also illustrative of incomplete segregation in the working life of the institution, as black and white women clearly worked together. Were her story to be pursued through the available sources and were the story of her childhood and marriage to be found, she would *become* extraordinary, at least in narrative.

Going to the narcissistic core of things, in a wry poem, Stevie Smith sketches the murderous rage of a child, after he is told he is 'only one of many / and of small account if any'.[56] This is the asylum case-study dilemma. There is something fundamentally difficult in the idea of personal suffering being regarded as a 'case'. It is equally problematic to dwell on the individual without keeping commonalities firmly in view. Psychoanalytic case studies have a significant contribution to make in this respect. In a theory and philosophy designed to study the nature of psychic conflict, it simultaneously celebrates the individual's suffering, and positions that suffering as the human condition. The historiographical art may lie in describing the collision of anomaly and institution, but also in giving the institution – especially one so saturated with human misery – the face of a person.[57]

The Intersubjective Archive

An intersubjective approach to asylums – colonial or not – confronts eventually writers' desire to reason about madness. Needless to say, there are a variety of potential motives, political and personal, and they range from reparative anxiety and hopes for solutions to one's own fragility, to voyeurism, to a quest for the 'divinest sense' that Emily Dickinson discerned in madness.

This chapter began with Bethlem, iconic of a particular intersubjective space; so it is to Bethlem that we return. As is well known, Bethlem used to host spectators who would come to stare at and observe the incarcerated. Modern readers think of this as barbarous, but we feed a popular culture that relishes films and confessional novels about madness, one that devours news reports about serial killers and psychopaths, and even fosters a small academic industry preoccupied with asylum histories. We have, in a sense, become virtual spectators. It is precisely because of this that the historiography of asylums needs such careful thought.

Institutions that care for those identified as mentally ill are placed between private misery and public gaze. They ambivalently protect both in their material traces. I am sympathetic to Parle's suggestion that colonial asylum histories might 'contribute to a lessening of the marginalization of the mentally ill'. However, the records both reveal and conceal private misery to the public. The erasure of patients' voices is partly to do with entrance into a private domain.[58] By contrast, asylums have always – and still do – institutionalize, name, count, categorize and make the private public. The private misery often can only be imagined. The public traces must be seen for what they are: stigmatizing in that they 'other' the insane; secretive in covering their professional traces; exhibitionist in their demands for money and thought and tales of anguish; violent, but containing violence; meeting it too, with violence of its own; but also ambivalently humane, standing by to be witness, as suffering that can only be imagined by the historian is endured.

There are from time to time reminders that these 'histories' are not simply for historians. Constructing family genealogies is a popular hobby, and requests come through both to the institution, and to those who have used this archive of patient files, for information about relatives known to have been in Valkenberg at some point. The causes of the hospitalization are often a mystery to the family and a source of intense curiosity, anxiety and dread. Negotiating this interface between the public and private, the living and the dead, with their linking strands of DNA and family relationships brings significance and aliveness to patients' narratives, in ways that are often beyond the reach of more neutral histories. To learn of great grandparents dying of tertiary neurosyphilis, the result of one's sexual betrayal of the other; or a grandfather who killed his son and then attempted suicide is weighty information indeed for a family to metabolize, and an important ethical check on the historians' ever-present urge to recover and uncover private spaces.

Conclusion

To share an agreed-upon reality, a history of ourselves, is a common-sense part of cohesive social functioning. Those societies, within which there is a disputed history and a contested archive, are inevitably at war with themselves.[59] It is profoundly disturbing both when history is challenged and when 'reality' turns out to be fantasy or delusion. So historians do the important ideological work of assuring us that history is discoverable, and that at some point there will be a past on which we must agree. In the same way, the insane – by being so patently out of touch with reality – assure us that there is one fairly solid reality in which we mostly participate, most of the time. Lunatic asylum archives neatly bring together these twin social concerns with a recoverable past and a sane and stable apprehension of reality.

Histories of colonial asylums are caught between two discursive structures: the one that underwrites 'the manufacture of madness', positioning colonial asylum doctors as agents of oppression, incarcerating and neglecting the black insane; and one that insists on both the inevitability of the asylum and its absent-minded, ambivalent disposition towards the sufferers within its walls. The colonial asylum archive has material that supports both and much more: the tension between the public and the private, tales of displacement and sea voyages, colonizers afraid of the sun, men and women struggling with their identities and skins, exploited peoples poorly understood and 'othered' even in their misery. Now seems the right moment to open the archive to this carnival of readings, and to use them to look outwards, beyond the history of ourselves. Colonial asylum histories interrupt the discursive formations into which western European asylum histories have fallen, offering new spaces and new words. They are histories that refract light between colony and 'home', the sane and the mad, local anxieties and the madness of Empire. They need to be carefully written so that their shadows and light continue to be alive.

11 DEATH AND EMPIRE: LEGAL MEDICINE IN THE COLONIZATION OF INDIA AND AFRICA

Jeffrey M. Jentzen

With the exception of the most primitive societies, the transmission of death investigation practices was a necessary component for the establishment of the rule of law. From the late sixteenth century through to the nineteenth century, as European states acquired political control over vast overseas territories, they had to determine whether to maintain existing indigenous legal systems or to replace them with the mechanism of European continental law and its agencies for the administration of colonial societies. This related to substantive as well as procedural law (i.e. the organization of courts and judges). Where states could establish direct rule, Europeans introduced their own laws. The introduction of European law could either mean the adoption of the legal code of the metropole or the development of new laws adapted to suit colonial rule, but built on European legal principals and procedures. In some instances, the indigenous culture required the amalgamation of European and indigenous legal systems. In short, European colonial expansion was also the expansion of European law.[1]

During the conquest and acquisition of New World colonies, England and the European powers required colonists to create legal systems of governance that would replicate the structure of Old World justice in the newly formed colonies. Medical jurisprudence, broadly defined as the use of medical knowledge by those who exercise legal authority, was an essential practice in the practice of law. The establishment of legal medicine, similar to the healing medical sciences, represented an empowering 'tool' in colonized lands, which provided for both the health and safety of the colonists and state control of indigenous peoples through the prosecution of crime and prevention of the epidemic spread of disease. In managing indigent populations, colonial governments required the application of science and the creation of integrated colonial and native institutions which also meant modernizing and governing them. Physicians, who provided medico-legal expertise, became valuable weapons of empire building and maintaining colonial control.[2] In some cases, indigenous populations employed these same institutions and medico-legal practices to provide legal protection for themselves against oppressive colonial governments. Colonies became medico-legal laboratories for the development of methods for the detection and prosecution of crime and public health epidemics – such as the development of the science of ballistics, fingerprints and pathological anatomy – but also in the advancement the medical science and public health.

The two major legal systems that shaped the development of forensic medicine from the medieval period were the European continental system, based on Roman and canon law, and the Anglo-American system, based on English common law. Every nation in the modern western world can trace the history of its civil, criminal law and medico-legal practices to one of these traditions. These legal systems also provided a foundation for modernization, imperial conquest, colonization and state creation, where the methods of legal and medical proof were necessary factors in defining and stimulating the need for the rule of law, and the reception of expert medical testimony during legal proceedings in distant imperial colonies.[3]

The British first established the East India Company in the sixteenth century for commercial purposes, which resulted in the subjugation of the Indian subcontinent under British rule of law after the fall of the Mughal empire. They ruled India for more than three centuries with a system which depended upon, first, the installation of a dual system of English common law in conjunction with indigenous judicial systems of India, and later, their amalgamation into a unified system of penal law.[4] The capitulation system allowed for the establishment of extraterritorial rights, which included death investigation practices and the right to a jury trial. These rights, which allowed colonial powers to have their own separate courts, protected subjects of the British empire in foreign lands under English law and became a source of friction between the colonists and the indigenous legal authorities. The abuse by colonial powers of extraterritorial courts served as a catalyst for the development of indigenous death investigation practices modelled on European and British law, on which all subsequent colonies operated and in many instances was the foundation for nationalism.[5]

European colonists established colonies similar to the model of the Dutch colonization of the South African Cape by the Dutch East India Company (VOC) in 1604. This was followed by the English occupation in the early nineteenth century that lead to the creation of a legal system consisting of a mixture of English and Dutch laws. The French invasion of Egypt in the late eighteenth century, and the 'Scramble for Africa' a hundred years later, allowed for the introduction of enlightened European legal principals, modernization and continental law into colonized lands, which lead to the eventual colonial state control. On each occasion, the colonizing force left the indelible marks of its unique system of law and death investigation practices, indicating the legal measures necessary to establish a colonial power and sustain the political control which has persisted until the present day.

In the context of European imperialism, medicine represented a 'tool of empire' as the European governments sought to replicate the Old World medicine in the territories. Medical science and its medical experts represented a powerful authority, in political, legal and cultural contexts. Physicians acted as front-line death investigators by examining bodies and performing autopsies in sudden, unexpected and suspicious deaths. They also functioned as medico-legal enforcers of imposed hygienic standards by the European colonial powers both in the medical control of epidemic disease and political control of colonized peoples. In addition, colonial physicians provided expert witness testimony in both indigenous courts of law for the native subjects and those under extraterritorial rules of law in support of colonists.

Medico-legal experts in far off lands were guided by a progressive medical science, coupled with their own empirical observations and experience, that projected Old World medical authority. By the late nineteenth century, the progress of scientific medicine labouring in extreme environments resulted in the creation of new medical specialists of tropical and military medicine – and, with it, the preservation of millions of lives.[6]

This chapter will examine the development of legal medicine and the use of medico-legal experts by English and European colonists and its impact on British India and South Africa. I will discuss the colonial medico-legal systems of death investigation and forensic medicine beginning in the sixteenth century under the English and Dutch colonists in India and South Africa, extending to decolonization and the integrated legal systems of the present.

Foundations of Criminal Justice

The Continental legal system and English common law provided the foundations for development of courts of justice by the state. In the medieval period there emerged two distinct trial procedures: the inquisitorial form in Europe and the accusatorial in England. In Europe, developing states acquired the *Corpus Juris Civilis*: a body of Roman civil law first codified between AD 529 and 534 by the Byzantine Emperor Justinian. The central attribute of the *Corpus* was its reliance on oral and written testimony which necessarily followed specified rules of evidence and standards of proof. The Roman system gave investigative or inquisitorial powers to academically trained judges who oversaw the fact finding investigation using written evidence obtained from university physicians. Developing states incorporated aspects of canon law with the *Corpus* to provide legal codes such as the Carolinian Code of Charlemagne in AD 950. Continental courts paid medical professionals to submit written reports, *consilia*, and relied on proof, written evidence and professional fact-finding that created medico-legal treatises which ultimately assisted in the creation of scientific thought in the developing states of Italy, France and Germany.[7]

English common law did not simply emerge from Continental law or existing customary or traditional laws of England. Instead, it was associated with the rise of the early English state and dependent on the consolidation of state power for its eventual dominance. Common law is law based on historical judicial opinions and local tradition. Common law relied on factual eye witness testimony that proceeded oral testimony given before a lay jury who in turn interpreted the evidence, decided upon matters of fact and determined the final outcome of the case.[8] The promulgation of a uniform common law across the whole of the English realm was the major vehicle for the expansion of English colonial power in the period following the Norman Conquest in 1066. English common law was particularly useful for the application of legal systems in colonial countries. A by-product of the common law is trial by lay jury and the coroner's inquest – recalled by early legal reformers as 'the bulwark of English liberties'.[9]

Hunnisett established the English coroner beginning in 1194 under Henry II, when the justices in Eyre required the election of three knights and one clerk in each county to be 'Keepers of the pleas of the crown' – the *custodies placitorum coronae*. These duties had been previously performed by other county officials such as the county justifier and serjeant or bailiff of the hundred. The serjeant, appointed under the direction of the sheriff, had many duties but was limited in jurisdiction to the hundred. The county coroner's sphere of activity was the entire country. The position originally was created to stop corruption and abuses of sheriffs. Coroners became increasingly important over the twelfth century; they were encumbered with many roles, including the investigation of sudden death and the collection of various fines for the King.[10]

The office of the coroner was at its zenith in the second half of the thirteenth century replacing the sheriff and justices of the peace who were not known to have performed the duties of the coroner after 1225. By 1250 the position of the coroner was firmly established and filled by influential men of the local community. Although coroners were originally established to act as a check against the power of the sheriff, sheriffs still maintained considerable influence on the election of the coroner. In shear political power, the coroner remained definitely below, and not equal to, the sheriff. The sheriff retained the ability to perform some coroner duties in the coroner's absence; whereas the coroner could only act as sheriff in financial or general administration matters or when specially authorized. The coroner retained the privilege of being the only political official able to arrest the sheriff, which persists to modern times. Both county and borough coroners declined in importance during the fourteenth and fifteenth centuries.[11]

The coroner arrived in distant colonies transplanted with the system of English common law. English colonists, appointed by colonial governors as coroners in far distant lands, were directed by elaborate oaths to the King to 'Doe all and everything done by any coroner of any county in England'.[12] American coroners, for example, adopted verbatim the statutory language from English law for inquest proceedings in the colonies. As the English became the dominant colonial power and expanded, they ultimately transported the system of common law and the coroner's inquest throughout their empire – America to Hong Kong and Singapore to Canada. Yet, whereas the duties, prestige and political power of coroners in England waned over the centuries, the power of the colonial coroners grew in legal and political stature.

British Transformation of Indian Law and Medicine

The establishment of the East India Company in 1600 and the conquest of Bengal by Robert Clive in 1757 brought the Indian subcontinent under English rule. The indigenous village democracy called the *panchayat* was the foundation of political and judicial order until the establishment of a British colonial administration. The British did not conquer a single homogenous country but a series of independent kingdoms that became the political state of India after they developed the important institutions of empire. According to historian Francis Fukyama, the institutions that bound India together as a nation polity – a civil service, an army, a common administrative language (English), a legal system of uniform and impersonal laws, i.e. democracy – were the result of Indians interacting with and accepting a British colonial regime.[13] In India, the criminal law was deeply rooted in religious law – Islamic and Hindu – rather than in policies of the state. Brahmanism religion, which developed contemporaneously with the period of Indian state formation, subordinated criminal investigations to the warrior class, the *Ksyatriyas* and priestly class, the Brahmin. More importantly, the earliest law tracts, the *Dharmasastras*, were written by the religious authorities, not emperors or magistrates. Prior to the arrival of the English, there were no formal legal institutions; disputes were settled through monetary payments, *diya* or blood money. One hundred cows was the price for killing a man.[14]

Initially, the English perceived India as a territory with two judicial systems, Islamic and Hindu. Jatis or castes subdivided all the *varnas* into hundreds of secondary occupational groups. The *varna* and *jati* formed the bedrock organization of society and limited the power of the states. Beginning with the Laws of Manu, Indian law developed out of religious rituals independent of political rulers. The Laws of Manu consisted of ritual Brahmin prayers developed through customary and oral traditions written down in the *Manava-Dharmasastra*. While Islamic law, the *šari'a* law established by Mohammad, was considered immutable in Arabic or Persian texts, Hindu law varied according to regional, status and caste boundaries. Their jurisprudence relied more often on the oral expertise of Brahmin jurists. As institutions grew, people met and appointed one man to maintain order from growing problems of theft, murder, adultery and other crimes.

The British ruled India for more than three centuries with the legal, medical and medico-legal systems of an extraterritorial law that began with a dual system of English common law for the English colonists and local laws for the local Hindu and Muslim populations in rural areas. This legal arrangement of indirect rule served as a model for other colonial states and in future English colonies. Initially, the British relied upon indigenous intermediaries to construct the legal bridges of law that allowed for the emergence of a blended legal structure, especially to assist with the administration of justice. They established both Crown courts and Company courts in the three presidential towns of Calcutta, Bombay and Delhi. These courts were not controlled by the English Parliament, but instead supervised by the East Indian Company, which itself was reluctant to become involved in matters of criminal justice, the *nizamat*. British reforms were influenced by two different systems: the Islamic criminal code and the contemporary British law. In 1790 the criminal justice system in Bengal was based entirely on Islamic law. With time, the English modified their attitude towards governance and the criminal law establishing a protectorate posture and reform through legislative reforms.[15]

Islamic law made the basic distinction between crimes against God šarī'a and crimes against human law. In modifying the legal system the British created a dual system which maintained šarī'a law and at the same time allowed extraordinary justice of English law. The punishments for crimes against God were fixed (the *hadd*), whereas other crimes were considered private justice subject to the desires of the victim's heirs. In Islamic law the family of the victim reserved the right to obtain blood money and even to pardon the murderer. The English considered the punishments for *šarī'a* to be excessively severe while they saw the treatment of other crimes too lenient owing to the amount of evidence required to convict under Islamic law. The *siyāsa*, that marked right of the ruler to interfere in the public interest, allowed for modifications of some laws. Under growing pressure from the British Parliament, culminating in the Regulating Act of 1773, the Company and its agents shifted from commercial plunder to more orderly governance and permanent forms of exploitation.[16]

Warren Hastings, Governor General of Bengal from 1772 to 1785, received orders from the Company Board of Directors in London to take over and directly control the whole administration of Bengal. The Company was now obliged to administer civil and criminal law in the newly acquired territories.[17] The reforms under Hastings from 1772 to 1774 consisted of reforming only the civil courts. While criminal courts remained under local jurisdiction, Hastings instigated changes some to the criminal law. With time the English became increasing repulsed by the mutilations allowed by Islamic law. They sought to change legal procedures and punishments by taking control of the criminal justice system, and in 1790 Indian judges were replaced by English judges, who in turn would be guided by the opinions (*fatwā*) of Islamic court officers attending the trial. The dual nature of the Indian criminal law allowed the British to control sentencing in a system they considered barbarous and inhuman, while at the same time respecting and maintaining šarī'a law. Ironically, as the English law strove to avoid mutilation as punishment for šarī'a law, the number of crimes that received capital punishment under English law increased.[18] The impact of the British on the Bengal criminal code was to allow the Indians to enjoy their own laws until their traditional relativism was supplemented with natural laws of English 'reason, humanity, and natural justice'.[19] Eventually the British completed the evolution of the dual system of British and Islamic law in the form of the presidential Penal Code, which was introduced by Thomas Babinton Macaulay in 1862 and was valid for all persons living in British India.

In India, English physicians performed the duties of police surgeons investigating deaths in the cities and towns; functioning as front-line medico-legal death investigators. They were encouraged to 'possess an intimate acquaintance with the dispositions, customs, prejudice and crimes of the people'.[20] In doing so, they developed racial profiles of the methods and motivation for criminal activity among the population. British death investigators encountered widespread perjury and false confessions from local natives which complicated criminal investigations. Medico-legal officials were stymied by the lack of oaths in testimony and common use of untruths by Indian perpetrators or accessories to crime. Police surgeons responded to the requests of local chiefs of police, the *darogah*, and magistrates charged with investigating sudden and suspicious deaths. These civic surgeons followed legal requirements for the examination of wound and death bodies according to the ancient methods of death investigation by coroners under English law.

> On receiving information of suspicious or unnatural deaths, the darogah, or some responsible person deputed by him, shall proceed to the spot and examine the wound, or other corporal injuries, but he shall not probe them, and he shall record the length, breadth and apparent depth of each, and the weapon by which the wounds appear to have been given, and whether the body appeared to have been brought and laid there.[21]

In cases of suspected murder, wounding or the endangerment of life, the body of the injured person would then have been sent to the local medical station without interference by police, except in cases of obvious lethal injuries where there was no doubt that they had died from their injuries. In cases of delayed death occurring days after the infliction of injuries where there was concern that medical treatment or other natural causes contributed to the death, the bodies were sent to be inspected by the police surgeon and the deposition invariably taken under oath before the magistrate or the sessions judge during the coroner's inquest. In such cases, 'the only certainty which we have in this country of the actual cause of death', cautioned the police surgeons, arose 'from the postmortem examination of the surgeon'.[22] Police surgeons were also required to examine the medicinal stocks of native traders under suspicion of providing deadly medications for the purpose of suicide or murder.

The moral sensitivities of the English encouraged the elimination of human sacrifice and other ancient practices as well as Islamic methods of punishment which the British saw as inhuman and barbarous.[23] With the moral revolution of the nineteenth century, English colonists were often offended by what they believed to be barbaric practices of indigenous peoples based on traditional or religious practices. Suicide was common, as self-sacrifice was considered an important feature of the Hindu, and thought to be the most acceptable sacrifice as a means of pleasing the gods. As severe as the traditional social practices may have been, English criminal laws focused on practices such as the sati, the immolation of the widow at her husband's funeral and other uncouth acts of public capital punishment. In a similar manner, infanticide – particularly of female infants – was commonly practised by some religious sects and formally abolished by the British by 1870.

Police surgeons, also known as civil surgeons, recognized the often insurmountable task of uncovering the cause of death in a country with a climate of interminable heat, difficulties of transportation, and innumerable exotic poisons. A major problem for the detection of sudden death was the rapid decomposition of the body. British statutes mandated that *darogahs* (local administrators, usually chiefs of police) prepare for the rapid removal of bodies from the scene by litter carriers to the sudder station for examination by the police surgeons. The Marsh test for detecting arsenic and other mineral poisons was known from English chemists.[24] However, isolated from advances in chemical testing taking place in Europe, they had few tools to detect the many plant poisons available in India. In investigating suspicious deaths caused by poisoning, British civil surgeons were ordered to keep the stomach and its contents intact and submit it to a chemical engineer in a distant laboratory for an examination and analysis of the contents for poisons. The police surgeons were expected

> to consider it to be their duty on all occasions of post mortem examination in which the signs are such as, in their opinion, to require that the contents of the stomach, or portion of the stomach itself, or of any other part of the body, should be transmitted to the Presidency to be tested by the Government Chemical Examiner, either to put up with their own hands theses suspected substances in a suitable vessel , or see them put up at once by an assistant or subordinates, and after affixing as many impression of their own seals as they may think necessary to guard, as far as possible, against the vessel being opened or tampered with without detection.[25]

In a distant and vast country, English physicians openly acknowledged the difficulties in maintaining any evidentiary value of biological evidence. 'I have long been of the opinion', admitted one English civil surgeon, 'that evidence derived from suspected substances, sent to Calcutta for examination, is of no value, and would not be admitted in any court of Justice on the Continent of Europe, were a greater degree of care and guardedness is required in all medico-legal cases than in England or India'.[26] Physicians called for increased security of retained specimens as well as improved training and preparation of the chemical examiners, many of which had not received sufficient training in the new field of toxicology now developing in continental Europe and America.

The Indian population quickly learned that the British chemists could detect mineral poisons (arsenic, mercuric chloride and strychnine) in minute quantities. As a result, they turned to a variety of indigenous biological, vegetable poisons.[27] In keeping with developments and their application to criminal justice in Europe and the United Kingdom, the British created Government Chemical Laboratories in India at Madras (1849), Calcutta (1853), Agra (1864) and Bombay (Mumbai) (1870). These small chemical laboratories assisted the civil surgeons with the medico-legal investigation of death. They were also used by the physicians as a method of evaluating exotic poisons, disease and methods of criminal deaths and detection. In addition, most European medical officers often experimented and studied the effects of exotic vegetal poisons as well as the use of snake venoms for medicinal purposes.

> Russell applied one drop of the poison of a cobra on his tongue and found it tasteless. It has commonly said that it may be swallowed with immunity, but Dr. Hering found, while residing at Surinam, that, on taking even small doses of it, much diluted with water, very perceptual effects were produced; such as pains through the body, abundant secretions of mucus from the nose and esophagus, and diarrhea.[28]

English physicians considered post-mortem examinations essential for the determination of the actual cause of death. Human dissection served other important causes of the state in the diagnosis and control of epidemics, investigating crime and providing the foundation for medical education. A majority of the indigenous population maintained a deep suspicion of the nature and methods of western medicine; dissection and contact with human corpses were considered taboo and derogatory topics. For most of the nineteenth century, hospitals and such practices as vaccination and post-mortems had given rise to fear, opposition and anger to the indigenous India population. Nineteenth-century British India reacted to the introduction of dissection and autopsy by engaging in acts of violence against British health officers – retaliation against the imposed legal sanctions of a colonial state eager to introduce a disciplinary measures by a recalcitrant peasantry constantly depicted and treated as different from their colonial masters.[29]

Although valued and approved in the early works of ancient Indian medicine, Ayurveda, dissection and the study of anatomy had been an important part of the early Hindu medical practices but had been abandoned and forgotten due in part to the social resistance against dissection. Autopsies carried a deep repugnance by almost all castes and creeds in India. Dealing with the disposal of the dead animals or humans was regarded as the most impure occupation and karma. The decay and polluting substances associated with death needed to be transcended. Only the lowest class and most despised Hindu could be recruited to assist with dissections. Doms or domes were among the lowest caste groups in India. Despised even by untouchables, they assisted at autopsies and became known indiscriminately as 'doms' or 'domes'.[30] They performed roles such as street cleaner, scavengers and other defiling tasks such as removing carcasses of dead animals and carrying dead bodies of humans to the burning grounds; often, they were employed by executioners.

Indians saw autopsies as representative of the vile nature of western medicine. On the other hand, Europeans saw this opposition as affirmation of Indian superstition and recalcitrance, and an obstacle for the advancement of scientific medicine in India. Since one of the principal criticisms of Indian medicine was its ignorance of anatomy, for the English and progressive native scientists, dissection epitomized the forward ascendancy of western medicine over their irrational, indigenous Indian rivals. At the Native Medical Institution in Calcutta dissections had never, for reasons of religion and caste, been performed on human corpses, only on sheep and other animals. In 1836, Pandit Madhusudan Gupta, himself of the vaidya caste (of hereditary physicians practising Ayurveda) and a former teacher at the Sanskrit College, became the first Indian in modern times to perform a human dissection. 'This day' declared the exuberant commentator, 'will forever be marked in the annals of western medicine in India as the moment when Indians rose superior to the prejudices of their earlier education and thus boldly flung open the gates of modern medical science to their countrymen'.[31] While this was cherished as a major accomplishment, the indigenous population continued to express suspicion about western practices. They avoided hospitals in part due to the fear of dissection. As a result there was a virtual ban by British doctors on performing autopsies on hospitalized Indian soldiers to avoid any misjudgement on their intentions for experimentation. Nevertheless, prison was the only place where medico-legal autopsies could be performed on natives and where British physicians continued to have unimpeded access to Indian corpses for research. By contrast, European solders, alive or dead, were seen one of the mainstays of medical research in India.[32]

Without the benefit of bacteriological methods and predating the general acceptance of the germ theory, English physicians considered post-mortems the only reliable method of diagnosing epidemic diseases. Post-mortem examinations performed on suspected plague victims were fiercely opposed by the local population on religious grounds. In the search for plague corpses, British civil surgeons and public health officials often encountered outright resistance, and more commonly evasion and concealment. Corpses were often buried clandestinely to avoid the intrusion of the medical officer and delay in burial, often in opposition of Islamic burial practices. The frequent delays of twelve to twenty-four hours elapsed before permission could be obtained to remove a body from houses, a practice condemned by both religion and the science of sanitation. In urging the inspection of corpses as the 'sheet-anchor' of plague detection, the Surgeon-Major saw nothing in it that 'hurt the sensibilities of the various races of India'. The government's decision to order the inspection of all corpses was sufficient to create widespread unrest, especially among Muslims, and resulted in a riot in Bombay in 1898. If a doctor persisted in the examination, local Indian leaders warned, 'he should not be allowed to do so even though our lives are sacrificed'.[33]

In addition to the medico-legal use of the autopsy and toxicology testing, India became the laboratory for pioneering research in the science of fingerprints. The use of fingerprinting for identification, known since antiquity, became highly developed for the scientific identification of criminals in India. Confronted with a large, homogenous and belligerent local population, British colonial officers sought methods of efficient social control and criminal investigation. Fingerprinting in India began as an effective technique for civil identification to combat widespread fraud and perjury. William Herschel, a chief administrator of Bengal district, initially used fingerprints to confirm proof of identity on contracts. Later, believing that tendency to commit crime was inherited and a common characteristic of lower social groups in India, the British sought to identify habitual criminals under the Criminal Tribes Act (1871) which called for the identification of criminals. In 1877 Herschel wrote to authorities in England regarding his use of fingerprints as a method of identification in prisons, pension registrations and the courts. Herschel's work attracted the attention of other prominent scientists including Sir Francis Galton, who expanded and refined the science. Thus was established he first fingerprint bureau was established in Calcutta in 1897 by Sir Edward Henry. In 1897, the manager of a tea house in the Bhutan district was stabbed to death. Police recovered a bloody fingerprint at the scene. They examined the print and when compared with the retained fingerprints of a suspicious employee, Kangli Charan, who had left the district, there were eighteen matching points of comparison. Charan was arrested, tried and convicted of burglary but acquitted of the murder. Despite the lesser charge, the Charan Case helped to lay the scientific foundation for the acceptance of fingerprint evidence in courts of law. In 1900 the Indian Evidence Act was enacted and marked the first endorsement of fingerprints as evidence. Initially developed for the control of civil population, law enforcement eventually employed fingerprints in criminal cases.[34]

The British also used their colonial territories to experiment with the forensic applications of ballistics. For instance, 'Dum-Dum' bullets were allegedly created by British soldiers as they attempted to neutralize Hashish-smoking mountain tribesman, a fanatical religious faction known as the Hashishins. Under the influence of the drugs and religious fervour, the Hashishins were able to withstand multiple direct hits from standard British .303 bullets without fatal effect. British soldiers reportedly made cruciform cuts in the tips of bullet to aid in the expansion of the bullet on impact and to increase the transmission of the bullet's energy or 'stopping power' of the ammunition. The practice was so successful the British began the large-scale manufacture of the altered projectiles at the Dum-Dum ammunition factory beginning in 1897 by Captain Bertie-Cla of the Indian Ammunition Works at Dum-Dum, India.[35]

The Indian Penal Code of 1862 mandated that inquests be convened in cases of sudden, unexpected deaths, homicides, suicides and accidents, infanticides, anaesthetic or medical deaths, poisonings, deaths in mental hospitals and any death under suspicious circumstances. Three types of inquests existed: the police inquest, the coroner inquest and Magistrate inquest. Initially mandated in 1861, the police inquest was the most prevalent method of inquiry, whereby the police officer acts as investigator and judge. This is by far the most common system throughout the country, and it follows the European system whereby the police and the judicial authorities control the medico-legal investigation and decide whether or not an autopsy is required. However, owing to India's great size and vast population, many problems arise with the implementation of this system. Any physician presumed to be sufficiently competent to perform an autopsy could be called upon to dissect bodies in even the most difficult forensic cases. Indeed, as a step towards greater professionalization among forensic sciences, the India Academy of Forensic Sciences was created in 1961.[36]

The coroner's inquest began in 1871 in the presidential cities of Calcutta, Delhi and Bombay. A remnant of the English system, a special officer known as the coroner was appointed by the government to inquire into cases of all unnatural or suspicious death. The coroner was usually an advocate, attorney, pleader, first-class magistrate with five years' experience or a metropolitan magistrate and presided over the coroner's court. He was of the rank of first-class judicial magistrate and his territorial jurisdiction extended to the city limit. The coroner system was similar to the English system in authority and governed by the Coroner's Act of 1871 which allowed the coroner to inquire into the cause of all unnatural or suspicious deaths and also deaths occurring in jails within the jurisdiction. The coroner's court had no authority to impose sentences or fines. The majority of autopsies were performed in hospitals attached to a coroner's court. Due to the bureaucratic nature of the procedure, the coroner's inquest resulted in numerous delays before the authorities handed the body over to the relatives. Despite the significant role played by the coroner, coroner's inquests have since ceased to be convened throughout the country.[37]

The magistrate inquest was present throughout the country except in Mumbai. The magistrate is a civil servant empowered by the state. Cases under magistrate inquest include: police custody deaths, police firings, prison deaths and dowry deaths. He had the authority to view a dead body and decide whether an autopsy or inquest is required. In order to perform the duties of the coroner, the magistrate could order an exhumation of a body or to conduct a post-mortem examination by any registered medical practitioner, usually the police surgeon, and require him to appear as an expert witness to give evidence court.

In 1947, at the time of independence, there were only thirty medical colleges; fifty years later the number had risen to 145. Legal medicine is now more commonly known as forensic medicine, medical jurisprudence or state medicine. Medical colleges eventually created separate forensic medicine departments and students were taught forensic medicine and toxicology in the later years of medical school.[38]

South Africa: English Law in Continental Courts

The introduction of legal medicine in Africa could be said to have started with the Dutch occupation of the South African cape during the seventeenth century. With the arrival of the British in the early nineteenth century, the legal system was transformed, becoming a mixed system that was part Dutch and part English common law. In Egypt, the process of legal change began, according to Khaled Fahmy, in the early nineteenth century with the introduction of European legal principals and forensic medicine practices by enlightened Egyptian Khedives of the Ottoman empire. With continued expansion, colonists reached out to the metropole for the medico-legal practices essential for control over the colonized societies and for providing justice and public health for its citizens. France occupied the central role in this process in the Magreb region beginning with Napoleon's Expedition and colonialization in 1798 and later by the many student educational missions and the transmission of European medico-legal practices through the translation of French legal codes into Arabic.[39]

The common law of Southern Africa was based on the Roman-Dutch law, which represented the system of laws that prevailed in the Netherlands from the fifteenth to eighteenth centuries. The Dutch brought this system of law to the Cape where it continued to develop in South Africa long after it was superseded by a Code in the Netherlands. It continues today as the foundation of the common law in the union of South African and all British African territories.[40]

Originally the fusion of Roman law with Dutch customs, Roman-Dutch law has been greatly influenced in various ways by Anglo-American law since the early part of the nineteenth century and later, after the Afrikaner republics became British colonies, during the Boer War 1899–1902. The most important contributions of the English common law are in the Laws of Evidence and Procedure, Criminal Law Procedure and Inquest Laws as applied in English Courts. Others included the procedures for post-mortem examination and dissection along with the designation of the legal next-of-kin, *naaste vrinden en bloedverwante*. Criminal trials in cases of murder, rape and serious assaults were conducted by a judge and a special jury. Post-mortem examinations performed by a physician, if possible, were mandated by the courts in all cases of homicide. South African judges did not hesitate to call upon other legal systems for guidance, particularly Anglo-American law, when the Roman-Dutch laws failed to meet the needs of society.[41]

Prior to Independence, south-west Africa and Southern Rhodesian had their own legislatures, with that of South Africa, all subject to the British Parliament. The Supreme Court of South Africa consisted of Appellate, Provincial and Local Divisions. Provincial courts had been established in Natal, Pretoria, Johannesburg (Witwatersrand), Durban and Kimberly, while inferior courts of South Africa are those controlled by the Magistrates and Justices of the Peace. Magistrate courts have jurisdiction over all criminal proceedings except murder, rape and treason which are referred to the Supreme Court. The whole of the Union and south-west Africa is policed by the South African Police with its administrative headquarters centred in Pretoria. This department has jurisdiction over and investigates all serious crimes.[42]

The state-employed district surgeons were mostly private medical practitioners who functioned on a part-time basis, appointed by district magistrates through the Department of Health. In south-west Africa they were under the control of the Medical Officer to the Administrate. Their principal duties were to investigate and examine complaints and assure persons in criminal matters as well as conduct post-mortem examinations and exhumations. Under the Inquests Act of 1914, British magistrates convened inquests and routinely requested assistance of physicians as medical experts.

Government pathologists performed official post-mortem examinations in Cape Town and Durban. In Johannesburg these examinations were carried out by trained medico-legal pathologists, assisted by district surgeons. In specialized specialties, such as toxicology examinations in the whole of the Union were performed by the Department of Agriculture at the Governmental Chemical Laboratory in Johannesburg. In Southern Rhodesia, government pathologists performed medico-legal autopsies at the public health laboratories in Salisbury and Bulawayo.[43] Under Public Health Acts, the public health officer could order compulsory autopsies in deaths from diseases which are suspected to be infectious or formidable epidemic diseases. In special cases, such as determining compensation for suspected silicosis deaths of native gold miners, medical practitioners were ordered to 'open the body of a deceased person whom he believes to have been a minor of native labourer ... preserve the respiratory organs of the deceased' and send them to the chemical laboratory for inspection.[44]

Roman-Dutch laws had little to say regarding the use of autopsies for medico-legal investigations. Instead, the laws were primarily concerned with the violation of graves and stealing of corpses. A very long tradition in Holland was to deliver the bodies of those who had been executed to the University of Leyden for anatomical studies and other scientific purposes.[45] In accordance with the Inquests Act, magistrates convene inquests and routinely request assistance of physicians as medical experts. Statutes authorized the performance of compulsory post-mortem examinations in cases of suspected homicide or unnatural death. 'The wishes of the deceased, the executor, or next-of-kin are clearly [to be] ignored', district surgeons were advised, 'and must be ignored'.[46]

For some medical observers, the existing medico-legal death investigation system fails to provide for adequate and consistent democratic justice. In South Africa, the forensic medical system of state-employed district surgeons and forensic pathologists is under the control of the South African Police Service (SAPS). The SAPS attend the death scene and is responsible for the physical infrastructure (morgues), and the district surgeons and forensic pathologists are required to use SAPS personnel. The intimate association of the SAPS with all aspects of the death investigation process has led to the perception of bias and manipulation within the system. Indeed, district surgeons are obligated to use and are bound to the facilities and staff of the SAPS, which has been implicated in the past for political killings.[47]

Most district surgeons have been forced to conduct autopsies under guiding control of the SAPS, and many believe that the police have hampered or attempted to influence their examinations in these cases. The incidence of torture is reported to occur in a high percentage of in-custody deaths. The majority of medico-legal autopsies carried out outside of South Africa's major cities are described as incomplete, superficial or inadequate, and purportedly performed by poorly trained district surgeons. Other problems include failure to maintain evidentiary chain of custody or to seek consultation with experienced regional forensic pathologists. Under these conditions, as a consequence, in South Africa, it is still believed by many medico-legal observers that a poor standard of death investigation is a continuing legacy of apartheid.[48]

As the European states acquired political control over vast overseas territories, they transported both their people and laws in the conquest of distant lands. With colonial expansion came the transmission of the European continental law and English common law across the globe. The goal was to develop new and productive countries under a western concept of the rule of law. Essential to maintaining the rule of law was the system of investigating sudden, unexpected and suspicious deaths. Colonists continued to function under the statutory laws developed for centuries under the foundation of Roman law and English common law. The latter was easily transported to distant lands where both colonist and indigenous peoples aspired for certainty and justice in the law. Medico-legal practices provided the protection of their colonists and the control of the indigenous peoples through the investigation of crime and surveillance and control of epidemics.

By the early 1850s, the connection between law and medicine had become well established in India, South Africa and other colonies with regard to the investigation of homicide cases. The physicians who responded to cases of sudden death had both public health and military backgrounds. They functioned as arms of the state controlling the local population and providing public health surveillance. Autopsies were an essential scientific tool for the police surgeon and aided in the administration of justice for both colonists and indigenous peoples. Colonies became medico-legal laboratories where physicians developed methods for the detection and prosecution of crime. Networks of colonial physicians were essential in the development of the science of ballistics, fingerprints, pathological anatomy and the control of public health epidemics and in their transmission to the metropole.

In recent years, nearly all of the previous colonial territories have undertaken efforts to reform their colonial death investigation systems mainly as the result of publicly humiliating errors. India, Australia, Canada, the United States and other prior colonies have abolished the coroner system or made major reforms to the system's legislation. In South Africa and other countries, modern reforms have not been successful in deterring the effects of the past colonial control of death investigation. In all former colonies, however, the foundations of past colonial death investigation practices are still visible in the courts and morgues.

NOTES

Bala, 'Introduction'

1. S. Marks and D. Engels (eds), *Contesting Colonial Hegemony: State and Society in Africa and India* (London: British Academic Press, 1994).
2. D. Ghosh and D. Kennedy (eds), *De-centering Empire: Britain, India and the Transcolonial World* (New Delhi: Orient Longman, 2006).
3. D. Arnold (ed.), *Imperial Medicine an Indigenous Societies* (Manchester: Manchester University Press, 1988); M. Vaughan, *Curing their Ills: Colonial Power and African Ilness* (Cambridge: Cambridge University Press, 1991); R. MacLeod and M. Lewis (eds), *Disease, Medicine and Empire* (London: Routledge, 1988).
4. H. Deacon, 'Racism and Medical Science in South Africa's Cape Colony in the Mid- to Late Nineteenth Century', *Osiris*, 27 (2000), pp. 190–206, on p. 190.
5. Ibid.
6. E. B. van Heyningen, 'Agents of Empire: The Medical Profession in the Cape Colony, 1880–1910', *Medical History*, 33 (1989), pp. 450–71, on p. 450.
7. A. Digby, *Diversity and Division in Medicine: Health Care in South Africa from the 1800s* (Oxford: Peter Lang, 2006), p. 27.
8. Ibid.
9. E. H. Burrows, *A History of Medicine in South Africa Up to the End of the Nineteenth Century* (A. A. Balkema, 1958). Burrows' study is a detailed portrayal of the contributions of surgeons and doctors who played a major role in establishing the medical profession, for instance, Dr William Stanger, D. H. Sauer and D. Poortsman.
10. A. A. Boahen, *African Perspectives on Colonialism* (Baltimore, MD: Johns Hopkins University Press, 1987).
11. Boahen, *African Perspectives*, p. 27. Variously explained, the sudden turn of events or the Scramble, or the Partition of Africa, is seen by some historians as being driven by the economy forces and the rising imperialism in Europe, or by political encounters between European powers or even by a combination of internal African situations and external European factors. For details the Scramble.
12. T. Ballantyne, 'Putting the Nation in its Place? World History and C. A. Bayly's *The Birth of the Modern World*', in A. Curthoys and M. Lake (eds), *Connected Worlds: History in Transnational Perspective* (Canberra: Australian National University E Press, 2005), pp. 23–44, on p. 30.
13. K. N. Chaudhuri, *Trade and Civilisation in the Indian Ocean: An Economic History from the Rise of Islam to 1750* (Cambridge: Cambridge University Press,1985). Other influ-

ential works include Curthoys and Lake (eds), *Connected Worlds*; S. Bose, 'Space and Time on the Indian Ocean Rim: Theory and History', in L. Fawaz and C. A. Bayly (eds), *Modernity and Culture: From the Mediterranean to the Indian Ocean, 1890–1920* (New York: Columbia University Press, 2002); for a more detailed account of global connections and the emergence of modernity, see C. A. Bayly, *The Birth of the Modern World, 1780-1914:Global Connections and Comparisons* (Malden: Blackwell, 2004).

14. A. Burton, 'Introduction', in A. Burton (ed.), *After the Imperial Turn: Thinking With and Through the Nation* (Durham, NC: Duke University Press, 2003), p. 2.

15. M. G. S. Hodgson, *Rethinking World History: Essays on Europe, Islam, and World History*, Edmund Burke 3rd edn (New York: Cambridge University Press, 1993).

16. B. Stutchey's remarkable study *Science Across the European Empires – 1800–1950* (London: Oxford University Press, 2005) offers useful insights into these engagements, and 'entangled histories' of the British, French, German and Dutch imperial powers, used by the colonized to resist colonial attempts at modernizing.

17. Ibid.

18. M. Harrison, *Medicine in the Age of Commerce and Empire: Britain and its Tropical Colonies, 1660–1830* (Oxford: Oxford University Press, 2010).

19. D. Arnold, *Colonizing the Body: State Medicine and Epidemic Disease in Nineteenth-Century India* (Berkeley, CA: University of California Press, 1993), pp. 8–10.

20. G. Prakash, *Another Reason: Science and the Imagination of Modern India* (Princeton, NJ: Princeton University Press), p. 199.

21. For a more detailed discussion on the concept, see J. C. Caldwell, P. Caldwell and P. Quiggen, 'The Social Context of Aids in Sub-Saharan Africa', *Population Development Review*, 15 (1989), pp. 185–235. For comparative histories, see P. W. Setel, 'Comparative Histories of Sexually Transmitted Diseases and HIV/AIDS in Africa: An Introduction', in P. Setel, M. Lewis and M. Lyons (eds), *Histories of Sexually Transmitted Diseases and HIV/AIDS in Sub-Saharan Africa* (Connecticut: Greenwood Press, 1999), pp.1–15, on p. 10.

22. For instance, a more recent study by M. U. Mushtaq, 'Public Health in British India: A Brief Account of the History of Medical Services and Disease Prevention in Colonial India', *Indian Journal of Community Medicine*, 34:1 (2009), pp. 6–14. Other key works include: J. Buckingham, *Leprosy in Colonial South India* (Basington: Palgrave, 2001); M. Harrison, *Public Health in British India: Anglo-Indian Preventive Medicine, 1859–1914* (Cambridge: Cambridge University Press, 1994).

23. R. Ramasubban, 'Imperial Health in British India, 1857–1900', in R. MacLeod and M. Lewis (eds), *Disease, Medicine and Empire* (London: Routledge, 1988), pp. 38–60.

24. I. Klein, 'Death in India, 1871–1921', *Journal of Asian Studies*, 22 (1973), pp. 639–59, on p. 656.

25. For details on exploratory travel account of various travellers, see S. Huigen, *Knowledge and Colonialism: Eighteenth-Century Travellers in South Africa* (Leiden: Brill, 2009). In this study, Huigen explores the ethnographic representations of travel accounts and in images during the period when the Cape Colony was under the Dutch East India Company and the Dutch State between 1652 and 1814. Several books were written on the indigenous population.

26. K. E. Flint, *Healing Traditions: African Medicine, Cultural Exchange, and Competition in South Africa, 1820–1948* (Athens, OH: Ohio University Press, 2008).

27. A. Ricardo Lopez and B. Weinstein (eds), *The Making of a Middle Class: Toward a Trans-National History* (Durham, NC: Duke University Press, 2012), p. 5.

28. Ibid., p. 11.
29. Ayurveda is one of the oldest medical systems practised in India. Its origins are documented in the oldest repositories of Indian culture, the Vedas. Besides, Unani medicine, or Unani-Tibb, is also being practised alongside Ayurveda. The two together constitute important knowledge systems of medical pluralism in India.
30. M. Echenberg's remarkable work, *Plague Ports: The Global Urban Impact of Bubonic Plague, 1894–1901* (New York: New York University Press, 2007) focusses on the third and largest plague epidemic (1894–1950) that unravels new patterns and analytical frameworks within which colonial transformations took place.
31. The divergence was also responsible for the political and social conflicts, aggravated by the professionalizing medicine and the nationalist reactions in the late nineteenth and early twentieth centuries. I have discussed this in my earlier works, especially *Imperialism and Medicine in Bengal: A Socio-Historical Perspective* (New Delhi: Sage, 1991).
32. Echenberg, *Plague Ports*, p. 3.
33. M. Few and Z. Tortorici (eds), *Centering Animals in Latin American History* (Durham, NC: Duke University Press, 2013). Their study focusses on animal–human interaction and the former's role in the colonizing process in Latin America – Mexico, Guatemala, the Dominican Republic, Puerto Rico, Cuba, Chile, Brazil, Peru and Argentina.
34. K. Soman, 'Women, Medicine and Politics of Gender: Institution of Traditional Midwives in Twentieth-Century Bengal' (Occasional Paper) November 2011 (Institute of Development Studies, Kolkata), pp. 1–36, on p. 1.
35. David Washbrook explains modernity in Max Weber's view of an 'ideal-typical set of qualities which he argues, may (or may not) be actually realised in any particular social and cultural setting'. See D. Washbrook, 'Intimations of Modernity in South India', *South Asian History and Culture*, 1:1 (2010), pp. 125–48, on pp. 125–6. This can be translated into 'coercive' aspects of colonial encounters with the colonized.
36. Colonial psychiatry has been discussed at length by Sally Swartz, 'Colonialism and the Production of Psychiatric Knowledge in the Cape, 1891–1920' (PhD thesis, University of Cape Town, 1996). Sally Swartz's work has been cited by H. Deacon, 'Racial Categories and Psychiatry in Africa: The Asylum on Robben Island in the Nineteenth Century', in W. Ernst and B. Harris, *Race, Science and Medicine, 1700–1960* (London and New York: Routledge, 1999), pp. 101–22, on p. 101.
37. Deacon, 'Racial Categories and Psychiatry in Africa'.
38. Ibid.
39. N. Stepan, 'Race, Science and Medicine: Citizenship and the Natural', Paper presented at the conference on Race, Science and Medicine, Southampton, September 1996, p. 8. Cited by W. Ernst. 'Introduction: Historical and Contemporary Perspectives on Race, Science and Medicine', in Ernst and Harris (eds), *Race, Science and Medicine*, pp. 1–28, on p. 4.
40. A. Digby's, *Diversity and Division in Medicine: Health Care in South Africa from the 1880s* (Oxford: Peter Lang, 2006), is, by far, the most comprehensive study on the social history of medicine in South Africa. Focussing on the Cape, Digby offers interesting insights into the role of patients/clientele and practitioners as enabling the emergence of new practices of 'healers', missionaries, doctors and nurses.
41. N. Rosenberg, *Inside the Black Box* (Cambridge: Cambridge University Press, 1982), p. 245. On a similar note Jan Todd provides an illustrative account of the transfer of technology in Australia, especially chapter 13. See J. Todd, *Colonial Technology: Science and the Transfer of Innovation to Australia* (Cambridge: Cambridge University Press, 1995).

1 Bala, '"Re-Constructing" Indian Medicine: The Role of Caste in Late Nineteenth- and Twentieth-Century India'

1. This includes Ayurveda and Unani.
2. Lord Montague was the Secretary of State for India from 1917 to 1922, and Lord Chelmsford was the Viceroy of India from 1916 to 1921.
3. G. Prakash, *Another Reason: Science and the Imagination of Modern India* (Princeton, NJ: Princeton University Press, 1998), p. 52.
4. M. N. Srinivas, *The Dominant Caste and Other Essays* (New York and London: Oxford University Press, 1987), p. 44.
5. See P. Bala (ed.), *Biomedicine as a Contested Site: Some Revelations in Imperial Contexts* (Lanham: Lexington, 2009).
6. For a detailed discussion, see D. Wujastyk and F. M. Smith (eds), *Modern and Global Ayurveda: Pluralism and Paradigms* (New York: State University of New York Press, 2008).
7. Ibid., p. 2.
8. The NMI was founded in 1822 but ceased to exist following a decision to introduce European sciences and English education. During his period, it had trained few medical men as Native Doctors.
9. The decision to introduce English as the official language followed the victory of those favouring this over education in Indian languages. This followed from Lord Macaulay's Minute on education which was endorsed by William Bentinck in 1835.
10. See details in R. Richardson, *Death, Dissection and the Destitute* (Harmondsworth: Penguin, 1988).
11. Gruesome murders were carried out in Edinburgh as a well in London. For details, see H. MacDonald, *Human Remains: Dissection and its Histories* (New Haven, CT: Yale University Press, 2006), pp. 23–7 (published in Australia as *Human Remains: Episodes in Human Dissection* (Carlton: Melbourne University Press, 2005).
12. H. MacDonald, 'Procuring Corpses: The English Anatomy Inspectorate, 1842 to 1858', *Medical History*, 53:3 (2009), pp. 379–96, on p. 379. The lingering doubts were confirmed by the 'unlawful' strategies adopted by the anatomy inspectorate, demonstrated by MacDonald. For a detailed discussion on this issue, see also the Organ Donation Taskforce's report, *Organs for Transplants: A Report* (London, Department of Health, January 2008); see also Macdonald, 'Procuring Corpses', note 2. It was the unpopularity of the series of murders carried out by Burke and Hare in the West Port of Edinburgh in 1828 that alarmed the public mind and the authorities, compelling the government to legislate medical practice in a more 'professional manner.' Besides, the discovery that 'sixteen persons were suffocated by William Burke and William Hare during eleven months, and that the bodies had been sold to the Edinburgh anatomist, Dr. Robert Knox, who "asked no questions", influenced the public so unfavourably'. See D. F. Harris, 'History of the Events which Led to the Passing of the British Anatomy Act, A.D. 1832', *Canadian Medical Association Journal*, 10:3 (1920), pp. 283–4, on p. 283. The impact of these activities was so severe and alarming that the term 'burking' came to be used in discussions on the Anatomy Bill in the House of the Commons; there was often a move to protect the poor from being 'burked'. See Harris, 'History of the Events', p. 24.
13. For a detailed discussion on the evolution of anatomical and surgical practices in England, see E. T. Hurren, *Dying for Victorian Medicine: English Anatomy and its Trade in the Dead Poor, c. 1834–1929* (New York: Palgrave Macmillan, 2011).

14. S. Alavi, *Islam and Healing*, cited by R. Berger, 'From the Biomoral to the Biopoliti-cal: Ayurveda's Political Histories,' *South Asian History and Culture* (December 2012), pp.1–17, on p. 4.

15. D. Kopf, *British Orientalism and the Bengal Renaissance: The Dynamics of Indian Mod-ernization, 1773–1835* (Berkeley, CA: University of California Press, 1969), p. 288.

16. Ibid., p. 257. I have also discussed the trajectory in one of my earlier works, *Medicine and Medical Polices in India: Social and Historical Perspectives* (Lanham: Lexington, 2007), p. 257. The College was founded in 1816 by Calcutta's influential patrons to provide their sons with an 'advantageous European knowledge.' Details on the history can also be found in *Presidency College Centenary Volume* (Alipore: West Bengal Government Press, 1955), pp. 301, 303.

17. He led a group of young men of Calcutta in developing a critical thinking of the cultural traditions of India, for which he was vehemently criticized, and led the Young Bengal movement that seemed drawn away from reinterpretation of Indian traditions. Details from Kopf, *British Orientalism and the Bengal Renaissance*, p. 254.

18. A majority of them came from the trader caste with 'obscure 'origins who adopted the cultural customs of higher castes, a process described by M. N. Srinivas as "Sanskritiza-tion'. For details, see M. N. Srinivas, 'Note on Sanskritization and Westernization,' *Far Eastern Quarterly*, 15:4 (August 1956), pp. 481–96.

19. Kopf, *British Orientalism and the Bengal Renaissance*, pp. 67–8.

20. T. Laffan, *The Medical Profession* (Dublin: Fannin, 1888), p. 131. For details on profes-sionalism and its location in social mobility, see N. Parry and J. Parry, *The Rise of the Medical Profession: A Study of Collective Social Mobility* (Cambridge: Croom Helm, 1976).

21. For details see, H. Singh, *Colonial Hegemony and Popular Resistance; Princes, Peasants and Paramount Power* (California: Alta Mira Press, 1998).

22. Prakash, *Another Reason*, pp. 57–9.

23. Ibid., p. 58.

24. A. Witz, 'Colonising Women: Female Medical Practice in Colonial India, 1880–1890', in A. Hardy and L. Conrad (eds), *Women and Modern Medicine* (Amsterdam: B. V. Rodopi, 2001), pp. 23–52, on p. 37.

25. N. Hassan, *Diagnosing Empire: Women, Medical Knowledge, and Colonial Mobility* (London: Ashgate, 2011), p. 89; L. Conrad and A. Hardy (eds), *Women and Modern Medicine* (Amsterdam: Rodopi B.V., 2001).

26. Hassan, *Diagnosing Empire*, p. 107.

27. Ibid.

28. M. F. Billington, *Woman in India*, with an Introduction by the Marchioness of Dufferin and Ava (London: Chapman and Hall, 1895).

29. A. Witz, 'Colonising Women: Female Medical Practice in Colonial India, 1880–1890', in Hardy and Conrad (eds), *Women and Modern Medicine*, pp. 23–52, on p. 37.

30. She was an ardent pioneer of female medical education, was one of the first five women to receive a license to practice medicine from the Kings' and Queens' Colleges of Physi-cians, Ireland in 1877. The others were Elizabeth Walker Dunbar, Louisa Atkins, Edith Pechey and Sophia Jex-Blake. See E. Lutzker, *Women Gain a Place in Medicine* (New York: McGraw-Hill, 1969).

31. Krupabai Satthianadhan lived from 1862 to 1896. Hailed as a prolific writer, and one of the first women to have been admitted to medical schools in India and Britain. More information can be obtained from Hassan, *Diagnosing Empire*.

32. Especially Hassan, *Diagnosing Empire*, ch. 4.
33. As reported in the 1901 Census, in 1891, the Anglo-native daily newspapers (i.e., papers written in English, but owned, edited and read by natives) had an estimated circulation of 3,400 copies. In 1900, the number of such papers had risen to five and the aggregate circulation to 16,800, whereas in 1881, there were six daily papers written in Bengali language had risen from twenty-four to thirty-four, and the circulation from 33,529 to 112,553, with none reported in Hindi, Urdu or Oriya. E. A. Gait, *Census of India* (Calcutta: Bengal Secretariat Press, 1902), vol. 6, p. 492.
34. S. Alavi, 'Unani Medicine in the Nineteenth-Century Public Sphere: Urdu Texts and the Oudh Akbar', cited in Berger, *Biomorality*, p. 4.
35. P. C. Ray, *Life and Experiences of a Bengali Chemist* (Calcutta: Chuckervetty, Chatterjee & Co., 1932).
36. Cited from Prakash, *Another Reason*, p. 54, fn 12. Details from P. Sinha, *Nneteenth Century Bengal: Aspects of Social History* (Calcutta: Firma K. L. Mukhopadhyaya, 1965).
37. They exist as the oldest repositories of Hindu society culture.
38. K. C. Mitra, *Hindu Medicine and Medical Education* (Calcutta: R. C. Lepage & Co., Metropolitan Press, 1865), p. 1.
39. For details on his life, see Ray, *Life and Experiences of a Bengali Chemist*.
40. R. Berger, 'Ayurveda and the Making of the Urban Middle Class in North India, 1900–1945', in Wujastyk and Smith (eds), *Modern and Global Ayurveda*, pp. 101–15, on p. 109.
41. *Indian Scientific Biographical Sketches* (Madras, 1929), p. 34. Cited from D. Arnold, *Science, Technology and Medicine in Colonial India* (Cambridge: Cambridge University Press, 2000), p. 158.
42. Arnold, *Science, Technology and Medicine in Colonial India*, p. 159.
43. Mahendralal Sircar, 'On the Desirability of Cultivation of the Sciences by the Natives of India', *Calcutta Journal of Medicine*, 2 (1869), pp. 286–91.
44. Hassan, *Diagnosing Empire*.
45. Z. Baber, 'Colonizing Nature: Scientific Knowledge, Colonial Power and the Incorporation of India into the Modern World-System', *British Journal of Sociology*, 52:1 (March 2001), pp. 37–58.
46. L. Carroll, 'Colonial Perceptions of Indian Society and the Emergence of Caste(s) Associations', *Journal of Asian Studies*, 37:2 (February 1978), pp. 233–50, on p. 250.
47. Ibid., p. 244.
48. Jean Langord provides an interesting account of the concept of medical 'mimicry' or adoption of western methods in indigenous medicine which she describes as the universality of European science. J. Langford. *Fluent Bodies: Ayurvedic Remedies for Postcolonial Imbalance* (Durham, NC: Duke University Press, 2002), p. 6.
49. A leading advocate of the Ayurvedic movement, he saw in this organization a new agenda for 'self-determination' and self-management of medical practice.
50. Practitioners of Ayurvedic medicine
51. With the idea of promoting indigenous knowledge in the local language, Varier wrote several medical books in the local language of Malyalam to make them accessible to the local population.
52. Bengal was divided along religious lines by the then Viceroy, Lord Curzon to manage administration of the country. This was a religious as well as geographical demarcation with a Hindu majority in the western and Muslim majority in the eastern half of Bengal.
53. Prakash, *Another Reason*, p. 199.

54. P. C., *The Nation and Its Fragments: Colonial and Postcolonial Histories* (Princeton, NJ: Princeton University Press, 1993)
55. Prakash, *Another Reason*, p. 89.
56. H. Singh, *Colonial Hegemony and Popular Resistance: Princes, Peasants, and Paramount Power* (Toronto: Canadian Scholars' Press, 1998), p. 165.
57. Arnold, *Science, Technology and Medicine in Colonial India*, p. 70.
58. P. Bala, *Contesting Colonial Authority: Medicine and Indigenous Responses in 19th and 20th-Century India* (Lanham: Lexington, 2012).
59. Bala, *Imperialism and Medicine in Bengal*, p. 90.
60. He wrote this in two volumes over a period of seven years, between 1902 and 1909.
61. P. Chakrabarti, 'Medical Marketplace beyond the West: Bazaar Medicine, Trade and the English Establishment in Eighteenth-Century India', in M. S. R. Jenner and P. Wallis (eds), *Medicine and the Market in England and its Colonies, c. 1450–1850* (Basingstoke: Palgrave Macmillan, 2007), pp. 196–215, on p. 204.
62. *Ayurveda Ka Vaigyanik Swaroop* (Kangri: Gurukul Yantralaya, 1918). See Prakash, *Another Reason*, pp. 256–7, n. 38.
63. H. Alavi, *Capitalism and Colonial Production* (London: Croom Helm, 1982), p.36.
64. C. Gordon (ed.), *Power/Knowledge: Selected Interviews and Other Writings 1972–1977*, by Michael Foucault, trans. Colin Gordon, Leo Marshall, John Mepham and Kate Soper (New York: Pantheon Books, 1977), pp. 170–1, on p. 170.
65. For details, see M. U. Mushtaq, 'Public Health in British India: A Brief Account of the History of Medical Services and Disease Prevention in Colonial India', *Indian Journal of Community Medcine*, 34:1 (January 2009), pp. 6–14.
66. R. Nair, 'The Construction of a "Population Problem" in Colonial India, 1919–1947', *Journal of Imperial Commonwealth History*, 39:2 (2011), pp. 227–47.
67. W. Halbfass, *India and Europe: An Essay in Understanding* (New York: State University of New Yorks Press, 1988), p. 399. See also Arnold, *Science, Technology and Medicine in Colonial India*, p.170.
68. Home Proceedings (Education), 5–9 February 1902, NAI.
69. This has been quoted with permission, from the Asiatic Society website, Kolkata, official communication, July 2013:
   'This was the first speech delivered in January 1784 prior to the establishment of the Society. Starting with 30 Europeans as members, The Asiatic Society was variously named as The Asiatic Society (1784–1825), The Asiatic Society (1825–1832), The Asiatic Society of Bengal (1832–1935), The Royal Asiatic Society of Bengal (1936–1951) and The Asiatic Society again since July 1951. It gradually opened membership to Indians in 1829, with opportunities for research and publications alongside. The earliest Indian members of the Society were Prasanna Kumar Tagore, Dwarkanath Tagore, Russamay Dutt and Ram Camul Sen. It was not until December 1832 that Radhakanta Deb was invited to become a member. Rajendra Lal Mitra (1822–1891) assumed responsibility as the first Indian President of the Society'.
70. Baber, 'Colonizing Nature', p. 47.
71. N. B. Dirks, *The Hollow Crown: Ethnohistory of an Indian Kingdom* (Cambridge: Cambridge University Press, 1987), p. 282.
72. Arnold, *Science, Technology and Medicine in Colonial India*, p. 35.
73. Ibid., p. 34.
74. He was a Tamil Brahmin Sanskrit scholar

75. He submitted the report in 1923 and in 1925 was appointed as the head of the Government School of Indian Medicine. See details in Dr G. Srinivasa Murti Foundation, *The Doctor G. Srinivasa Murti Birth Centenary* (Madras and Bangalore: Dr G. Srinivasa Murti Foundation, 1987), pp. 2-4. See also Prakash, *Another Reason*.

76. The college was an amalgamation of the extant Ayurvedic Colleges – Astanga Ayurvedic College, Baidyashastrapith and the Govinda Sundari Ayurvedic College; G. Mukhopadhyaya, *History of Indian Medicine* (Calcutta: University of Calcutta, 1926), vol. 2.

77. Kopf, *British Orientalism and Bengal Renaissance*, p. 5. Bengal is characterized by the existence of a middle class which resulted from various policies governing the land system simultaneous with the destruction of Indian industries. As rent-receivers and with an increasing income, they amassed huge fortunes which enabled them to respond to British calls for western and English education. "The entire socio-economic and cultural context, thus, created a new social category, identified neither with the class owning the means of production nor with those selling labour for survival." The latter quote is drawn from For B. Chakrabarty, *The Partition of Bengal and Assam, 1932–1947: Contour of Freedom* (London: RoutledgeCurzon, 2004), p. 244.

78. A. Irwin and B. Wynne (eds), *Misunderstanding Science? The Public Reconstruction of Science and Technology* (Cambridge: Cambridge University Press, 1996); R. A. Harris (ed.), *Landmark Essays on Rhetoric of Science: Case Studies* (New Jersey: Lawrence Erlbaum Associates, 2004).

79. S. Locke, 'Sociology and the Public Understanding of Science: From Rationlisation to Rhetoric,' *British Journal of Sociology*, 52:1 (March 2001), pp. 1–18, on p. 14.

80. Prakash, *Another Reason*, p. 129.

81. Prakash discusses this at length in *Another Reason*, ch. 5.

82. See notes 59 and 60 in Sarkar's essay in this volume.

2 Phatlane, 'The Resurgence of Indigenous Medicine in the Age of the HIV/AIDS Pandemic: South Africa beyond the "Miracle"'

1. S. Dubow, *South Africa's Struggle for Human Rights: A Jacana Pocket History* (Johannesburg: Jacana Media, 2012), p. 9.

2. A. Carlsson, 'Controversy between Politics and Science when South Africa Handles the AIDS Epidemic', online at http://www.axess.se/english//currentissue/essay.php (2004), p. 2. [accessed 10 March 2009].

3. D. M. Tutu, 'Foreword', K. D. Kauffman and D. L. Lindauer, *AIDS and South Africa: The Social Expression of a Pandemic* (New York: Palgrave Macmillan, 2004), p. xi.

4. A. Whiteside and C. Sunter, *AIDS: The Challenge for South Africa* (Cape Town: Human and Rousseau, 2000), p. 118.

5. J. N. Hays, *The Burdens of Disease: Epidemics and Human Response in Western History* (London: Rutgers university Press, 1998), p. 240.

6. T. Mbeki, Remarks at the first meeting of the Presidential Advisory Panel on AIDS, online at http://www.anc.org.za (2000a) [accessed 16 April 2009].

7. A. Jeeves, 'Introduction', *South African Historical Journal*, 45 (2001), pp. 1–10, on p. 9.

8. M. Jacobs, 'The Role of Traditional Medicine in a Changing South Africa', *Critical Health*, 43 (1993), p. 73.

9. P. W. Setel, M. Lewis and M. Lyons (eds), *Histories of Sexually Transmitted Diseases and HIV/AIDS in sub-Saharan Africa* (London: Greenwood Press, 1999), p. 31.

10. 'WHO Says African Herbs are Crucial', *Business Day Newspaper*, 1 September 2003, p. 3.

11. B. Stein, *A History of India* (United Kingdom: Wiley Blackwell, 2010), p. 253.

12. M. L. Arthur, 'A Fundamental Pedagogical Perspective on Multicultural Education with Special Reference to Tertiary Institutions' (M.Ed dissertation, Unisa, 1992), p. 1.

13. F. Capra, *The Turning Point: Science, Society and the Rising Culture* (London: Flamingo, 1983), p. 12.

14. H. Holland, *African Magic: Traditional Ideas that Heal a Continent* (Durban: Viking, 2001), p. 7.

15. S. N. Phatlane, 'Poverty, Health and Disease in the Era of High Apartheid: South Africa 1948–1976' (PhD thesis, Unisa, 2006), p. 234.

16. Personal communication with Ngaka Conrad Tsiane on March 21, 2008. 'Ngaka' is a Sepedi word which refers to a practitioner of indigenous medicine without distinction as to herbalist, sangoma, diviner etc.

17. Personal communication with Ngaka Mmamoraka Phalane on 25 February 2007.

18. Personal communication with Ngaka Tsiane on 21 March 2008.

19. K. L. Fontaine, *Healing Practices: Alternative Therapies for Nursing* (New Jersey: Prentice-Hall, 2000), p. 12.

20. R. E. Spector, *Cultural Diversity in Health and Illness* (Connecticut: Appleton Century, 1985), p. xi.

21. M. Green, 'Africa Unlocks Herbal Secrets to Fight AIDS', *Citizen Newspaper*, 16 April 2002, p. 22.

22. N. Motlana, quoted in M. Freeman and M. Motsei, 'Planning Health Care in South Africa – Is there a Role for Traditional Healers?', *Social Science & Medicine*, 34:11 (1992), pp. 1183–90, on p. 1186.

23. Personal communication with Dr Philimon Maepa on 10 February 2007.

24. E. E. Evans-Pritchard, *Witchcraft, Oracles and Magic among the Azande* (London: Oxford University Press, 1937), p. 12.

25. F. Staugård, *Traditional Medicine in Botswana* (Gaborone: Ipelegeng Publishers, 1985), p. 68.

26. R. Jeffrey, *The Politics of Health in India* (Berkeley, CA: University of California Press, 1988), p. 19. For more on this topic, see, P. Bala, '"Defying" Medical Autonomy: Indigenous Elites and Medicine in Colonial India', in P. Bala (ed.), *Biomedicine as a Contested Site: Some Revelations in Imperial Contexts* (Lanham: Lexington Books, 2009), p. 39.

27. P. Bala, *Imperialism and Medicine in Bengal: A Socio-Historical Perspective* (New Delhi: Sage Publications, 1991).

28. R. S. Viljoen, 'Medicine, Medical Knowledge and Healing at the Cape of Good Hope: Khoikhoi, Slaves and Colonists', in P. Bala (ed.), *Medicine and Colonialism: Historical Perspectives in India and South Africa* (forthcoming, 2014), p. 1.

29. D. Arnold, *Colonizing the Body: State Medicine and Epidemic Disease in Nineteenth Century India* (California: University of California Press, 1993), p. 7. See also, D. Arnold, *Imperial Medicine and Indigenous Societies* (Manchester: Manchester University Press, 1988) and for a comprehensive history, one may also see, P. Bala, *Imperialism and Medicine in Bengal: A Socio-Historical Perspective*.

30. D. Arnold, *Science, Technology and Medicine in Colonial India* (Cambridge: Cambridge University Press, 2000), p. 15.

31. RSA, Department of Information, *Report from South Africa* (1972), p. 27.

32. Bala, '"Defying" Medical Autonomy', p. 30.

33. Arnold, *Colonizing the Body*.

34. NASA, TES 7159 56/76 the witch-doctors in Natal and Zululand.
35. A. Jeeves, 'Introduction', *South African Historical Journal*, 45 (2001), pp. 1–10.
36. NASA, TES 7159 56/76, the witch-doctors in Natal and Zululand.
37. Ibid.
38. Personal communication with Msongelwa. Ntuli, on 20 February 2010.
39. See, S. Warshaw and C. D. Bromwell, *A Concise History of India from its Origins to the Present* (San Francisco, CA: Canfield Press, 1974), p. 47.
40. E. C. Green and L. Makhubu, 'Traditional Healers in Swaziland: Towards Improved Cooperation between Traditional and Modern Health Sectors', *Social Science & Medicine*, 18:12 (1984), pp. 1071–9, on p. 1074.
41. Heyl, quoted in T. Sodi, 'Towards Recognition of Indigenous Healing: Prospects and Constraints', *CHASA: Journal of Comprehensive Health*, 7:1 (1996), p. 7.
42. T. Sodi, 'Towards Recognition of Indigenous Healing: Prospects and Constraints', *Chasa: Journal of Comprehensive Health*, 7:1 (1996), pp. 5–9, on pp. 7–8.
43. T. Masemola, 'Legislating Traditional Ways', *Sunday Tribune Newspaper*, 5 October 2003, p. 10.
44. Holland, *African Magic: Traditional Ideas that Heal a Continent*, p. 12.
45. N. Nattrass, *Mortal Combat: AIDS Denialism and the Struggle for Antiretrovirals in South Africa* (Scottsville: University of Kwazulu Natal Press, 2007), p. 44. See also, C. Terreblanche, 'Minister Withholds Details of HIV/AIDS Treatment Options', *Cape Times Newspaper*, 14 May 2003, p. 6.
46. K. Foss, 'Traditional Medicine Needs Recognition', *Star Newspaper*, 21 May 2009, p. 2.
47. S. Terreblanche, *A History of Inequality in South Africa, 1652–2002* (Pietermaritzburg: University of Kwazulu Natal Press, 2002), p. 3.
48. J. E. Bereda, 'Traditional Healing as a Health Care Delivery System in a Trans-cultural Society' (MA dissertation: Unisa, 2002); F. M. Mulaudzi, 'Women and Sexually Transmitted Diseases: An Exploration of Indigenous Knowledge and Health Practices Among the Vhavenda' (PhD thesis: Unisa, 2003); S. N. Shai-Mahoko, 'The Role of Indigenous Healers in Disease Prevention and Health Promotion Among Black South Africans: A Case Study of the North West Province' (PhD thesis: Unisa, 1997).
49. A. Jeeves, 'Public Health in the Era of South Africa's Syphilis Epidemic of the 1930s and 1940s', *South African Historical Journal*, 45 (2001), 79–102, on pp. 82–3.
50. IADJ, SGJ Box 201 File 59/5, *Star Newspaper* 20/6/1946.
51. P. J. Furlong, 'Improper Intimacy: Afrikaner Churches, the National Party and the Anti-Miscegenation Laws', *South African Historical Journal*, 31 (1994), pp. 55–71, on p. 67.
52. Shai-Mahoko, *The Role of Indigenous Healers in Disease Prevention and Health Promotion Among Black South Africans*, p. 30.
53. Mulaudzi, *Women and Sexually Transmitted Diseases*. p. 57.
54. Personal communication with Sop Ntuli, on 13 March 2009.
55. Personal communication with Ngaka Enicar Mkhonto on 16 May 2009.
56. Personal communication with Ngaka Hlathikhulu Ngobeni on 13 March 2008.
57. Mulaudzi, *Women and Sexually Transmitted Diseases*, p. 61.
58. Personal communication with Ngaka Tsiane, on 21 March 2008.
59. C. Smith, 'Calling all Sangomas', *Business Day Newspaper*, 6 July 2001, p. 9.
60. L. Clark, 'I was on the Way Out: Now I am Working', *Sunday Independent Newspaper*, 26 May 2002, p. 5.
61. Z. Mkhuma, 'Sole Survivor of "Aids Cure" Charmer ... But They Were Not So Lucky', *Star*, 24 July 2003, p. 19.

62. Masemola, 'Legislating Traditional Ways' *Sunday Tribune*, 5 October 2003, pp. 9–10.

63. M. Zondi, 'Drug from Traditional Herb Offers Help to AIDS Patients', *Saturday Star Newspaper*, 13 January 2001, p. 10.

64. K. Van Rijn, 'The Politics of Uncertainty: The AIDS Debate, Thabo Mbeki and the South African Government', *Social History of Medicine*, 19:3 (2006), pp. 521–38, on p. 522.

65. M. Green, 'Africa Unlocks Herbal Secrets to Fight AIDS', *Citizen*, 16 April 2002, p. 22. See also, R. Thornton, 'The Transmission of Knowledge in South African Traditional Healing', *Africa*, 79:1 (2009), pp. 17–34.

66. F. Peete, 'Plea for State, Traditional Healers to Work Together', *Pretoria News*, 15 March 2001, p. 2.

67. Z. Mapumulo, 'Traditional Medicine Not Taboo', *Sowetan Newspaper*, 23 February 2004, p. 6.

68. ANC, *National Health Plan for South Africa* (Johannesburg, ANC, 2004), p. 10.

69. RSA, 'Draft Policy on African Traditional Medicine for South Africa', *Government Gazette*, 517: 31271 (2008), p. 12.

70. S. N. Phatlane, 'Poverty and HIV/AIDS in Apartheid South Africa', *Social Identities: Journal for the Study of Race, Nation and Culture*, 9:1 (2003), p. 87.

71. R. L. Ostergard and C. Barcelo, 'Personalist Regimes and the Insecurity Dilemma: Prioritizing AIDS as a National Security Threat in Uganda', in *The African State and the AIDS Crisis*, ed. A. S. Patterson (Aldershot: Ashgate, 2005), pp. 155–69.

72. H. Phillips, 'AIDS in the Context of South Africa's Epidemic History: Preliminary Historical Thoughts', *South African Historical Journal*, 45 (2001), pp. 11–26.

73. T. Mbeki, 'Speech at the Opening Session of the 13th International AIDS Conference in Durban (SA)', online at http://www.anc.org.za (2000b) [accessed 16 April 2009].

74. S. P. Molakeng, 'First Traditional Hospital Opens in Mpumalanga', *Sowetan*, 6 October 1998.

75. K. Sunker, 'Traditional Healers Pool Skills', *Pretoria News*, 2 October 2001, p. 8.

76. T. Kahn, 'Call for Traditional Cure for AIDS-Sufferers Rises', *Business Day*, 3 September 2003, p. 4.

77. J. De Beer, 'A Forward View of Health Services in South Africa', *South African Medical Journal*, 50 (1976), p. 433.

78. E. M. Mankazana, 'The Case for the Traditional Healer in South Africa', *South African Medical Journal*, 56:23 (1979), pp. 1003–7.

79. T. Asuni, 'The Dilemma of Traditional Healing with Special Reference to Nigeria', *Social Science and Medicine*, 13 (1979), pp. 33–9, on p. 37.

80. D. Wujastyk and F. M. Smith (eds), *Modern and Global Ayurveda: Pluralism and Paradigms* (New York: State University of New York Press, 2008), p. 246.

3 Viljoen, 'Medicine, Medical Knowledge and Healing at the Cape of Good Hope: Khoikhoi, Slaves and Colonists'

1. See R. Viljoen, 'Medicine, Health and Medical Practice in Precolonial Society: An Anthropological-Historical Perspective', *History and Anthropology*, 11:4 (1999), pp. 552–3; G. Scott and M. L. Hewett, 'Pioneers in Ethnopharmacology: The Dutch East India Company (VOC) at the Cape from 1650–1800', *Journal of Ethnopharmacology*, 115:13 (2008), pp. 339–60.

2. O. F. Mentzel, *A Geographical and Topographical Description of the Cape of Good Hope, Part 1.* (Van Riebeeck Society: Cape Town, no.4, 1921), p. 113.

3. C. P. Thunberg, *Travels in Europe, Africa and Asia, 1770–1779, Vol. 1* (London, 1795), p. 225.

4. H. Leibbrandt, *Precis of the Archives of the Cape of Good Hope: Letters Despatched from the Cape, 1652–1662, Vol. 3* (Cape Town, 1900), p. 116.

5. Ibid., p. 153.

6. R. Raven-Hart, *Cape Good Hope 1652–1707: The First Fifty Years of Dutch Colonisation as seen by Callers. Vol. 1* (Cape Town: A. A. Balkema, 1971), p. 193.

7. I. Bruijn, *Ship's Surgeons of the Dutch East India Company* (Leiden: Leiden University Press, 2009), pp. 91, 112.

8. Ibid., pp. 104–6.

9. Ibid., pp. 109–12.

10. G. C. Botha, *History of Law, Medicine and Place Names in the Cape of Good Hope* (Cape Town: C. Struik, 1962), pp. 180–4. See also J. Franken, 'Die Hugenote aan die Kaap', in *Argiefjaarboek vir Suid-Afrikaanse Geskiedenis* (Pretoria, 1978), pp. 154–7, 163, 170.

11. J. Hoge, 'Personalia of the Germans at the Cape, 1652–1806', in *Archives Year Book for South African History* (Cape Town, 1946), pp. 9, 12, 21 22, 31, 33, 34, 108.

12. C. Price, 'Medicine and Pharmacy at the Cape of Good Hope, 1652–1807', *Medical History*, 6 (1962), p. 169.

13. A. Sparrman, *A Voyage to the Cape of Good Hope towards the Antartic Polar Circle round the world and to the Country of the Hottentots and Caffres from the year 1772–1776, Vol. 1*, 2nd series, no. 6 (Cape Town: Van Riebeeck Society, 1975), p. 93.

14. W. McNeill, *Plagues and Peoples* (Oxford: Basil Blackwell, 1976), p. 239.

15. D. Moodie, *The Record or Series of Official papers relative to the Condition and Treatment of the Native Tribes of South Africa* (Cape Town: A. A. Balkema, 1959), p. 46.

16. Ibid., p. 347 for more examples.

17. Raven-Hart, *Cape Good Hope 1652–1702*, vol. 1, p. 68.

18. Ibid., vol. 2, pp. 436–7.

19. P. Kolb, *The Present State of the Cape of Good Hope, Vol. 1* (New York: Reprint, 1968), pp. 302–11.

20. Moodie, *The Record*, p. 46.

21. Raven-Hart, *Cape Good Hope 1652–1702*, vol. 1, pp. 21–2.

22. Moodie, *The Record*, p. 317.

23. Ibid., p. 347 note at the bottom of page.

24. See *Suid-Afrikaanse Argiefstukke, Kaap no.2; Resolusies van die Politieke Raad, Deel 2, 1670–1680* (Cape Town, 1959), pp. 72, 73, 75.

25. McNeill, *Plagues and Peoples*, p. 199.

26. E. Le Roy Ladurie, *The Mind and Method of the Historian* (Chicago, IL: University of Chicago Press, 1984), p. 29.

27. According to Thunberg the following diseases were identified on board ships: spotted fevers, putrid fevers, catarrhal fevers, malignant ulcers, abscess, scurvy, rheumatism, coughs, diarrhoea, dysentery and venereal diseases. Thunberg, *Travels in Europe, Africa and Asia*, 91. See also M. Boucher, *The Cape of Good Hope and Foreign Contacts 1735–1755* (Pretoria: Unisa Press, 1985), pp. 12–13.

28. R. Elphick, *Kraal and Castle: Khoikhoi and the Founding of White South Africa* (Johannesburg: Ravan, 1985), p. 125.

29. J. Grevenbroek, 'An Elegant and Accurate Account of The African Race living around the Cape of Good Hope commonly called the Hottentots', in I. Schapera and B. Farrington (eds), *The Early Cape Hottentots* (Cape Town: Van Riebeeck Society, 1933), p. 241.

30. *The Dictionary of Medicine* (London: Galley Press, 1989), p. 97. Impetigo is a contagious skin disease caused by bacteria. It forms a sore that are soon covered with thick yellow crusts. It is initially treated with antiseptic or antibiotic cream or lotion.

31. P. Speed, *Social Problems of the Industrial Revolution* (London: Arnold-Wheaton, 1985), p. 18.

32. S. Marks and N. Andersson, 'Typhus and Social Control: South Africa, 1917–50', in R. Macleod and L. Milton (eds), *Disease, Medicine and the Empire* (London: Routledge, 1988), p. 265.

33. Cape Archives (hereafter CA) Verbatim Copies (VC) 27 Daghregister, 20 May 1755.

34. Thunberg, *Travels in Europe, Africa and Asia*, p. 199.

35. Sparrmann, *A Voyage to the Cape of Good Hope*, vol. 1, pp. 175–6.

36. Erysipelas was a painful skin infection caused by streptococcal bacteria. *The Dictionary of Medicine*, p. 68.

37. Thunberg, *Travels in Europe, Africa and Asia*, p. 303. His description of *erysipelas* corresponds with the modern description of the disease. See *Dictionary of Medicine*, p. 68. This once again proves how valuable and reliable travel accounts are in reconstructing the history of pre-colonial societies.

38. H. Deacon, 'Leprosy and Racism at Robben Island', in E. van Heyningen (ed.) *Studies in the History of Cape Town, Vol. 7* (Cape Town: UCT Press, 1994), pp. 64ff. Metcalf, 'A History of Tuberculosis', in H. Coovadia and S. Benatar, *A Century of Tuberculosis: South African Perspectives* (Cape Town: Oxford University Press, 1991), p. 21.

39. R. Viljoen, 'Disease and Society: VOC Cape Town, its People and the Smallpox epidemics of 1713, 1755 and 1767', *Kleio*, 27 (1995), pp. 29ff.

40. Ibid., pp. 29–31.

41. CA C 652 Personal Letters to and from Governors of the Cape, 31 March 1757. S de Monchy from Rotterdam to Governor Rijk Tulbagh.

42. McNeill, *Plagues and Peoples*, p. 251.

43. See Viljoen, 'Medicine, Health and Medical Practice in Precolonial Society', pp. 552–3.

44. F. Valentijn, *Description of the Cape of Good Hope, Vol.1*, 2nd series, no. 2 (Cape Town: Van Riebeeck Society, 1971), pp. 217–9.

45. Valentijn, *Description of the Cape of Good Hope*, p. 219. For a detailed discussion on religion and epidemics see T. Ranger, 'Plagues of beasts and men: Prophetic responses to epidemic in eastern and southern Africa', in T. Ranger and P. Slack (eds), *Epidemics and Ideas: Essays on the historical perception of pestilence* (London: Cambridge University Press, 1992), pp. 241–68.

46. CA VC 20 Daghregister, 14 February, 1714, pp. 39, 45–6. Elphick, *Kraal and Castle*, p. 233.

47. McNeill, *Plagues and Peoples*, p. 251.

48. Ibid.

49. D. R, Hopkins, *The Greatest Killer: Smallpox in History* (Chicago, IL and London: University of Chicago Press, 2002), pp. 139ff; G. Williams, *Angel of Death: The Story of Smallpox* (London: Palgrave MacMillan, 2010), p. 6.

50. Ibid., pp. 144–6.

51. Viljoen, 'Medicine, Health and Medical Practice in Precolonial Khoikhoi Society', p. 523.
52. CA C 492 Letters Received, 20 August 1755, pp. 57–9.
53. J. Peires, *The Dead Will Arise: Nongqawuse and the Great Xhosa Cattle-killing Movement of 1856–7* (Johannesburg: Ravan: 1989), p. 31.
54. CA C 520 Letters Received, 22 Feb. 1769, pp. 58–9.
55. CA C 517 Letters Received, 20 November 1767, pp. 292–5.
56. Viljoen, 'Disease and Society', p. 42.
57. V. Bickford-Smith, *Ethnic Pride and Racial Prejudice in Victorian Cape Town* (Johannesburg: Witwatersrand University Press, 1995), p. 84; M. Swanson, 'The Sanitation Syndrome: Bubonic Plague and Urban Policy in the Cape Colony, 1900–1909', *Journal of African History*, 18:3 (1977), pp. 387–410.
58. Viljoen, 'Disease and Society', p. 44.
59. Thunberg, *Travels in Europe, Africa and Asia*, p. 293.
60. Ibid., p. 225.
61. Sparrman, *A Voyage to the Cape of Good Hope*, vol. 1, p. 160.
62. Grevenbroek, 'The African Race ... Commonly Called Hottentots', p. 267.
63. Sparrman, *A Voyage to the Cape of Good Hope*, vol .2, p. 217.
64. Ibid., p. 217; Thunberg, *Travels in Europe, Africa and Asia*, p. 246.
65. CA 1/STB 10/166 Letters Received from Private Individuals 1686–1797, 25 March 1777.
66. CA 1/SWM 3/14 Sworn Statements, 11 July 1780.
67. Kolb, *The Present State*, vol. 2, p. 337.
68. E. Burrows, *A History of Medicine in South Africa* (Cape Town: A. A. Balkema, 1958), p. 77. A certain doctor Joseph Mackrill who practised medicine at the Cape was apparently responsible for introducing *buchu* as a medicinal herb into England.
69. Burrows, *A History of Medicine*, p. 67.
70. F. Bradlow and M. Cairns, *The Early Cape Muslims: A Study of their Mosques, Genealogy and Origin* (Cape Town: A. A. Balkema, 1978), p. 89.
71. M. Vink, '"The World Oldest Trade": Dutch Slavery and Slave Trade in the Indian Ocean in the Seventeenth Century', *Journal of World History*, 14:2 (2003), pp. 131–77, p. 160.
72. A. Dick, 'The Notebook of Johannes Smiesing (1697–1734), Writing and Reading in the Cape Slave Lodge', *Quarterly Bulletin of the National Library of South Africa*, 64:4 (2010), pp. 167–70.
73. Sparrman, *Voyage to the Cape of Good Hope*, vol. 2, p. 251.
74. Semple. R, *Walks and Sketches at the Cape of Good Hope* (Cape Town and Amsterdam: A. A. Balkema, 1968), p. 49. See also M. Harrison, *Climates and Constitutions: Health, Race, Environment and British Imperialism in India, 1600–1850* (New Delhi, 1999).
75. N. Jensen, 'Texts and Documents: The Medical Skills of the Malabar Doctors in Tranquebar, India as Recorded by Surgeon TLF Folly, 1798', *Medical History*, 49 (2005), pp. 489–515.
76. R. Carruba and J. Bowers, 'Engelbrecht Kaempfer's First Report of the Torpedo Fish of the Persion Gulf in the Late Seventeenth Century', *Journal of the History of Biology*, 15:2 (1982), pp. 263–74, on p. 266.
77. V. S. Forbes (ed.), *Carl Peter Thunberg at the Cape of Good Hope 1772–1775*, 2nd series, no. 17 (Cape Town: Van Riebeeck Society, 1986), p. 64.
78. Ibid.

79. V. De Kock, *Those in Bondage: An Account of the Life of the slave at the Cape of Good Hope in the days of the Dutch East India Company* (Pretoria: Union Book Sellers, 1963), p. 135.

80. Sparrman, *Voyage to the Cape of Good Hope*, vol. 1, p. 276.

81. A. Smith, 'Different Facets of the Crystal: Early European images of the Khoikhoi at the Cape, South Africa', *South African Archaeological Society Goodwin Series*, 7:8–20 (1993), pp. 16ff.

82. Sparrman, *Voyage to the Cape of Good Hope*, vol. 1, pp. 181–5.

83. Ibid., 'With regard to their persons, they are as tall as most *Europeans*. The root of the nose is mostly very low, by which means the distance of the eyes from each other appears to be greater than in *Europeans*. In like manner, the tip of the nose is pretty flat. The head would appear to be covered with a black, though not very close, frizzled kind of wool, if the natural harshness of it did not show, that it was hair, if possible, more woolly than that of the negroes. If in other respects there should, by a great chance, be observed any traces of a beard or hair in any parts of the body, such as are seen on the *Europeans*', pp. 181–2 (emphasis added).

84. S. J. Gould, *The Flamingo's Smile: Reflections in Natural History* (New York: Norton, 1985); S. J. Gould, *The Mismeasure of Man* (New York: Norton, 1996).

85. R. Holmes, *The Hottentot Venus: The Life and Death of Saartjie Baartman, Born 1789-Buried 2002* (Johannesburg and Cape Town: Jonathan Ball Publishers, 2007); C. Crais and P. Scully, *Sara Baartman and the Hottentot Venus: A Ghost Story and a Biography* (Johannesburg: Wits University Press, 2009).

86. Sparrman, *Voyage to the Cape of Good Hope*, vol. 1, p. 154. For more information on scientific racism in colonial and modern South Africa, see S. Dubow, *Illicit Union: Scientific Racism in Modern South Africa* (Johannesburg,: Witwatersrand University Press, 1995).

87. Ibid., p. 154.

88. Ibid.

89. Ibid., p. 176.

90. Ibid., pp. 318–9. On this occasion, besides the tobacco, he administered *vinum emeticum* medicine which he prepared according the *Dispensary of the London College for 1762*, along with two ounces of *croc. antim.* lot in a bottle of common Cape wine to bring them to vomit.

91. Ibid., p. 320.

92. M. Harrison, '"The Tender Frame of Man": Disease, Climate and Racial Difference in India and the West Indies, 1760–1860', *Bulletin of the History of Medicine*, 70:1 (1996), pp. 68–93; D. Arnold, *Colonizing the Body: State Medicine and Epidemic Disease in 19th Century India* (Berkeley, CA: California, 1999).

93. B. Arnold, 'Race, Place and Bodily Difference in Early Nineteenth-Century India', *Historical Research*, 77:196 (2004), pp. 257–8.

94. Ibid., p. 257.

95. Ibid., p. 258.

96. Ibid., p. 261.

97. Sparrman, *Voyage to the Cape of Good Hope*, vol. 1, p. 276.

98. Ibid., pp. 276–7.

99. Ibid., p. 276.

100. Viljoen, 'Disease and Society', p. 42.

101. CA 1/SWM 7/8 Civil Cases, 1760–1772, 7 August 1769.

102. Burrows, *History of Medicine*, p. 60.

103. CA 1/SWM 11/26 Letters Received from Fiscal, 1795–1797, 11 November 1796.
104. CA 1/SWM 3/16 Sworn Statements, 8 February 1791.
105. CA CJ 3173 Notebooks of inquests held on bodies of drowned, injured and other persons who died in accidents 1757–1766, 15 April 1764.
106. CA CJ 3173 Notebooks of inquests held on bodies of drowned, injured and other persons who died in accidents, 1757–1766, 7 October 1757, pp. 19ff.
107. K. Ward, 'Monitoring Death at the Cape of Good Hope', *South African Historical Journal*, 59 (2007), pp. 155–6.
108. H. Heese and R. Viljoen, 'Trial and Sentence of Hans Jurgen Kettner: A German Scapegoat at the Cape?', *Asien, Afrika Lateinamerika*, 23 (1995), pp. 587–96.
109. A German by descent, Georg Carl Ludwig Geering from Hohe Geisz, Germany arrived at the Cape in 1764 and practiced medicine in Stellenbosch. See Hoge, 'Personalia of the Germans at the Cape, 1652–1806', p. 108.
110. Heese and Viljoen, 'Trial and Sentence of Hans Jurgen Kettner', pp. 591–2.
111. CA 1/SWM 3/14 Sworn Statements, 16 March 1783.
112. CA CJ 796 Criminal Sentences, no. 3, 22 July 1790, pp. 19–25.
113. Arnold, 'Race, Place and the Bodily Difference in Early Nineteenth-Century India', p. 257.
114. M. Harrison, *Medicine in an Age of Commerce and Empire: Britain and its Tropical Colonies, 1660–1830* (Oxford: Oxford University Press, 2010), p. 4.

4 Samanta, 'Dealing with Disease: Epizootics, Veterinarians and Public Health in Colonial Bengal, 1850–1920'

1. Captain John Gregory, Deputy Commissioner of Luckimpore to the Commissioner of Assam, No. 346, Debrooghur, 30 June 1869. West Bengal State Archive (hereafter, WBSA). Political department (Medical Branch), 27 July 1869. Pro No. 66 and 67.
2. Shree Manicklal Mallik, 'Niramish Bhojon' (Vegetarian Diet), *Swasthya-Samachar*, 5 (1916).
3. John Stalkartt to Colonel H. C James, Private Secretary to the Lieutenant Governor of Bengal, 3 February 1864. WBSA. General Department (Medical Branch), February 1864. No. 20–3.
4. European accounts often referred to rinderpest as cattle plague. The disease affects all cloven-hoofed animals, including domestic cattle, African buffalo, and various species of antelope. It is the most lethal plague known in cattle. See P. A. Koolmees, 'Epizootic Diseases in the Netherlands, 1713–2002: Veterinary Science, Agricultural Policy and Public Response', in K. Brown and D. Gilfoyle (eds), *Healing the Herds: Disease, Livestock Economies and the Globalization of Veterinary Medicine* (Athens, OH: Ohio University Press, 2010).
5. An epizootic is the equivalent in animal population of a human epidemic, i.e. high mortality due to a disease that is normally not present in that region.
6. In the Victorian era, the boundary between animal and human health was not so secure; indeed the pioneering work after 1870s on how germs caused infection began with studies of diseases that crossed species barriers – anthrax, tuberculosis and rabies. See N. Pemberton and M. Worboys, *Mad Dogs and Englishmen: Rabies in Britain, 1830–2000* (New York: Palgrave Macmillan, 2007).

7. The numerous letters and official correspondence can be found in West Bengal State Archive (WBSA), Kolkata. Major Agnew, Officiating Commissioner of Assam to the Junior Secretary to the Government of Bengal, March 1864. WBSA. General Department (Medical Branch), March 1864, No. 6–20.

8. K. Waddington, *The Bovine Scourge: Meat, Tuberculosis and Public Health 1850–1914* (Woodbridge: Boydell Press, 2006).

9. The idea of contagion has had a complicated history within the medical traditions of the world. Christopher Hamlin has demonstrated in the context of Victorian England that seeing disease causation merely in terms of a binarism between contagionism and anticontagionism is unhelpful. See C. Hamlin, *Public Health and Social Justice in the Age of Chadwick: Britain, 1800–1854*, Cambridge Studies in the History of Medicine (London: Cambridge University Press, 2009).

10. This question preoccupied the veterinarians and authorities in different parts of the globe, wherever cattle plague broke out. Martine Barwegen argued in the context of nineteenth century Java that resolving this question was considered the only way to combat the cattle plague. Berwegen, 'For Better or for Worse', in K. Brown and D. Gilfoyle (eds), *Healing the Herds: Disease, Livestock Economies and the Globalization of Veterinary Medicine*, p. 102.

11. John Stalkartt to E. C. Craster, Magistrate of Howrah, December 1863. General Department (Medical Branch), March 1864. WBSA. Stalkartt was convinced it were the *chamars* because he noted that, by not permitting them to have the animal skin buried in the compound, no animal of that year was affected.

12. In miasma theory, diseases were caused by the presence in the air of a miasma, a poisonous vapor characterized by its foul smell. See S. Halliday, 'Death and Miasma in Victorian London: An Obstinate Belief', *British Medical Journal*, 323:7327 (2001), pp. 1469–71.

13. *Report on the Calcutta Epizootic or Cattle Disease of 1864*. Letter from Dr. C. Palmer, Presidency Surgeon to S. C. Bayley, Junior Secretary to the Government of Bengal, 7 October, 1865. WBSA. General (Medical Branch), November 1865. No.71.

14. Ibid.

15. Ibid.

16. Ibid.

17. Henry H. Purves, Civil Assistant Surgeon of Gowhatty to the Deputy Commissioner of Kamroop, Gowhatty, 30 August 1868. WBSA. Medical (General Branch), October 1868, F.N. 73, No. 50.

18. K. McLeod, Civil Assistant Surgeon, Jessore to H.L Harrison, Junior Secretary to the Government of Bengal, 8 October, 1868. WBSA. Medical (General Branch), October 1868, F.N. 582, No.51.

19. H. L. Harrison, Junior Secretary to the Government of Bengal to the Officiating Commissioner of the Presidency Division, Fort William, 16 May 1868. WBSA. Medical (General Branch), July 1868, F.N., 2426, No. 50.

20. *Krishi-Gazette*, no. 1 (1886), Calcutta; Copies of Reports from the Divisional Commissioners and from the Agricultural and Horticultural Society containing information regarding the nature of the disease prevalent among Cattle in the Bengal Presidency forwarded to the Govt., with a request to furnish any further information that may be available relating to the disease in that Presidency. WBSA, General Department (Medical Branch), March 1864. Pro. No, 6–20, No. 15.

21. J. A. Voelkar, *Report on the Improvement of Indian Agriculture*, 1897. Paragraph 271, p. 213 at http://www.archive.org/stream/cu31924001039324#page/n4/mode/thumb [accessed on 7 January 2012].

22. J. H. B Hallen, *Manual of the More Deadly Forms of Cattle Disease in India* (Calcutta: 1885). The correspondences can be found in Municipal Department (Medical Branch), November 1884. WBSA. File no. 2. Pro. No. B31–62.

23. On a history of animals diseases and veterinary research in South Africa see Karen Brown, 'Tropical Medicine and Animal Diseases: Onderstepoort and the Development of Veterinary Science in South Africa 1908–1950', *Journal of Southern African Studies*, 31: 3 (Sept 2005), pp. 513–29.

24. H. Farrell, Veterinary Surgeon on special duty to Ashley Eden, Secretary to the Government of Bengal, Judicial Dept., Calcutta Hastings, 2 April 1870. WBSA. Political Department (Medical Branch), May 1870.

25. J. R. Fisher, 'Not Quite a Profession: The Aspirations of Veterinary Surgeons in England in the Mid-Nineteenth Century', *Historical Research*, 66 (1993), pp. 284–302.

26. M. Worboys, *Spreading Germs: Disease Theories and Medical Practice in Britain, 1865–1900* (Cambridge: Cambridge University Press, 2000), p. 46.

27. W. G. Clarence-Smith, 'Diseases of Equids in Southeast Asia, c. 1800–1945: Apocalypse or Progress?', in K. Brown and D. Gilfoyle (ed.), *Healing the Herds: Disease, Livestock Economies and the Globalization of Veterinary Medicine*.

28. C. S. Wills, Surgeon-Major of Barrackpore to Deputy Surgeon-General, Presidency District, 29 December 1881, Proceedings of the Lieutenant-Governor of Bengal, Medical and Municipal Dept. (Medical Branch) WBSA.

29. Ibid.

30. *London Times/Evening Mail*, Calcutta, 21 August 1885.

31. D. Arnold, *Colonizing the Body: State Medicine and Epidemic Disease in Nineteenth-Century India* (London: University of California Press, 1993).

32. Captain A. E. Campbell, Deputy Commissioner, Seebsaugor, to the Personal Assistant to the Commissioner of Assam, Seebsaugor, 22 June 1869. WBSA, Political Department (Medical Branch), 27 July 1869, Proceedings 66 and 67, No. 384.

33. See M. Vaughan, *Curing Their Ills: Colonial Power and African Illness* (Stanford, CA: Stanford University Press, 1991); J. Iliffe, *East African Doctors: A History of the Medical Profession.* (Cambridge: Cambridge University Press, 1998).

34. M. Ramanna, *Western Medicine and Public Health in Colonial Bombay, 1845–1895* (Delhi: Orient Longman, 2002); K. Ray, *History of Public Health in Colonial Bengal 1921–1947* (Calcutta: K. P. Bagchi & Co., 1998); P. Bala, *Medicine and Medical Policies in India: Social and Historical Perspectives* (Lexington Books, 2007).

35. P. B. Mukharji, *Nationalizing the Body: The Medical Market, Print and Daktari Medicine* (London: Anthem Press, 2009).

36. Ibid., p. 150. For an overview on the introduction of western science in Bengal see, D. Kumar, *Science and the Raj: A Study of British India* (Delhi: Oxford University Press, 2006).

37. In 1886, the Bengali periodical *Krishi-Gazette* lamented the lack of adequate agriculture periodicals and pamphlets composed by the Bengali literati.

38. K. Waddington, *The Bovine Scourge: Meat, Tuberculosis and Public Health 1850–1914*, p. 3, p. 175.

39. Municipal Department (Medical Branch), July 1889. Pro No., 66–7.

40. Industry and Science Department, March 1900. File no., 4C/4, Pro No., 52–6.

41. Political Department (Medical Branch), 27 July 1869. Pro No. 66, 67, July 1869.
42. I am using the term *bhadralok* very loosely to indicate the educated, Bengali middle class. In reality, it was an extremely diverse group marked by huge heterogeneity in terms of its social position, relationship to commerce, bureaucracy, intellectual or cultural values. The *bhadralok* can thus be very broadly defined as the Bengali middle income group, characterized by English education, professional occupation and overwhelming Hindu and upper caste. For an overview on the role and shifting identities of the *bhadralok* in colonial Bengal, see Tapan Raychaudhuri, *Europe Reconsidered: Perceptions of the West in Nineteenth-Century Bengal* (Delhi: Oxford University Press, 1988); Sumit Sarkar, *Writing Social History* (Delhi: Oxford University Press, 1997); Sumanta Banerjee, *The Parlour and the Streets: Elite and Popular Culture in Nineteenth Century Calcutta* (Calcutta: Seagull, 1989); Partha Chatterjee, *The Nation and its Fragments: Colonial and Postcolonial Histories* (Princeton, NJ: Princeton University Press, 1993).
43. M. Sinha, *Colonial Masculinity: The 'Manly Englishman' and the 'Effeminate Bengali' in the Late Nineteenth Century* (Manchester and New York: Manchester University Press, 1995); J. Sengupta, 'Nation on a Platter: the Culture and Politics of Food and Cuisine in Colonial Bengal', *Modern Asian Studies*, 44 (2010), pp. 81–98; S. Prasad, 'Crisis, Identity, and Social Distinction: Cultural Politics of Food, Taste, and Consumption in Late Colonial Bengal', *Journal of Historical Sociology*, 19:3 (2006), pp. 245–65.
44. Several such examples can be found in the *Swashthyo-Samachar* during this period.
45. For a history of vegetarianism in India see, K. T Acharya, *A Historical Dictionary of Indian Food* (Delhi: Oxford University Press, 1998).
46. For an analysis of Bengali medical printing as it emerged in the nineteenth century, see P. B. Mukharji, *Nationalizing the Body*, ch. 2: 'Daktari Prints: The World of Bengali Printing and the Multiple Inscriptions of *Daktari* Medicine'.
47. Anonymous writer, *Bangabashi*, 1916.
48. Sree M. Mallick, 'Niramish-Bhojon', *Swasthyo-Samachar*, vol. 5 (1916) (emphasis added).
49. J. Sengupta, 'Nation on a Platter: the Culture and Politics of Food and Cuisine in Colonial Bengal', *Modern Asian Studies*, 44 (2010), pp. 81–98; S. Prasad, 'Crisis, Identity, and Social Distinction: Cultural Politics of Food, Taste, and Consumption in Late Colonial Bengal', *Journal of Historical Sociology*, 19:3 (2006), pp. 245–65.
50. U. Ray, 'Eating "Modernity": Changing Dietary Practices in Colonial Bengal', *Modern Asian Studies*, 46 (2012), pp. 703–29.
51. Ramendra Shundor Tribedi, 'Amish Bhojon' (Meat Diet), *Punya*, 8 (1899).
52. S. Marks, 'What is Colonial about Colonial Medicine? And What has Happened to Imperialism and Health?' *Social History of Medicine*, 10 (1997).
53. Some scholars have hinted at the Bengali *bhadralok*'s attempt to internalize modern science and medicine. Arnold's *Colonizing the Body* had ended with comments about how Indian middle classes had appropriated 'modern science' and integrated these into the latter's rhetoric of legitimation. Jayanta Sengupta has argued that by the turn of the twentieth century the scientific quest for a suitable diet had become linked with the cultural politics of *bhadralok* identity. These studies however have not developed fully the extent of the middle-class scientific appropriation and dilemma.
54. Mukharji, *Nationalizing the Body*, p. 9.
55. Pande makes a similar argument as she demonstrates that by the end of the 19th century the Bengali *bhadralok* was no longer the passive object of a medical gaze because 'he

refused to be pathologized as the other'. I. Pande, *Medicine, Race and Liberalism in British Bengal: Symptoms of Empire* (New York: Routledge, 2010), p.16.

56. K. Waddington, *The Bovine Scourge: Meat, Tuberculosis and Public Health 1850–1914*, p. 38.

57. M. Worboys, 'Germ Theories of Disease and British Veterinary Medicine, 1860–1890', *Medical History*, 15 (1991), pp. 308–27.

58. On the nature of tropical medicine, see M. Worboys, 'Manson, Ross and Colonial Medical Policy: Tropical Medicine in London and Liverpool, 1819–1914', in R. MacLeod and M. Lewis (eds), *Disease, Medicine and Empire: Perspectives on Western Medicine and the Experience and European Expansion* (London: Routledge, 1988), pp. 21–37.

59. P. F. Cranefield, *Science and Empire: East Coast Fever in Rhodesia and the Transvaal* (New York: Cambridge University Press, 1991); K. Brown, 'Tropical Medicine and Animal Diseases: Onderstepoort and the Development of Veterinary Science in South Africa 1908–1950', *Journal of Southern African Studies*, 31:3 (September 2005), pp. 513–29.

60. K. Brown, 'Tropical Medicine and Animal Diseases: Onderstepoort and the Development of Veterinary Science in South Africa 1908–1950', *Journal of Southern African Studies*, 31:3 (September 2005), pp. 513–29.

61. R. MacLeod, 'On Visiting the "Moving Metropolis": Reflections on the Architecture of Imperial Science', *Historical Records of Australian Science*, 5:3 (1982), pp. 1–6.

62. Brown, 'Tropical Medicine and Animal Diseases'.

63. *Vedas* and *Puranas* are ancient Hindu texts that were composed during 1500–1000 BC The Sanskrit word 'Veda' means knowledge. The four major Vedas were orally transmitted for over generations, and formed the basis of Hindu scriptural authority.

64. For a historiographical sketch on the centrality of disease in environmental history, see Gregg Mitman, 'In Search of Health: Landscape and Disease in American Environmental History', *Environmental History*, 10:2 (April 2005), pp. 184–210.

65. T. Mitchell, *Rule of Experts: Egypt, Techno-Politics, Modernity* (Berkeley, CA: University of California Press, 2002).

66. J. R. McNeill, *Mosquito Empires: Ecology and War in the Greater Caribbean, 1620–1914* (New York: Cambridge University Press, 2010).

67. M. Few and Z. Tortorici (eds), *Centering Animals in Latin American History: Writing Animals in History* (Durham, NC: Duke University Press, 2013).

68. Erica Fudge has argued that animals appear in archives and libraries as 'absent-presences: there, but not speaking'. E. Fudge, 'A Left-Handed Blow: Writing the History of Animals', in N. Rothfels (ed.), *Representing Animals* (Bloomington, IN: Indiana University Press, 2006), p. 6.

5 Phillips, 'Mahatma Gandhi under the Plague Spotlight'

1. M. K. Gandhi, *An Autobiography or The Story of My Experiments with Truth* (London: Penguin Books, 2001), p. 268.

2. M. W. Dols, 'The Comparative Communal Responses to the Black Death in Muslim and Christian Societies', *Viator*, 5 (1974), pp. 269–87, at p. 275.

3. Swami Dwiroopanand, *Mahatma Gandhi: Ambassador of God for Mankind in the 21ˢᵗ Century* (Ahmedabad: Adhyatma Vignan Prakashan, 1992); K. Kripalani (ed.), *All Men Are Brothers: Life and Thoughts of Mahatma Gandhi As Told In His Own Words* (New York: Columbia University Press, 1958).

4. *The Collected Works of Mahatma Gandhi* (New Delhi: Publication Division Government of India, Electronic Book, 1999) at http://www.gandhiserve.org/*cwmg*/*cwmg*.htm (hereafter *CWMG*), vol. 76, document 454, *Harijan*, 30 September 1939 [accessed 12 December 2012].

5. The *Yersinia pestis* bacillus had been identified as the causative pathogen of plague by two bacteriologists working independently in Hong Kong in 1894, Alexandre Yersin and Shibasaburo Kitasato, while a French bacteriologist working in Bombay, Paul Louis Simond, had put forward the argument in 1898 that the rat flea was the vector of the disease. However, it took over a decade for this to be generally accepted by the medical profession, let alone by laypeople like Gandhi. For a more detailed discussion of the by-no-means uncontested manner in which this new explanation gained dominance and the considerable historiographical consequences of this, see the chapter in this volume by K. Royer, 'The Blind Men and the Elephant: Imperial Medicine, Medieval Historians, and the Role of Rats in the Historiography of Plague'.

6. *CWMG*, vol. 4, document 407, *Indian Opinion*, 14 October 1905.

7. Gandhi, *An Autobiography or The Story of My Experiments with Truth*, p. 179.

8. Ibid., p. 205.

9. The version in J. J. Doke, *M. K. Gandhi: An Indian Patriot in South Africa* (London: Indian Chronicle, 1909), ch. 15 is presumably based on Gandhi's own oral account, as given to Doke. The versions by F. Meer, *Apprenticeship of a Mahatma: A Biography of M. K. Gandhi 1869–1914*, 2nd edn (Durban: Institute for Black Research, 1994), by S. Wolpert, *Gandhi's Passion: The Life and Legacy of Mahatma Gandhi* (New York: Oxford University Press, 2001) and by R. Gandhi, *Gandhi: The Man, His People, and the Empire* (Berkeley, CA: University of California Press, 2007) largely mirror that given by Gandhi himself in Gandhi, *An Autobiography or The Story of My Experiments with Truth*, pp. 266–72.

10. S. Khilnani, 'Introduction', in Gandhi, *An Autobiography or The Story of My Experiments with Truth*, p. 5.

11. Gandhi, *An Autobiography or The Story of My Experiments with Truth*, p. 149.

12. D. Arnold, *Gandhi* (Harlow: Longman, 2001), p. 49.

13. *Rand Daily Mail*, 22 March 1904, p. 8.

14. Gandhi, *An Autobiography or The Story of My Experiments with Truth*, p. 267.

15. *Rand Daily Mail*, 22 March 1904, p. 8.

16. Gandhi, *An Autobiography or The Story of My Experiments with Truth*, pp. 267, 268.

17. Ibid., p. 268.

18. Ibid., p. 272.

19. Ibid., p. 269.

20. *Rand Daily Mail*, 6 April 1904, p. 8.

21. *Rand Daily Mail*, 6 April 1904, p. 8.

22. *CWMG*, vol. 3, document 303, *Indian Opinion*, 9 April 1904.

23. Ibid.

24. 'Report of the Medical Officer of Health for July 1904 to June 1906' in Johannesburg Municipality, *Minute of the Mayor for Year Ending October 1906*, p. 133.

25. *CWMG*, vol. 3, document 298, *Indian Opinion*, 24 March 1904.

26. *CWMG*, vol. 3, document 300, *Indian Opinion*, 2 April 1904.

27. Gandhi, *An Autobiography or The Story of My Experiments with Truth*, p. 271.

28. Ibid., p. 272.

29. *CWMG*, vol. 3, document 299, *Indian Opinion*, 9 April 1904.

30. E. Itzkin, *Gandhi's Johannesburg: Birthplace of Satyagraha* (Johannesburg: Witwatersrand University Press in association with Museum Africa, 2000), p. 13.
31. *CWMG*, vol. 3, document 309, *Indian Opinion*, 16 April, 1904.
32. *CWMG*, vol. 3, document 299, *Indian Opinion*, 9 April 1904.
33. *CWMG*, vol. 3, document 296, *Star*, 21 March 1904.
34. *CWMG*, vol. 3, document 299, *Indian Opinion*, 2 April 1904.
35. *CWMG*, vol. 4, document 103, *Indian Opinion*, 26 November 1904. On responses to the bubonic plague pandemic in other cities, see M. Echenberg, *Plague Ports: The Global Urban Impact of Bubonic Plague, 1894–1901* (New York: New York University Press, 2007).
36. *Rand Daily Mail*, 22 March 1904, p. 8. See too Transvaal (Colony), *Rand Plague Committee: Report upon the Outbreak of Plague on the Witwatersrand March 18th to July 31st, 1904* (Johannesburg, 1905), p. 76; and 'Report of the Medical Officer of Health for July 1904 to June 1906', in *Johannesburg Municipality, Minute of the Mayor for Year Ending October 1906*, p. 34.
37. *CWMG*, vol. 3, document 313, *Indian Opinion*, 23 April 1904.
38. *CWMG*, vol. 4, document 108, *Indian Opinion*, 10 December 1904.
39. *CWMG*, vol. 4, document 70, *Indian Opinion*, 8 October 1904.
40. Gandhi, *An Autobiography or The Story of My Experiments with Truth*, p. 272.
41. *CWMG*, vol. 3, document 309, *Indian Opinion*, 16 April 1904.
42. Gandhi, *An Autobiography or The Story of My Experiments with Truth*, p. 272.
43. *CWMG*, vol. 3, document 317, *Indian Opinion*, 30 April 1904.
44. *CWMG*, vol. 3, document 316, *Indian Opinion*, 30 April 1904.
45. *CWMG*, vol. 3, document 312, *Indian Opinion*, 23 April 1904.
46. Ibid.
47. *CWMG*, vol. 4, document 48, Letter to Dr Porter cited in *Indian Opinion*, 3 September 1904.
48. Ibid. Gandhi's use of the objectionable label 'Kaffir' has embarrassed some admiring editors of his writings into silently replacing this term with 'Native' (e.g. F. Meer (ed.), *The South African Gandhi – An Abstract of the Speeches and Writings of M.K. Gandhi 1893–1914* (Pietermaritzburg: Madiba Publishers in association with Gandhi Memorial Committee, 1995), pp. 808–9 and has excited critical comment from other authors – e.g. M. Swan, *Gandhi: The South African Experience* (Johannesburg: Ravan Press, 1985), p. 84; G. B. Singh, *Gandhi Behind the Mask of Divinity* (Amherst: Prometheus Books, 2004), passim; J. Lelyveld, *Great Soul: Mahatma Gandhi and His Struggle with India* (New York: Knopf, 2011), p. 53, 57–8; Penn and Teller TV show 'The Dark Side of Gandhi' (2007) at http://www.youtube.com/watch?v=9WezyyL5j2U [accessed 16 January 2013] – and the storm of responses to this. None realizes that the term was not quite as pejorative in 1904 as it was to become. For instance, see its use at this time by the pioneering African politician, Isaac Dyobha Williams Wauchope – J. Opland and A. Nyamende (eds), *Isaac Williams Wauchope, Selected Writings 1874–1916* (Cape Town: Van Riebeeck Society, 2008), p. xxxiv.
49. *CWMG*, vol. 4, document 75, *Indian Opinion*, 22 October 1904.
50. *CWMG*, vol. 4, document 153, *Indian Opinion*, 25 February 1905.
51. Transvaal (Colony), Rand Plague Committee: *Report upon the Outbreak of Plague on the Witwatersrand March 18th to July 31st, 1904* (Johannesburg, 1905), p. 86.
52. *CWMG*, vol. 3, document 305, *Indian Opinion*, 9 April 1904.

53. By January 1905 almost all the former Coolie Location Indian residents had moved to Malay Location near the now blackened site of Coolie Location. Swan (*Gandhi: The South African Experience*, pp. 107–8, p. 114) hints that Gandhi wished to see them return to Johannesburg as soon as possible mainly to ensure that they did not default on paying their debts to well-off Indian merchants whose agent, she avers, he then was.

54. 'Report of the Medical Officer of Health for July 1904 to June 1906' in Johannesburg Municipality, *Minute of the Mayor for Year Ending October 1906*, p. 132.

55. *CWMG*, vol. 5, document 11, *Indian Opinion*, 18 November 1905.

56. *Star*, 13 October 1904, p. 10; Union of South Africa, *Report of the Transvaal Asiatic Land Tenure Act Commission*, U.G. 7–1934, p. 88, paras. 29–30.

57. Swan, *Gandhi: The South African Experience*, p. 112.

58. Gandhi, *An Autobiography or The Story of My Experiments with Truth*, p. 273.

59. *CWMG*, vol. 4, document 165, *Indian Opinion*, 18 March 1905.

60. S. Khilnani, 'Introduction' in Gandhi, *An Autobiography or The Story of My Experiments with Truth*, p. 2.

61. Ibid., p. 258.

6 Sarkar, 'Plague Hits the Colonies: India and South Africa at the Turn of the Twentieth Century'

1. Assistant US Surgeon-General J. M. Eager, *Eradicating Plague from San Francisco: Report of the Citizens' Health Committee and an Account of its Work* (San Francisco, CA: Press of C.A. Murdock & Co., 1909), p. 28. The list of regions affected by the third plague pandemic included: Arabia, Asiatic Russia, Asiatic Turkey, China, Chinese Turkestan, French Indo-China, India, Japan, Persia, Persian Turkestan, Siam, Straits Settlements, Algeria, British East Africa, British South Africa, Egypt, French Ivory Coast, German East Africa, Liberia, Madagascar, Portuguese East Africa, Reunion, Tunis, Zanzibar, Australia, Hawaii, New Caledonia, New Zealand, Philippines, Sumatra, Austria, France, Germany, England, Scotland, Italy, Portugal, Russia, Turkey, Argentina, Brazil, Chile, Mexico, Panama, Paraguay, Peru, Trinidad, United States, and Uruguay.

2. Wu Lien-teh, Chun, J. W. H., Pollitzer, R. and Wu, C. Y., *Plague: A Manual for Medical and Public Health Workers* (Shanghai: National Quarantine Service, 1936).

3. R. Pollitzer, *Plague* (Geneva: World Health Organization, 1954), p. 16.

4. P. Curson and K. McCracken, *Plague in Sydney: The Anatomy of an Epidemic* (New South Wales: New South Wales University Press, 1940), p. 3.

5. M. Echenberg, 'Pestis Redux: The initial Years of the Third Bubonic Plague Pandemic, 1894–1901', *Journal of World History*, 13:2 (2002), p. 433.

6. M. Echenberg, *Plague Ports: The Global Urban Impact of Bubonic Plague, 1894–1901* (New York: New York University Press, 2007), pp. 270–4.

7. W. M. Haffkine, *The Bombay Plague* (Bombay: Education Society's Steam Press, 1900), p. 68.

8. Report on the Outbreak of Bubonic Plague, P. C. H. Snow, Municipal Commissioner for the City of Bombay, 2 October 1897, p. 2.

9. Report on Native Newspapers (NNR hereafter) – Bengal, *Hitavadi*, 30 December 1898.

10. Maharashtra State Archives (MSA), G.D. (Plague), vol. 332, 1898, T.S. Weir, Health Officer, Bombay, 27 September 1897 to P. C. H. Snow, Municipal Commissioner, pp. 46–7.

11. *Bombay Gazette*, 7 October 1896.
12. Ibid., p. 6.
13. Members of the Suryavanshi Kshatriya clan known to have originated in the region of Punjab and having migrated to Sindh and Gujarat at some point.
14. Occupational caste of traders and money-lenders from western and central India.
15. *Bombay Gazette*, 26 September 1896.
16. Kalpish Ratna, *Uncertain Life and Sure Death: Medicine and Mahamari in Maritime Mumbai* (Bombay: Maritime History Society, 2008), pp. 274–5. The Hong Kong plague of 1894 raged for five months with a death toll of 2,550. Its recurrence in 1896 was milder, with 700 reported deaths. It was believed that it was this 'contained' outbreak which arrived at Bombay's shore.
17. W. J. Simpson, *Treatise on Plague dealing with the Historical, Epidemiological, Clinical, Therapeutic and Preventive aspects of the Disease* (Cambridge: Cambridge University Press, 1905), p. 71.
18. Ibid., p. 266.
19. *Natal Mercury*, 3 December 1900.
20. Ibid.
21. *Publications of the South African Institute of Medical Research*, March 1927, p. 89.
22. *Indian Opinion*, 9 July 1903.
23. *Publications of the South African Institute of Medical Research*, March 1927, p. 91.
24. L. Fabian Hirst, *The Conquest of Plague: A Study of the Evolution of Epidemiology* (Oxford: Clarendon Press, 1953), p. 174. The period that marked the discovery of the specific plague micro-organism in the summer of 1894 and ended with the final proof in 1908 that it was transmitted by rat fleas, has been acknowledged as the 'pioneer phase' of modern plague research.
25. R. E. McGrew, *Encyclopedia of Medical History* (London: Macmillan Press, 1985), p. 44. It was in Hong Kong in 1893–4 that a team of scientists worked on the bacteriological origins of the plague. Alexandre Emil Jean Yersin and Shibasaburo Kitasato simultaneously discovered the bacillus that caused plague.
26. Fabian Hirst, *The Conquest of Plague*, p. 180.
27. See Arthur Henry Moorhead's 'Plague in India: Sketch of its Cause and Spread' in *Eradicating Plague from San Francisco: Report of the Citizens' Health Committee and an account of its work*, San Francisco Citizens' Health Committee, March, 1909, for the transference mechanism.
28. B. K. Natarajan, *Social Work and the City in Bombay Today and Tomorrow* (Bombay: D. B. Taraporewalla Sen and Co., 1930), p. 35.
29. Gillian Tindall, *City of Gold* (London: Temple Smith, 1982), p. 245.
30. Gillian Tindall, *City of Gold: The Biography of Bombay* (Bombay: Penguin Books Ltd., 1982), pp. 246–7. Mandvi was the area where Jains formed an appreciable population. They suffered heavily from plague. In 1891, they constituted three per cent of the island's population, while in 1901 they formed only one per cent of it. Cited in *Census of India*, part 5, vol. 11, 1901.
31. *Report of the Bombay Plague Committee*, J. N. Campbell (1898), pp. 52–3.
32. MSA, General Department (Plague) Vol. 332,1898, T.S. Weir, Municipal Health Officer, Bombay, to P.C.H. Snow, Municipal Commissioner, 27 September 1897, p. 138.
33. NNR-Bombay, *Rast Goftar*, 10 January 1897.
34. Cape Town *Mayor's Minutes* (MM), 1900–1901, pp. 169–73.
35. MM, 1901, pp. 172–3.

36. MM, 1899–1900, p. 53; MM, 1900–1, pp. 179–80.
37. Public Health Act No.4 of 1883 as amended by Act No.23 of 1897. Section 15: 'In cases of urgent necessity arising from the prevalence or threatened outbreak in any district of infectious disease … it shall be lawful for the Minister to make and proclaim such regulations to be in force within such districts as may be required to prevent the outbreak, or check the progress of, or eradicate such disease'.
38. MM, 1900–1, p. 180.
39. Alan Mabin, 'The Rise and Decline of Port Elizabeth, 1850–1900', International Journal of African Historical Studies, 19 (1986), pp. 275–303.
40. See Sheila T. Van der Horst, *Native Labour in South Africa* (Oxford: Oxford University Press, 1942), pp. 114–6.
41. E. J. Inggs, 'Mfengu beach labour and Port Elizabeth harbor development, 1835–1870', Contree 21, Journal for South African Urban and Regional History, January 1987, p. 12.
42. Sheila T. Van der Horst, *Native Labour in South Africa*, p. 120.
43. R. Pollitzer, *Plague*, pp. 46–50.
44. A. Sawant (ed.), *India and South Africa: A Fresh Start* (Delhi: Kalinga Publications, 1994), p. 198.
45. When plague broke out in the Indian Location at Johannesburg, Gandhi took energetic and prompt measures for the care of the sick and for arresting the spread of the disease. Every effort was made to prove beyond doubt that the neglect of the Town Council was the main cause of the plague outbreak. The *Indian Opinion* had, in Gandhi's hands, become an instrument of increasing influence. Especially through the Gujarati columns, he tried to educate the Indians in South Africa in self-discipline, sanitation and good citizenship.
46. *Indian Opinion*, 2 April 1904, p. 155.
47. Ibid.
48. *Indian Opinion*, 25 May 1904, p. 16.
49. *Report by Surgeon-Major Lyons*, President of the Plague Research Committee, 1897.
50. Ibid.
51. *Report of the Bombay Plague Committee*, p. 55.
52. Ibid., pp. 55–6.
53. *Report of the Bombay Plague Committee on the Plague in Bombay for the period extending from the 1st July, 1897 to the 30th April, 1898.*
54. Ibid.
55. NAI, *Proceedings, Home: Medical and Sanitary*, 19 (June 1898), p. 3.
56. Ibid. Number 276 B, p. 20. Also, Major E. Inglis, *Plague in Jullundur and Hoshiarpur 1897–98*, p. 81.
57. *Indian Opinion*, 18 February 1905, p. 357. In this context, Howard Phillips, in his chapter in this volume, 'Mahatma Gandhi under the Plague Spotlight', highlights Gandhi's perceptions of the epidemic plague as not being devoid of 'political aspirations' in the wake of the rising political consciousness in India at the time.
58. *Indian Opinion*, 25 February 1905, pp. 361–4.
59. *Report of the Bombay Plague Committee on the Plague in Bombay for the period extending from the 1st July, 1897 to the 30th April, 1898*, p. 53.
60. *Bombay Gazette*, 15 October 1896, p. 6.
61. NNR-Punjab, *Gurakhi*, 19 February 1897.
62. M. E. Couchman, *Account of the Plague Administration in the Bombay Presidency from Sept. 1896–May 1897* (Bombay, 1897), p. 6.

63. NNR-Bombay, *Native Opinion*, 21 February 1897, p.90.

64. NAI, *Proceedings, Home: Medical and Sanitary*, 17–27 (May 1904), p. 2.

65. Ibid.

66. *Indian Opinion*, 16 July 1904, p. 224.

67. *Times of India*, 16 June 1897, p. 3.

68. *Bombay Gazette*, 16 November 1896, p. 5.

69. *Bombay Gazette*, 24 February 1897, p. 6.

70. NAI, *Proceedings, Home: Medical and Sanitary*, 398–405B (April 1898), p. 2.

71. Narayani Gupta, *Between Two Empires, 1803–1931, Society, Government and Urban Growth* (Oxford: Oxford University Press, 1998), p. 137.

72. NAI, *Proceedings, Home: Medical and Sanitary*, 279B (April 1898), pp. 1–2.

73. NAI, *Proceedings, Home: Medical and Sanitary*, 39–51 (June 1898), p. 3.

74. *Cape Times*, 27 July 1899.

75. *Indian Opinion*, 9 April 1904.

76. *Indian Opinion*, 9 July 1903, p. 360.

77. Ibid., p. 361.

78. *Purdah* referred to the practice of concealing women from men. Women were required to observe complete seclusion and avoid contact with people other than their family members. The women covered their bodies in an effort to conceal their form. Both Hindu and Muslim women from especially northern and central India followed this practice, and continue to do so.

79. NNR-Bombay, *Gulzar-i-Hind*, 27 September 1902.

80. Trading community that originated from Malwa and Majha regions of Punjab.

81. E. Wilkinson, *Report on the Inoculation in Jullundur and Hoshiarpur Districts of the Punjab October 1899–September 1900* (Punjab Government Press, Lahore, 1901), pp. 50–1.

82. Inglis, *Plague in Jullundur and Hoshiarpur 1897–98*, p. 20.

83. Wilkinson, *Inoculation in Jullundur and Hoshiarpur 1899–1900*, pp. vi–vii.

84. Ibid., pp. 47–9.

85. Ibid.

86. *Tribune*, 24 March 1904, pp. 2–3.

87. *Indian Opinion*, 17 June 1905.

88. *Indian Opinion*, 5 July 1913. Some of these measures: a plague case was to be segregated and those who nursed him were not to come in contact with others; the house was to be sprinkled with lime and left unoccupied for ten days; a wet sheet pack for fever; a thick mud pack for application on the buboes/swollen glands; a clean, wholesome and spare diet; regular exercise; patient to lie in an open space with plenty of fresh air; in areas where plague cases had occurred, houses were to be cleared of gain to avoid rats; rat-holes were to be filled in. Dead rats were to be removed with a pair of tongs to a distant place and burnt with the help of hay or kerosene or even buried in a deep pit at a great distance from human habitation. The place where a dead rat was found was to be covered with ash and whitewashed. The ensuing debates on the association of rats with the transmission of epidemic plague and the role of the Plague Research Commission have been discussed by Katherine Royer in her chapter in this volume, 'The Blind Men and the Elephant: Imperial Medicine, Medieval Historians and the Role of Rats in the History of Plague.'

89. R. Carstairs, *The Little World of an Indian District Officer* (London: Macmillan and Co., Ltd, 1912), pp. 154–5. As per this official report, on an average, one doctor was available for every two thousand people in Bengal. This was hopelessly inadequate. The poor in the countryside could not afford costly European drugs. The colonial government was

unwilling to provide the required staff trained in western medicine for rural areas. The skeletal Health Services only served governmental establishments in the urban areas.

90. M. Prem Behari Mathur, *Plague-Panacea or A Pamphlet on Plague and its Remedies* (Agra Cantonment: Damodar Printing Works, 1911), p. 48.

91. Practitioners of Ayurveda.

92. Rajvaid Sri Bamandasji Kaviraj, *Short Treatise on Plague*, pp. 8–12.

7 Royer, 'The Blind Men and the Elephant: Imperial Medicine, Medieval Historians and the Role of Rats in the Historiography of Plague'

1. *Indian Plague Commission* (hereafter *IPC*), 5 vols (London: HMSO by Eyre and Spottiswoode, 1900–1).

2. *IPC*, vol. 1, p. 20.

3. *IPC*, vol. 1, p. 29.

4. *IPC*, vol. 1, pp. 29–30, and W. J. Simpson, *A Treatise on the Plague Dealing with the Historical, Epidemiological, Clinical, Therapeutic and Preventive Aspects of the Disease* (Cambridge: Cambridge University Press, 1905), p. 97.

5. *IPC*, vol. 5, pp. 68–75, and Paul-Louis Simond, 'La propagation de la peste', *Annales de L'Institute Pasteur*, 12 (October 1898), pp. 625–87. This theory posits that epidemic plague is primarily a disease of rats that only secondarily infects humans. The bacillus *Yersinia pestis* is passed from rats to humans through the rat flea, *Xenopsylla cheopsis*. Since fleas tend to be species specific, a rat flea only feeds on a human host if it cannot find a live rat. Therefore, epidemics of plague among rats have to reduce the number of rodents first before the disease moves on to humans. When the animal dies, its fleas search for a new source of food, which can be a nearby human. According to this theory, an epidemic among the animal host must exist prior to the transmission of the disease to large numbers of humans.

6. There were three major British colonial research commissions dedicated to plague. The first was the committee appointed by the Presidency of Bombay in 1896, then the Indian Plague Commission, which took testimony between 1898 and 1899, and finally the Plague Research Commission, which began its work in 1905. The research of the Plague Research Commission was published in a series of articles in the *Journal of Hygiene* beginning in 1906. See Brigadier-General W. F. Gatacre, *Report on the Bubonic Plague in Bombay, 1896–1897*, 2 vols (Bombay, 1897); *IPC*; and 'Plague Research Commission', *Journal of Hygiene*, 6:4 (September 1906).

7. Kuhn argues that the dominant paradigm of the moment is always resistant to change and during its period of 'normal science' attributes the failure of a result to conform to the paradigm to mistakes of the researcher rather than to problems with the paradigm. T. Kuhn, *The Structure of Scientific Revolutions* (Chicago, IL: University of Chicago Press, 1996).

8. J. F. D. Shrewsbury, *A History of Bubonic Plague in the British Isles* (Cambridge: Cambridge University Press, 1970), p. 6.

9. *The Black Death*, ed. and trans. R. Horrox (Manchester: Manchester University Press, 1994), p. 5.

10. As Robert Lerner points out in 'Fleas: Some Scratchy Issues Concerning the Black Death', *Journal of the Historical Society*, 8:2 (June, 2008), p. 214, the few accounts that describe

rodent mortality during the Black Death are formulaic and also say that it rained vermin along with earthquakes, locusts and lightening.

11. P. Slack, *The Impact of the Plague in Tudor and Stuart England* (Oxford: Clarendon Press, 1985), pp. 11–12.

12. Many of the revisionists arguments center on the observation that the Black Death moved quickly and was exceptionally lethal; whereas, the third pandemic traveled slowly and killed a smaller percentage of the population. See G. Twigg, *The Black Death: A Biological Reappraisal* (New York: Schocken Books, 1985); S. Scott and C. Duncan, *Biology of Plagues: Evidence from Historical Populations* (Cambridge: Cambridge University Press, 2001) and *The Return of the Black Death: The World's Greatest Serial Killer* (Chichester: Wiley and Sons, Ltd, 2004); G. Christakos, R. A. Olea, M. L. Serre, Hwa-Lung Yu, and Lin-Lin Wang, *Interdisciplinary Public Health Reasoning and Epidemic Modeling: The Case of the Black Death* (Berlin: Springer-Verlag, 2005); Lerner; and S. Cohn, Jr, *The Black Death Transformed: Disease and Culture in Early Renaissance Europe* (London: Hodder Headline Group, 2002).

13. There were three major plague pandemics. The Justinian plague that began in North Africa in 541 coursing as far as Britain and Persia, the Black Death, which primarily impacted Europe and the Middle East in the fourteenth century, and a third pandemic that is believed to have started in China in the eighteen the century and then moved to India, Australia, Hawaii, and the Americas, with a few sporadic cases reported in Europe.

14. G. Mandel (ed.), *Principles and Practice of Infectious Disease* (New York: Churchill Livingstone, 1990), p. 1748; and A. Fauci et al. (ed.), *Harrison's The Principles of Internal Medicine* (New York: McGraw, 2008), pp. 980–5.

15. In 'Ecology, Evolution and the Epidemiology of Plague' in *Plague and the End of Antiquity: The Pandemic of 541–750*, ed. L. Little (Cambridge: Cambridge University Press, 2007), Robert Sallares argues that the rat was the source of the disease in the Justinian plague.

16. M. Ogata, 'Ueber die Pestepidemie in Formosa', *Centralblatt für Bakteriologie*, 21 (June 1897), p. 769.

17. Simond, 'La propagation de la peste', pp. 625–87.

18. L. Fabian Hirst, *The Conquest of Plague: A Study of the Evolution of Epidemiology* (Oxford: Clarendon Press, 1953), pp. 28 and 158–9, and P. Manson-Bahr (ed.), *Manson's Tropical Disease: A Manual of the Diseases of Warm Climates*, 7th edn (New York: William Wood and Co., 1921), p. 258.

19. 'Papers Relating to the Outbreak of Bubonic Plague in India with Statements Showing the Quarantines and Other Restrictions Recently Placed Upon Indian Trade up to March 1897', *House of Commons Parliamentary Papers 1897*, vol. 63, pp. 35–6; *Bombay Medical and Physical Society's Transactions*, vol. 2 (1839), and vols 2–3 (1855–6), p. xxvii; and E. H. Hankin, 'On the Epidemiology of Plague', *Journal of Hygiene*, 5:1 (January 1905), pp. 54–63.

20. Simpson's *Treatise on Plague* was published in 1905 and E. H. Hankin's article was published the same year in the *Journal of Hygiene*.

21. Ibid., p. 219.

22. Hirst, *The Conquest of Plague*, p. 159, and W. Hunter, *A Research into Epidemic and Epizootic Plague* (Hong Kong: Noronha, 1904).

23. Hankin, , 'On the Epidemiology of Plague', pp. 64–6.

24. Ibid., pp. 64–6.

25. Ibid., pp. 64–83.

26. Ibid., pp. 82–3.
27. Hirst, *The Conquest of Plague*, p. 236, and Alexandre Yersin, Calmette and Borrel, 'La peste bubonique', *Annales de L'Institute de Pasteur*, 9 (1895), p. 589.
28. D. Arnold, *Colonizing the Body: State Medicine and Epidemic Disease in Nineteenth-Century India* (Berkeley, CA: University of California Press, 1993), pp. 207–32; and 'Disease, Medicine, and the Empire', in *Imperial Medicine and Indigenous Societies*, ed. D. Arnold (Manchester: Manchester University Press, 1988), p. 158. As Howard Phillips demonstrates in his essay in this volume, Gandhi shared the view that plague was a disease of dirt and this influenced his role in the 1904 epidemic in Johannesburg.
29. Michael Worboys, *Spreading Germs: Disease Theories and Medical Practice in Britain 1865–1900* (Cambridge: Cambridge University Press, 2000), pp. 1–7, pp. 282–90.
30. Simpson, *Treatise on Plague*, p. 144.
31. Ibid., pp. 168–79.
32. Ibid., pp. x–xi, and 'The Need of a Sanitary Service for India', *Transactions of the First Indian Medical Congress* (Calcutta: Caledonian Steam Printing Works, 1895), pp. 222–7.
33. Hankin, 'On the Epidemiology of Plague', pp. 48, 68.
34. Ibid., p. 80.
35. Ibid., p. 83, and W. G. Liston, *Indian Medical Gazette*, 40 (1905), p. 43.
36. Hirst, *The Conquest of Plague*, pp. 145–51, and J. Ashburton Thompson, 'A Contribution to the Aetiology of Plague', *Journal of Hygiene*, 1:2 (April 1901), pp. 153–62.
37. Ashburton Thompson, 'A Contribution to the Aetiology of Plague'
38. Thompson, 'On the Epidemiology of Plague', *Journal of Hygiene*, 6:5 (October 1906), p. 568.
39. Ibid.
40. Ibid., pp. 537–8.
41. Ibid., pp. 567–8.
42. Ibid., p. 568, and Thompson, 'A Contribution to the Aetiology of Plague', p. 162.
43. Hirst, *The Conquest of Plague*, p. 145, calls Thompson's reports a model of 'cogent reasoning' and repeats the Chief Medical Officer's contention that the 'civilized' population in Australia justified privileging the observations made there over those from India.
44. C .C. Baxter-Tyrie, 'Report of an Outbreak of Plague in Queensland during the First Six Months of 1904', *Journal of Hygiene*, 5:3 (July, 1905): pp. 312–4.
45. 'Plague Research Commission', *Journal of Hygiene*, 6:4 (September 1906), p. 422.
46. Hirst, *The Conquest of Plague*, p. 236, wrote that the Plague Research Commission ignored human ectoparasites in general in their research.
47. In its introductory article published in the *Journal of Hygiene* in 1906 the Plague Research Commission stated that 'from an epidemiological point of view one must regard plague as essentially a rat disease in which human beings participate'. The Commission went on to report that its mission was to study how the epizootic spread among rats and the precise means by which the disease was communicated from rat to man. 'Plague Research Commission', *Journal of Hygiene*, pp. 422–30.
48. Hirst, *The Conquest of Plague*, p. 236.
49. G. Blanc and M. Baltazard, *C. R. Academie Science* (1941), pp. 813–49; M. Baltazard, 'Novelles donnes sur la transmission interhumaine de la peste', *Bulletin de L'Académie Nationale de Médecine* (1959), pp. 517–22; and G. Blanc, 'Une opinion non conformiste sur le mode de transmission de la peste', *Revue Hyg. Med. Société*, 4 (1956), p. 535. They

believed the rat was the natural reservoir of the disease, but that human ectoparasites were the vector in the North African epidemics.

50. Some Continental scientists such as G. Girard, *Bulletin Acad. Médicine*, 114 (1935) and *Bulletin Soc. Path. exotic*, 36 (1943), p. 4, criticized Blanc and Balthazard because they did not have a suitable method for collecting *Xenopsylla cheopis* in the specimens that contained large numbers of *Pulex irritans*. There remained, however, a contingent of Continental scientists and historians who continued to give *Pulex irritans* serious consideration as the vector in the second pandemic. For example, see Jean Noel Biraben, *Les Hommes et la Peste en france et dans les Pays Européens et Méditerranéen* (Paris: Mouton and Co., 1975) and E. Rodendwalt, *Pest in Venedig 1575–1577 Ein Beitrag zu der Frageder Infektkette bei den Pest-epidemien Westeuropas* (Heidelberg, 1953), pp. 102–3. There were also a few works in the English literature that looked at a possible role for the human flea. See Stephen Ell, 'Interhuman Transmission of Medieval Plague', *Bulletin of the History of Medicine* 54: 4 (1980), pp. 497–510, and John Norris, 'East or West? The Geographic Origin of the Black Death', *Bulletin of the History of Medicine* 51: 1 (Spring 1977), p. 17. However, the majority of the English literature discounted the potential of *Pulex irritans* as a significant vector largely because of the work of Bacot and Martin on blocked fleas, which demonstrated that in order for a flea to be able to transmit *Yersinia pestis* through a flea bite, the insect had to first become 'blocked'. This meant its foregut was blocked by the rapidly reproducing bacillus so that it kept eating because food could not get into its stomach, which also made the flea regurgitate the bacillus into the mammal upon which it was feeding. *Xenopsylla cheopis* blocks very quickly, within five days, which makes it the supposed ideal vector; whereas, *Pulex irritans* does not block as quickly. It was also argued that if human ectoparasites were the vector, the disease would be much more prevalent and have a more uniform footprint. See Hirst, 239–46, and A. W. Bacot and C. J. Martin, *Plague Supplement*, 3 (1914), p. 423.

51. It was the fact that rats become bacteremic at a higher level than humans, and so could more easily block their fleas, that became the cornerstone of most arguments against *Pulex irritans* as a significant vector. Humans were not believed to become sufficiently bacteremic to cause their fleas to block. This is why Hirst, p. 244, believed the human flea was too weak a transmitter of plague to lead to an epidemic. However, Hirst, p. 237, did acknowledge that this conclusion was drawn from patients with bubonic plague and so may not have been true for patients with septicemic plague, which would have led to higher levels of bacteremia.

52. Hirst, *The Conquest of Plague*, p. 246.

53. Ibid., p. 133.

54. R. Pollitzer, *Plague* (Geneva: World Health Organization, 1954), p. 7.

55. M. Worboys, 'Germs, Malaria, and the Invention of Mansonian Tropical Medicine: From "Diseases in the Tropics" to "Tropical Diseases"', *Warm Climates and Western Medicine*, ed. D. Arnold (Amsterdam: Rodopi, 1996). Many of the other essays in this collection also address this topic. See also M. Harrison, *Climates and Constitutions: Health, Race, Environment and British Imperialism in India 1600–1850* (Oxford: Oxford University Press, 1999); *Public Health in British India: Anglo-Indian Preventative Medicine 1859–1914* (Cambridge: Cambridge University Press, 1994); *Imperial Medicine and Indigenous Societies*, ed. D. Arnold (Amsterdam: Rodopi, 1996); and S. Marks, 'What is Colonial About Colonial Medicine? And What Has Happened to Imperialism and Health', *Social History of Medicine*, 10 (1997), pp. 205–19. More recently, historians

such as Mark Harrison have demonstrated the important and long standing influence of imperial science on the center.

56. The history of colonial medicine in India is bound up in the epistemological debates regarding infectious disease in the nineteenth century, the changes in the medical profession, both at the periphery and the center, and the use of science as an instrument of empire. See M. Harrison, 'Towards a Sanitary Utopia? Professional Visions and Public Health in India, 1880–1914', *Climates and Constitutions: Health, Race, Environment and British Imperialism in India 1600–1850* (Oxford: Oxford University Press, 1999), pp. 25–6; *Medicine in An Age of Commerce and Empire: Britain and Its Tropical Colonies 1660–1830* (Oxford: Oxford University Press, 2010); 'Quarantine, Pilgrimage and Colonial Trade: India 1886–1900', *The Indian Economic and Social History Review*, 29:2 (1992): pp. 117–44; and D. Arnold, 'Cholera and Colonialism and British India', *Past and Present*, 113 (1986), pp. 118–51; D. Arnold, *Colonizing the Body: State Medicine and Epidemic Disease in Nineteenth-Century India*; and D. Arnold, *Medicine in An Age of Commerce and Empire: Britain and Its Tropical Colonies 1660–1830* (Oxford: Oxford University Press, 2010).

57. Hirst devotes the first hundred pages of *The Conquest of Plague* to the rise of the germ theory of disease.

58. Hirst, *The Conquest of Plague*, pp. 121–6, and Pollitzer, *Plague*, p. 13.

59. Pollitzer, *Plague*, pp. 11–18; Wu Lien-Teh, *A Treatise on Pneumonic Plague* (Geneva: World Health Organization, 1926); Hirst, pp. 163–72; and F. Eberson and W. Lien-Teh, 'Transmission of Plague Among Marmots', *Journal of Infectious Disease*, 20 (1917), p. 170; and Hirst, pp. 189–99.

60. Pollitzer, *Plague*, pp. 30–3, and 251–401, and Hirst, *The Conquest of Plague*, pp. 189–219

61. Hirst, *The Conquest of Plague*, pp. 228–31.

62. Ibid., pp. 121–8.

63. Pollitzer, *Plague*, p. 13.

64. Scott and Duncan, *The Biology of Plagues*, p. 53; Christakos, et al., *Interdisciplinary Public Health Reasoning and Epidemic Modeling*, p. 110; and Twigg, *The Black Death*, p. 16.

65. Shrewsbury, *A History of Bubonic Plague*, pp. 123–6.

66. Because of the descriptions of carbuncles in the Black Death, a clinical feature not often found in the third pandemic, some revisionists went on to posit that the Great Mortality was caused instead by anthrax or a viral hemorrhagic fever like Ebola. Twigg, *The Black Death*, pp. 200–21, argues for anthrax, Scott and Duncan, *Return of the Black Death*, pp. 225–6, favour viral hemorrhagic fever, and Samuel Cohn, Jr does not really commit to a specific disease, but contends that the Black Death was not caused by plague. However, carbuncles are a nonspecific clinical finding that can be present in a myriad of diseases, both viral and bacterial, because they are the result of disseminated intravascular coagulation, which is seen with septic shock. So they would be found in viral hemorrhagic fevers like Ebola, as well as plague.

67. B. Bramanti et al., 'Distinct Clones of *Yersinia pestis* Caused the Black Death', *PLoS Pathogens*, 6 (October 2010).

68. V. Schuenemann, H. Poinar et al., 'Targeted Enrichment of Ancient Pathogens Yielding the pPP1 Plasmid of *Yersinia pestis* from Victims of the Black Death', *Proceedings of the National Academy of Science* (2011).

69. Mandel (ed.), *Principles and Practice of Infectious Disease*; Fauci, et al. (eds), *Harrison's The Principles of Internal Medicine*, pp. 980–5; R. E. Thomas et al., 'Experimentally

Induced Plague Infection in the Northern Grasshopper Mouse Acquired by Consumption of Infected Prey', *Journal of Wildlife Disease*, 25:4 (1989), p. 477; and L. Houhamdi, H. Lepidi, M. Drancourt and D. Raoult, 'Experimental Model to Evaluate the Human Body Louse as a Vector of Plague', *Journal of Infectious Disease*, 194:11 (2006), pp. 1589–96.

70. N. C. Stenseth et al., 'Plague: Past, Present and Future', *PLoS Medicine* (15 January 2008), pp. 1–12. This group of plague scientists cautioned that there is a lack of understanding of the disease even in the best studied foci.

71. A. Laudisoit et al., 'Plague and the Human Flea, Tanzania', *Emerging Infectious Diseases*, 13:5 (13 May 2007), pp. 687–93, and R. J. Eisen et al., 'Early-Phase Transmission of *Yersinia pestis* by Unblocked Fleas as a Mechanism Explaining Rapidly Spreading Plague Epizootics', *Proceedings of the National Academy of Sciences*, 103:42 (17 October 2006), pp. 15380–5.

72. S. Ayyadurai, F. Sebbane, D. Raoult and M. Drancourt, 'Body Lice, *Yersinia Pestis* Orientalis, and Black Death', *Emerging Infectious Diseases*, 16:5 (2010), pp. 892–3.

73. O. Benedictow, *The Black Death 1346–1353: The Complete History* (Woodbridge: Boydell Press, 2004).

74. P. Manson-Bahr, p. 264. This position was also taken in an article on plague in *JAMA* in 1903. 'The Plague', *Journal of the American Medical Association*, 41 (June 1903), p. 322.

75. Of course, the distinction was been made by the second generation of plague scientists between the occasional case of plague or small localized outbreaks, which they believe could be transmitted by disparate vectors, and epidemic plague which they contended always required a preceding rat epizootic. Yet it cannot be overlooked that their evidence for the essential nature of a rat epizootic to epidemic plague came primarily from Asia during an epidemic that had no significant impact on Europe.

76. Simpson, *Treatise on Plague* p. 179.

77. Ibid., pp. 161, 46.

78. Ibid., pp. 179, 126–44.

79. Ibid., pp. 90–5, 150.

80. Hankin, 'On the Epidemiology of Plague', pp. 63–4.

81. Ibid., pp. 71–7.

82. Hirst, *The Conquest of Plague*, p. 241.

83. Hankin, 'On the Epidemiology of Plague', p. 71, and Simpson, *Treatise on Plague*, p. 69, disagreed on the impact of the extensive anti-plague measures employed by the colonial government at the onset of the epidemic in India. Simpson felt they had limited the spread of the disease and Hankin believed they led the Indians to conceal cases. Either way, these measures are one reason why the Indian plague experience in the late nineteenth century cannot be used as a control group for untreated plague.

84. In the last several years, both scientists and historians have begun to consider the possibility of vectors other than the black rat in plague transmission and they have also begun to take into consideration the influence of environmental factors on the history of the disease, so the Plague Research Commission's tight grip on plague historiography has begun to loosen, although the rat is still usually given primacy of place in its transmission. See P. D. Buell, '*Qubilai* and the Rats', *Sudhoffs Archiv*, 96:2 (2012), pp. 127–43, and B. Campbell, 'Panzootics, Pandemics and Climate Anomalies in the Fourteenth Century', in *Beiträge zum Göttinger Umwelthistorischen Kolloquium 2010–2011*, ed. B. Herrman (Göttingen: Universitäts verlag Göttingen, 2011), pp. 177–215.

85. 'Targeted Enrichment of Ancient Pathogens Yielding the pPP1 Plasmid of *Yersinia pestis* from Victims of the Black Death'.

8 Samanta, 'Physicians, Forceps and Childbirth: Technological Intervention in Reproductive Health in Colonial Bengal'

1. Some of the recent writings on the theme include S. Mukherjee, 'Disciplining the Body: Healthcare for Women and Children in Early 20th Century Bengal', in D. Kumar (ed.), *Disease and Medicine in India: A Historical Overview* (New Delhi: Tulika Publication, 2001); S. Mukherjee, 'Women, Medicine and Empire: Female Practitioners and Patterns of Healthcare in Colonial Bengal', *Modern Historical Studies,* Journal of the Department of History, RabindraBharati University, vol. 2, 2001; S. Mukherjee, 'Medical Education for Female Doctors in Colonial Bengal: Genesis and Social Importance', Paper Presented at *IAHA,* JNU, 14–17 November 2008; S. Hodges (ed.), *Reproductive Health in India: History, Politics Controversies* (New Delhi: Orient Longman, 2006); G. Forbes, 'Managing Midwifery in India', in *Women in Colonial India: Essays on Politics, Medicine and Historiography* (New Delhi: Chronicle Books, 2005); G. Forbes, 'No Science for Lady Doctors: The Education and Medical Practice of Vernacular Women Doctors in Nineteenth Century Bengal', in N. Kumar (ed.), *Women and Science in India: A Reader* (New Delhi: Oxford University Press, 2009); S. Guha, 'A History of the Medicalization of Childbirth in Bengal in the Late Nineteenth and Early Twentieth Centuries' (PhD Thesis: University of Calcutta, 1996); M. Borthwick, *The Changing Role of Women in Bengal, 1849–1905* (Princeton, NJ: Princeton University Press, 1984)
2. G. H. Forbes, *Women in Colonial India: Essays on Politics, Medicine and Historiography* (New Delhi: Chronicle Books, 2005), p. 86
3. C. Van Hollen; *Birth on the Threshold: Child birth and Modernity in South India* (New Delhi: Zubaan, 2003), p. 36.
4. P. Mukharji, *Nationalizing the Body: The Medical Market, Print, and Daktari Medicine* (New York: Anthem Press, 2009), pp. 77–83.
5. Ibid., pp. 36–7.
6. Hodges (ed.), *Reproductive Health in India,* p. 5.
7. Forbes, *Women in Colonial India,* p. 80.
8. P. Branca, *Silent Sisterhood; Middle Class Women in the Victorian Home* (London: Croom. Helm, 1975), p. 63
9. For a more detailed study one might look up Branca, *Silent Sisterhood,* p. 63.
10. A. Dhar, 'Bengali Male Physicians in the Domain of Women's Reproductive Health in Colonial Bengal', in A. Samanta et al. (eds), *Life and Culture in Bengal: Colonial and Post-Colonial Experiences* (Kolkata: Progressive Publishers, 2011), pp. 52–73.
11. M. Murmu, 'Unshackling Bamalekhani: The Emergence of Bengali Women Authors in the Second half of the Nineteenth Century' (PhD Dissertation submitted to the Jawaharlal Nehru University, New Delhi, 2011).
12. S. Mukherjee; 'Women Medicine and Empire: Female Practitioners and Patterns of Health Care in Colonial Bengal', *Modern Historical Studies,* 2 (2001), pp. 188–204.
13. Dhar, 'Bengali Male Physicians in the Domain of Women's Reproductive Health in Colonial Bengal', p. 55
14. D. Arnold, *Colonizing the Body: State Medicine and Epidemic Disease in Nineteenth-Century India* (Berkeley, CA: University of California Press, 1993), p. 6.
15. S. Guha, 'The Best Swadeshi' in *Reproductive Health in Bengal 1840–1940,* in Hodges (ed.), *Reproductive Health in India,* p. 149.

16. Borthwick, *The Changing Role of Women in Bengal*, p. 161–2. Also Aparajita Dhar in Samanta et al. (eds), *Life and Culture in Bengal: Colonial and Post-Colonial Experiences*, pp. 64–5

17. *Amritabazar Patrika*, 25 May 1869, p. 5

18. *Report of the General Committee of the Fever Hospital and Municipal Improvements*, Appendix D, pp. 88–9. West Bengal State Archives.

19. *British Medical Journal* (28 March 1936), pp. 670–1.

20. *Obstetric Forceps: Its History and Evolution* (St Louis: VV Mosby Company, 1929).

21. Dhar, 'Bengali Male Physicians in the Domain of Reproductive Health in Colonial Bengal', pp. 61–2.

22. See www.indiandoctors.com/OBGYN/.../Procedures_in_OBGYN_03.htm [accessed 5 May 2012].

23. The Sanskrit word 'Ankush' denotes a stick with a spike or prong at one end that is used in India for goading elephants. But here it indicates a forceps designed to induce safe and less painful delivery.

24. 'Ancient India', *Medical History*, Albert S. Lyons, http://www.healthguidance.org/entry/6311/1/Ancient-India.html [accessed 8 May 2012].

25. Simpson forceps, devised by Professor Donald Simpson, sometime in 1848, are surgical forceps that are used during childbirth. They are comprised of two metal handles for the physician to grip, a pelvic blade, a cephalic blade and the shank, where the blades meet the handles. Simpson forceps are often used when the child's head becomes elongated as he or she passes through the birth canal. See www.wisegeek.com/what-are-simpson-forceps.html [accessed 4 January 2011].

26. Dr V. Sudhakaram, 'Institutional Deliveries in India: A Socio-Economic and Cultural View'. Source: http://www.articlesbase.com/womens-health-articles/institutional-deliveries-in-india-a-socio-economic-and-cultural-view--808672.html [accessed 10 May 2011].

27. P. Fajans, R. Simmons and L. Ghiron, 'Helping Public Sector Health Systems Innovate: The Strategic Approaches to Strengthening Reproductive Health Policies Program', *American Journal of Public Health*, 96:3 (March 2006), pp. 435–40.

28. C. P. McCormack (ed.), Preface, in *Ethnography of Fertility and Birth* (London: Academic Press, 1982). Referred to by S. Guha, 'From Dias to Doctors: The Medicalization of childbirth in Colonial India'. URL: http://www.hsph.harvard.edu/Organizations/healthnet/SAsia/suchana/0603/guha.html [accessed 10 May 2011].

29. J. Donnison, *Midwives and Medical Men: A History of the Struggle for the Control of Childbirth* (London: New Barnet Historical Publications, 1988), p. 17.

30. For an interesting discussion on 'natural childbirth' and its transformation in Britain see, O. Moscucci, 'Holistic Obstetrics: The Origins of "Natural Childbirth" in Britain', *Postgrad Medical Journal*, 79 (2003), pp. 168–73.

31. Cecil G. Helman, 'Introduction: The Scope of Medical Anthropology', in *Culture, Health and Illness* (London: Hodder Arnold, 2007); see also, chapter 6: 'Gender and Reproduction'.

32. P. A. Treichler, 'Feminism, Medicine, and the Meaning of Childbirth', in *Body/Politics: Women and the Discourses of Science*, ed. M. Jacobus, E. Fox Keller and S. Shuttleworth (New York: Routledge, 1990), pp. 113–38.

33. A. Digby and H. Sweet, 'Nurses as Culture Brokers in Twentieth-Century South Africa', in W. Ernst (ed.), *Plural Medicine, Tradition and Modernity, 1800–2000* (London and New York: Routledge, 2002), p. 113.

34. Ibid., p. 120.

35. H. Deacon, 'Midwives and Medical Men in the Cape Colony before 1860', *Journal of African History*, 39:2 (1998), pp. 271–94.

36. A. Schriefer, *Shifting the Medical Gaze: Towards a Feminist Ethic of Childbirth*. URL: http://www2.gwu.edu/~medusa/articles.html [accessed 16 November 2011]. Also R. Davis-Floyd, 'The Technocratic, Humanistic, and Holistic Paradigms of Childbirth' in *Medical Anthropology Quarterly* 2001; 20 (2, 3 and 4), pp. 105–39. It is a special issue on theme of 'Daughters of Time: The Shifting Identities of Contemporary Midwives'.

37. This section is heavily drawn on Jayanta Bhattacharya's paper 'Modernity and Indigenization: A Study into Biomedical Discourses in India'. URL: ftp://ftp.solutionexchange.net.in/public/mch/.../res-07-271106-24.doc [accessed 22 February 2011].

38. LokSwaasthyaParamparaSamvardhanSamithi (LSPSS), *Mother and Child Care in Traditional Medicine,* Parts I and II. URL: http://www.healthlibrary.com/reading/ncure/mother/ [accessed 20 January 2005].

39. R. A. Aronowitz, *Making Sense of Illness; Science, Society, and Disease* (New York: Cambridge University Press, 1998), pp. 166–71.

40. W. Stephenson, 'A Criticism of the Midwifery Forceps in General Use', *British Medical Journal*, 1:1422 (31 March 1888), pp. 684–5.

41. Dr Henry Jellett, Correspondence, *British Medical Journal*, 2:1916 (18 September 1897), p. 746.

42. W. Legge, 'The Use of the Forceps in Midwifery', Correspondence, *British Medical Journal*, 2:1915 (11 September 1897), p. 682.

43. *Report of the Health Survey and Development Committee*, 1 (Delhi: Manager of Publications, 1946), p. 9.

44. *Report of the Health Survey and Development Committee*, 2: 487. D. Arnold, 'Official Attitudes to Population, Birth Control and Reproductive Health in India, 1921–1946', in Hodges (ed.), *Reproductive Health in India: History, Politics, Controversies*, p. 46.

45. M. Sharma, 'Creating a Consumer: Exploring Medical Advertisements in Colonial India', in B. Pati and M. Harrison (eds), *The Social History of Health and Medicine in Colonial India* (London and New York: Routledge, 2009), pp. 223–4.

46. C. Jaffrelot, *The Hindu Nationalist Movement and Indian Politics 1925 to the 1990s* (London: Hurst & Company, 1996), p. 14.

9 Saha, 'Not Fit for Punishment: Diagnosing Criminal Lunatics in Late Nineteenth-Century British India'

1. Major J. M. Woolley, 'Appendix A: Insanity in the Andamans', in R. F. Lowis (ed.), *Census of India, 1911, Volume II: The Andaman and Nicobar Islands* (Calcutta: Superintendent Government Printing, 1912), pp. 106–7.

2. Major J. M. Woolley, 'Suicide among Indian Convicts under Transportation', *British Journal of Psychiatry*, 59 (1913), pp. 335–43.

3. A. Appadurai, 'Number in the Colonial Imagination', in C. A. Breckenridge and P. Van Der Veer (eds), *Orientalism and the Postcolonial Predicament: Perspectives on South Asia* (Philadelphia, PA: University of Pennsylvania Press, 1993), pp. 114–35.

4. For a relevant example, see J. H. Mills, *Madness, Cannabis and Colonialism: The 'Native-Only' Lunatic Asylums of British India, 1857–1900* (Basingstoke: Palgrave Macmillan, 2000), pp. 43–65.

5. Woolley, 'Appendix A: Insanity in the Andamans', pp. 107–9.

6. Particularly in comparison with French North Africa: R. Keller, 'Madness and Colonization: Psychiatry in the British and French Empires, 1800–1962', *Journal of Social History*, 35:2 (2001), pp. 295–326.

7. W. Ernst, *Mad Tales From the Raj: Colonial Psychiatry in South Asia, 1800–58* (London; New York: Anthem, 2010); Mills, *Madness, Cannabis and Colonialism*.

8. M. Foucault, *Madness and Civilisation*, trans. R. Howard (London; New York: Routledge, 2005).

9. W. Ernst, 'Idioms of Madness and Colonial Boundaries: The Case of European and "Native" Mentally Ill in Early Nineteenth-Century British India', *Comparative Studies in Society and History*, 37:1 (1997), pp. 153–81.

10. J. H. Mills, 'Body as Target, Violence as Treatment: Psychiatric Regimes in Colonial and Post-Colonial India', in J. H. Mills and S. Sen (eds), *Confronting the Body: The Politics of Physicality in Colonial and Post-Colonial India* (London: Anthem, 2004), pp. 80–101.

11. S. Kapila, 'Masculinity and Madness: Princely Personhood and Colonial Sciences of the Mind in Western India, 1871–1940', *Past & Present*, 187 (2005), pp. 121–56; S. Kapila, 'The "Godless" Freud and his Indian Friends: An Indian Agenda for Psychoanalysis', in S. Mahone and M. Vaughan (eds), *Psychiatry and Empire* (Basingstoke: Palgrave Macmillan, 2007), pp. 124–52.

12. T. Sherman, *State Violence and Punishment in India* (Abingdon: Routledge, 2010), pp. 1–13.

13. J. Saha, 'Madness and the Making of a Colonial Order in Burma', *Modern Asian Studies*, 47:2 (2013), pp. 406–35.

14. A. A. Yang, 'Disciplining "Natives": Prisons and Prisoners in Early Nineteenth-Century India', *South Asia*, 10:2 (1987), pp. 29–45; D. Arnold, 'The Colonial Prison: Power, Knowledge and Penology in Nineteenth-Century India', in D. Arnold and D. Hardiman (eds), *Subaltern Studies VIII: Essays in Honour of Ranajit Guha* (New Delhi: Oxford University Press, 1994), pp. 148–87.

15. M. Foucault, *Discipline and Punish: The Birth of the Prison*, trans. Alan Sheridan (London: Penguin Books, 1991).

16. S. B. Frietag, 'Crime in the Social Order of Colonial North India', *Modern Asian Studies*, 25:2 (1991), pp. 227–61; A. J. Major, 'State and Criminal Tribes in Colonial Punjab: Surveillance, Control and Reclamation of the "Dangerous Classes"', *Modern Asian Studies*, 33:3 (1999), pp. 657–88; R. Singha, '"Providential Circumstances": The Thuggee Campaign of the 1830s and Legal Innovation', *Modern Asian Studies*, 27:1 (1993), pp. 83–146; V. Lal, 'Everyday Crime, Native Mendacity and the Cultural Psychology of Justice in Colonial India', *Studies in History*, 15:1 (1999), pp. 145–66.

17. Arnold, 'Colonial Prison'.

18. Mills, *Madness, Cannabis and Colonialism*, pp. 90–7.

19. A. Scull, *The Most Solitary of Afflictions: Madness and Society in Britain, 1700–1900* (New Haven, CT and London: Yale University Press, 1993).

20. Arnold, 'Colonial Prison'.

21. J. Sadowsky, *Imperial Bedlam: Institutions of Madness in Colonial Southwest Nigeria* (Berkley, CA and London: University of California Press, 1999), pp. 78–96; M. McKittrick, 'Faithful Daughter, Murdering Mother: Transgression and Social Control in Colonial Namibia', *Journal of African History*, 40:2 (1999), pp. 265–83.

22. M. Vaughan, 'Idioms of Madness: Zomba Lunatic Asylum, Nyasaland, in the Colonial Period', *Journal of Southern African Studies*, 9:2 (1983), pp. 218–38; L. Jackson, *Surfac-*

ing Up: Psychiatry and Social Order in Colonial Zimbabwe, 1908–1968 (Ithaca, NY and London: Cornell University Press, 2005).

23. J. L. Comaroff, 'Reflection on the Colonial State, in South Africa and Elsewhere: Factions, Fragments, Facts and Fictions', *Social Identities*, 4:3 (1998), pp. 321–61.

24. Also noted recently in a study on French Indochina: C. Edington, 'Getting in and Getting out of the Colonial Asylum: Families and Psychiatric Care in French Indochina', *Comparative Studies in Society and History*, 55:3 (2013), pp. 725–55.

25. S. Sen, *Disciplining Punishment: Colonialism and Convict Society in the Andaman Islands* (New Delhi and Oxford: Oxford University Press, 2000), pp. 158–60.

26. G. F. W. Ewens, *Insanity in India: Its Symptoms and Diagnosis with Reference to the Relation of Crime and Insanity* (Thacker: Calcutta, 1908), pp. 16–18. For more on the use of nasal feeding as both treatment and punishment, see I. Miller, 'Necessary Torture? Vivisection, Suffragette Force-Feeding, and Responses to Scientific Medicine in Britain, c. 1870–1920', *Journal of the History of Medicine & Allied Sciences*, 64:3 (2008), pp. 333–72; J. Saha, '"Uncivilized Practitioners": Medical Subordinates, Medico-Legal Evidence and Misconduct in Colonial Burma, c.1875–1907', *South East Asia Research*, 20:3 (2012), pp. 423–7.

27. Mills, 'Body as Target, Violence as Treatment'.

28. S. Swartz, 'The Regulation of British Colonial Lunatic Asylums and the Origins of Colonial Psychiatry, 1860–1864', *History of Psychology*, 13:2 (2010), pp. 160–77.

29. India Office Records, British Library, hereafter IOR, P/1006, *Government of India, hereafter GoI, Home Department (Port Blair)*, August 1876.

30. Sen, *Disciplining Punishment*, 131–65.

31. IOR, P/1006, *GoI, Home Dept. (Port Blair)*, November 1878, Part B.

32. Ibid., August 1876.

33. IOR, V/24/3875, *Andaman and Nicobar Islands, Medical Department: Annual sanitary and medical report on the settlement of Port Blair* (Andamans, 1869); and the following year's report, IOR, P/697C, *GoI, Dept. of Agriculture, Revenue and Commerce (Port Blair)*, November 1871.

34. These concerns had long precedence in transportation procedures, see: C. Anderson, '"The Ferringees are Flying – the Ship is Ours!" The Convict Middle Passage in Colonial South and Southeast Asia', *Indian Economic and Social History Review*, 42:3 (2005), pp. 143–86. IOR, MSS Eur F98/37, *Chief Commissioner's Office, Port Blair, Selections From Correspondence (1970–75) of Late Field Marshall Sir D. M. Stewart* (1900), No. 145.

35. IOR, P/528, *GoI, Home Dept. (Port Blair)*, June 1875.

36. Ibid., August 1874.

37. On the changing role of Alipore jail in penal transportation, see: A. A. Yang, 'Indian Convict Workers in Southeast Asia in the Late Eighteenth and Early Nineteenth Centuries', *Journal of World History*, 14:2 (2003), pp. 193–5, p. 206.

38. IOR, P/256, *Government of Bengal, Jails Dept.*, April 1873.

39. IOR, MSS Eur F98/37, *Correspondence of Stewart*, No. 145.

40. B. Anderson, *Legible Bodies: Race, Criminality and Colonialism in South Asia* (Oxford: Anthem, 2004), pp. 32–6.

41. IOR, P/697C, *GoI, Dept. of Agriculture, Revenue and Commerce (Port Blair)*, January 1873.

42. IOR, V/10/589, *Andaman and Nicobar Islands Administration Report, 1872–1873*, p. 14.

43. IOR, P/528, *GoI, Home Dept. (Port Blair)*, January 1874.

44. Sen, *Disciplining Punishment*, 58–61.
45. IOR, P/528, *GoI, Home Dept. (Port Blair)*, January 1874.
46. Ibid.
47. Ibid.
48. Ibid.
49. Ibid., March 1875.
50. Ibid., June 1875.
51. IOR, P/1006, *GoI, Home Dept. (Port Blair)*, November 1876.
52. These started as temporary committees convened when necessary, but they became permanent in the 1880s: Ibid., March 1877; and IOR, P/2246, *Government of Bengal, Jails Dept.*, July 1885.
53. IOR, P/1670, *GoI, Home Dept. (Port Blair)*, September 1882.
54. IOR, P/2512, *GoI, Home Dept. (Port Blair)*, March 1885.
55. IOR, P/1670, *GoI, Home Dept. (Port Blair)*, September 1882.
56. IOR, P/2263, *GoI, Home Dept. (Port Blair)*, December 1884.
57. Ibid., June 1884, Part B.
58. IOR, P/2512, *GoI, Home Dept. (Port Blair)*, May 1885.
59. Ibid.
60. IOR, P/2961, *GoI, Home Dept. (Port Blair)*, January 1887, Part B.
61. A, Skaria, 'Shades of Wildness: Tribe, Caste and Gender in Western India', *Journal of Asia Studies*, 56:3 (1997), pp. 726–45; for Bengali views of the Santal see, P. Banerjee, 'Historic Acts? Santal Rebellion and the Temporality of Practice', *Studies in History*, 15:2 (1999), pp. 209–46.
62. IOR, P/2263, *GoI, Home Dept. (Port Blair)*, December 1884, Part B.
63. On its use in colonial India see, Kapila, 'Masculinity and Madness', p. 148.
64. IOR, P/6, *British Burma, Home Dept.*, 30 September 1874.
65. Ibid., 2 November 1874.
66. For Burma, see: P. Edwards, 'Bitter Pills: Colonialism, Medicine and Nationalism in Burma, 1870–1940', *Journal of Burma Studies*, 14 (2010), pp. 21–58; A. Naono, 'Inoculators, the Indigenous Obstacle to Vaccination in Colonial Burma', *Journal of Burma Studies*, 14 (2010), pp. 91–114; J. Saha, '"Uncivilized Practitioners"', pp. 423–43. And for British India as a whole, see: D. Arnold, *Colonizing the Body: State Medicine and Epidemic Disease in Nineteenth-Century India* (California: University of California Press, 1993), pp. 11–60; M. Harrison, '"The Tender Frame of Man": Disease, Climate and Racial Difference in India and the West Indies, 1760–1860', *Bulletin of the History of Medicine* 70:1 (1996), pp. 68–93.
67. IOR, P/5, *British Burma, Home Dept.*, 5 March 1874.
68. IOR, P/3, *British Burma, Home Dept.*, 26 May 1873.
69. K. N. MacDonald, *The Practice of Medicine Among the Burmese, Translated From Original Manuscripts with an Historical Sketch of the Progress of Medicine, from the Earliest Times* (Edinburgh: Maclachlan and Stewart, 1873), p. 26, pp. 30–1, p. 36.
70. J. G. Scott, *The Burman: His Life and Notions* (London: Macmillan, 1882), pp. 414–20.
71. IOR, P/5, *British Burma, Home Dept.*, 22 June 1874.
72. I. Brown, 'South East Asia: Reform and the Colonial Prison', in F. Dikotter and I. Brown (eds), *Cultures of Confinement: A History of the Prison in Africa, Asia and Latin America* (Ithaca: Cornell University Press, 2007), pp. 221–68; I. Brown, 'A Commissioner Calls: Alexander Paterson and Colonial Burma's Prisons', *Journal of Southeast Asian Studies*, 38:2 (2007), pp. 293-308; J. Warren, 'The Rangoon Jail Riot of 1930 and the Prison

Administration of British Burma', *South East Asia Research*, 10:1 (2002), pp. 5–29; J. Saha, 'Colonization, Criminality, and Corruption: Policing Gambling in Burma, c.1880–1920', *South East Asia Research* (Forthcoming).

73. *Annual Report of the Rangoon Lunatic Asylum, for the Year 1888*.

74. IOR, P/4, *British Burma, Home Dept.*, 22 February 1873.

75. Ibid.

76. Ibid., 29 May 1873.

77. Ibid., 31 October 1873.

78. IOR, P/779, *British Burma, Home Dept.*, 17 February 1876.

79. S. Gilman, *Seeing the Insane: A Cultural History of Madness and Art in the Western World* (New York: Wiley, 1982).

80. IOR, P/4, *British Burma, Home Dept.*, 22 February 1873.

81. Ibid., 7 August 1873.

82. IOR, P/4, *British Burma, Home Dept.*, 7 August 1873; *Annual Report of the Rangoon Lunatic Asylum, for the year 1884*.

83. IOR, P/2, *British Burma, Home Dept.*, 30 October 1871.

84. C. Ikeya, 'The "Traditional" High Status of Women in Burma', *Journal of Burma Studies*, 10 (2005), 51–81; J. Saha, 'The Male State: Colonialism, Corruption and Rape Investigations in the Irrawaddy Delta c.1900', *Indian Economic and Social History Review*, 47:3 (2010), pp. 343–76; *Report on Criminal and Civil Justice in British Burma, for the Year 1870–71*.

85. IOR, P/1272, *British Burma, Home Dept.*, 4 February 1879.

86. Ibid., 9 July 1879.

87. Arnold, *Colonizing the Body*, pp. 1–10.

88. I make a similar point regarding medicine in British Burma more broadly in Saha, '"Uncivilized Practitioners"' and J. Saha, 'State Medicine or Medical State? A Prison Epidemic in Colonial Burma, 1881', in R. Deb Roy and G. Attewell (eds), *Locating the 'Medical' in Histories of South Asia* (New Delhi: Oxford University Press, forthcoming).

89. Kapila, 'The "Godless" Freud and his Indian Friends'.

90. D. G. Crawford, *A History of the Indian Medical Service 1600–1913* (London: W Thacker, 1914).

10 Swartz, 'Multiple Voices and Plausible Claims: Historiography and Colonial Lunatic Asylum Archives'

1. A version of this chapter appeared as 'Colonial Lunatic Asylums: Challenges to Historiography', *Kronos*, 34 (2008), pp. 285–302.

2. P. Allderidge, 'Bedlam: Fact or Fantasy?' in W. Bynum, R. Porter, and M Shepherd (eds), *Anatomy of Madness*, vol. 1 (London: Tavistock, 1985), p. 17.

3. J. Derrida, *Archive Fever* (Chicago, IL: University of Chicago Press, 1996).

4. A. Stoler, 'Colonial Archives and the Arts of Governance: On the Content in the Form', in *Refiguring the Archive*, ed. C. Hamilton, V. Harris, J. Taylor, M. Pickover, G. Reid and R. Saleh (Cape Town: David Philip, 2002), p. 92, p. 100.

5. See F. Fanon, *Black Skins, White Masks* (Grove Press, 1967), and M. Foucault, *Madness and Civilization: A History of Insanity in the Age of Reason* (Vintage, 1988). R. Keller, 'Madness and Colonization: Psychiatry in the British and French empires, 1800–1962',

Journal of Social History, 35 (2001), pp. 295–326 gives a succinct essential history of scholarship on African colonial psychiatry.

6.   M. Vaughan, *Curing Their Ills: Colonial Power and African Illness* (Oxford: Polity Press, 1991) ch. 5; J. McCulloch, *Colonial Psychiatry and 'The African Mind* (Cambridge, Cambridge University Press, 1995); J. Sadowsky, *Imperial Bedlam: Institutions of Madness in Colonial Southwest Nigeria* (Berkeley: University of California Press, 1999); R. Edgar and H. Sapire, *African Apocalypse: The Story of NontethaNkwenkwe, a Twentieth-Century South African Prophet* (Johannesburg: Witwatersrand University Press, 2000); L.Jackson, *Surfacing Up: Psychiatry and Social Order in Colonial Zimbabwe, 1908–1968* (Ithaca, NY and London: Cornell University Press, 2005); J. Parle, *States of Mind: Mental Illness and the Quest for Mental Health in Natal and Zululand, 1868–1918* (Scottsville: University of KwaZulu-Natal Press, 2007).

7.   For example, H. Deacon, 'Madness, Race and Moral Treatment: Robben Island Lunatic Asylum, 1846–1890', *History of Psychiatry*, 7 (1996), pp. 287–97; F. Swanson, '"Of Unsound Mind": A History of Three Eastern Cape Mental Institutions, 1875–1910' (M.A (History) thesis, University of Cape Town, 2001); S. Swartz, 'Colonizing the Insane: Causes of Insanity in the Cape, 1891–1920', *History of the Human Sciences*, 8 (1995), pp. 39–57; S. Swartz, 'The Black Insane in the Cape, 1891–1920', *Journal of Southern African Studies*, 21 (1995), pp. 399–415; S. Marks, '"Every Facility That Modern Science and Enlightened Humanity Have Devised": Race and Progress in a Colonial Hospital, Valkenberg Mental Asylum, Cape Colony, 1894–1910', in J. Melling and B. Forsythe (eds), *Insanity, Institutions and Society, 1800–1914: A Social History of Madness in Comparative Perspective* (London: Routledge, 1999); H. Deacon, E. van Heyningen, S. Swartz, and F. Swanson, 'Mineral Wealth and Medical Opportunity', in H. Deacon, H. Phillips, and E. van Heyningen (eds), *The Cape Doctor in the Nineteenth Century: A Social History* (Amsterdam: Rodopi, 2004). Wellcome Series in the History of Medicine. See also the valuable collection of S. Mahone, and M. Vaughan (eds), *Psychiatry and Empire* (Basingstoke: Palgrave Macmillan, 2007).

8.   See A. Lambert and D. Lester, 'Introduction: Imperial Spaces, Imperial Subjects', in A. Lambert and D. Lester (eds), *Colonia Lives across the British Empire: Imperial Careering in the Long Nineteenth Century* (Cambridge University Press: Cambridge, 2006) for a description of the 'new imperial studies' agenda.

9.   W. Ernst, *Mad Tales from the Raj: the European Insane in British India, 1800–1858* (London: Routledge, 1991); J. Mills, *Madness, Cannabis and Colonialism: The 'Native-Only' Asylums of British India, 1857–1900* (Basingstoke: Palgrave Macmillan, 2000); C. Coleborne, *Madness in the Family: Insanity and Institutions in the Australasian Colonial World, 1860–1914* (New York: Palgrave Macmillan, 2010); J. Saha, 'Madness and the Making of a Colonial Order in Burma', *Modern Asian Studies*, 47 (2013), pp. 406–35. and H. Pols, 'Psychological Knowledge in a Colonial Context: Theories on the Nature of the "Native Mind" in the Former Dutch East Indies', *History of Psychology*, 10 (2007), pp. 111–31. For a transcolonial perspective on colonial psychiatry, see S. Swartz, 'The Regulation of British Colonial Lunatic Asylums and the Origins of Colonial Psychiatry, 1860–1864', *History of Psychology*, 13 (2010), pp. 160–77.

10. For a summary of the kinds of justifications used, see Swartz, 'The Black Insane', and 'Colonizing the Insane'.

11. See M. Foucault, *The Archaeology of Knowledge* (London: Tavistock, 1972), ch. 5.

12. *Curing Their Ills*, p. 118. For a very illuminating comparison with British officials' construction of otherness in the Burmese insane, see J. Saha, 'Not Fit for Punishment', Chapter 9 in this volume.

13. For a description of the late nineteenth century South African history of this particular discourse, see Swartz, 'Colonizing the Insane'. It was repeated in similar forms throughout Africa in the first part of the twentieth century.

14. T. D. Greenlees, 'Insanity among the Natives of South Africa', *Journal of Mental Science*, 41 (1895), pp. 71–8; J. Conry, 'Insanity among Natives in Cape Colony', *South African Medical Record*, 5 (1907), pp. 33–6.

15. Swartz, 'Colonizing the Insane'.

16. Cape Archives (CA), CO 7542 February 1899; Parle, *States of Mind*, chs 3 and 4.

17. *Imperial Bedlam*, p. 116; *States of Mind*, p. 304.

18. *Curing Their Ills*, p. 125.

19. *African Apocalypse*, p. 34.

20. Swartz, 'Colonizing the Insane'; Parle, *States of Mind*, Ch 1.

21. *Surfacing Up*, p. 14.

22. Ibid., p. 127.

23. Ibid., p. 110.

24. For example, Sadowsky's treatment of the colonial psychiatry/oppression link is very sophisticated and careful, and yet the title of his book, *Imperial Bedlam*, rehearses this genealogy.

25. M. Foucault, *The Archaeology of Knowledge*, p. 129.

26. The history of this term is obscure, but appears to have been widely used in colonial contexts.

27. For a full description of the remaining buildings, and their original functions, see H. Deacon, unpublished historical research report on Oude Molen, March 2003. J. Louw and S. Swartz, 'An English Asylum in Africa: Space and Order in Valkenberg Asylum', *History of Psychology*, 4 (2001), pp. 3–23, gives a description of the relationship between spaces and social functioning.

28. S. Brand, *How Buildings Learn: What Happens After They're Built* (New York: Penguin, 1994). The heavy doors with inset observation hatches and century-old iron keys of these 'offices' have been known to 'forget' themselves, and slam shut on clinicians (myself among them), who are then obliged to shout for their release.

29. S. Swartz, 'The Third voice: Writing Case Notes', *Feminism and Psychology*, 16 (2006), pp. 427–44; Swartz, 'Can the Clinical Subject Speak?' *Theory and Psychology*, 15 (2005), pp. 505–25.

30. *Curing their Ills*, p. 102.

31. For an extended treatment of the South African 'archive' see *Refiguring the Archive*.

32. CO 7826.

33. For example, The *Journal of Mental Science*, copies of which from this period are housed in the archive of University of Cape Town's Medical Library, are annotated.

34. For an analysis of Valkenberg's buildings, see Louw and Swartz, 'An English Asylum in Africa'.

35. See for example E. Spooner, '"The Mind Is Thoroughly Unhinged": Reading the Auckland Asylum Archive, New Zealand, 1900–1910', *Health and History* (2005), pp. 56–79; S. Piddock, 'A Space of Their Own: Nineteenth Century Lunatic Asylums in Britain, South Australia and Tasmania', *Australian Archaeology*, 56 (2003), p. 58; S. Piddock, '"An Irregular and Inconvenient Pile of Buildings": The Destitute Asylum of

Adelaide, South Australia and the English Workhouse', *International Journal of Historical Archaeology*, 5 (2001), pp. 73–95. *Medicine and Magnificence: British Hospital and Asylum Architecture, 1660–1815* (Paul Mellon Centre for Studies in British Art, 2000); S. Spencer-Wood and S. Baugher, 'Introduction and Historical Context for the Archaeology of Institutions of Reform. Part I: Asylums', *International Journal of Historical Archaeology*, 5 (2001), pp. 3–17.

36. A. Stoler, '"In Cold Blood": Hierarchies of Credibility and the Politics of Colonial Narratives', *Representations*, 37 (1992), pp. 151–89.

37. Ibid., p. 183.

38. Ibid., p. 184.

39. Swartz, 'The Black Insane'.

40. For example he is on record as dismissing a nurse for hitting a patient with a slipper 'during a scuffle'. 'She has forfeited my confidence. She has been spoken to before for her sharp way of speaking to patients and I do not think she has the qualities necessary for a good mental nurse'. CO 7975, 30th August, 1905.

41. CO 7178.

42. *Select Committee*, p. 16, p. 9.

43. See F. Jensz, 'Missionaries and Indigenous Education in the 19thj Century British Empire. Part II: Race, Class, and Gender'. *History Compass* 10 (2012), pp. 306–17. See also the ongoing research project of R. Swartz on native education in Natal and Western Australia, History Department of Royal Holloway, University College London.

44. FC 201, 2 March, 1918.

45. Phillip D, MC 67.

46. E. Dickinson, 'Much Madness is Divinest Sense', in *Selected Poems*, ed. J. Reeves (London: Heinemann, 1963).

47. S. Swartz, 'Lost Lives: Gender, History and Mental Illness in the Cape, 1891–1910', *Feminism and Psychology*, 9 (1999), pp. 152–8; and 'Can the Clinical Subject Speak?'

48. David Wright sets out a programme for this kind of panoptical treatment of the insane subject in 'Getting Out of the Asylum: Understanding the Confinement of the Insane in the Nineteenth Century', *Social History of Medicine*, 10 (1997), pp. 137–55.

49. H. Deacon, 'Madness, Race and Moral Treatment'; H. Deacon, H. Phillips and E. van Heyningen, *The Cape Doctor in the Nineteenth Century*.

50. See for example, C. Stevenson, *Medicine and Magnificence: British Hospital and Asylum Architecture, 1660–1815* (New Haven, CT: Yale University Press, 2000); D. Sibley, *Geographies of Exclusion* (London: Routledge, 1995); C. Philo, 'Foucault's Geography', *Environment and Planning D: Society and Space*, 10 (1992), pp. 137 – 161; H. Ngubane, *Body and Mind in Zulu Medicine: An Ethnography of Health and Disease in Nyuswa-Zulu Thought and Practice* (London: Academic Press, 1977).

51. Jackson, *Surfacing Up*, p. 170.

52. For sensitive descriptions of the tensions between social historical analyses of colonial asylums and the reality of psychiatric illness, see Sadowsky, *Imperial Bedlam*, ch 4; and Parle, *States of Mind*, ch 2.

53. See P. Allderidge, 'Bedlam: Fact or Fantasy'; M. Jay, *The Air Loom Gang: The Strange and True Story of James Tilly Matthews and His Visionary Madness* (London: Bantam Press, 2003); S. Plath, *The Bell Jar* (London: Heinemann, 1963).

54. C. Van Onselen, *The Fox and the Flies, the World of Joseph Silver, Racketeer and Psychopath* (London: Jonathan Cape, 2007).

55. Valkenberg case records, UCT Manuscripts and Archives. 'Malay tricked' is a term of unclear original that surfaces occasionally in the case records, referring to patients' suspicion that their insanity was brought about by magical powers superstitiously attributed to the religious practices of the Cape Malay community.
56. S. Smith, *Selected Poems*, ed. J. MacGibbon (Harmondsworth: Penguin, 1975), p. 65.
57. An excellent example of this strategy is Sadowsky's description of the extraordinary case of Isaac O, *Imperial Bedlam*, pp. 78–96.
58. Parle, *States of Mind*.
59. Nations emerging from the effects of colonialism are in this position. The effects of colonialism on the construction of archives and the need to embed readings of them in contexts that illuminate their production has attracted a great deal of attention both before and after Derrida's *Archive Fever*. A cross-disciplinary perspective on this can be found in Ann Stoler, 'Colonial Archives and the Arts of Governance'.

11 Jentzen, 'Death and Empire: Legal Medicine in the Colonization of India and Africa'

1. J. Fisch, *Cheap Lives and Dear Limbs: The British Transformation of the Bengal Criminal Law, 1769–1817* (Wiesbarden: Franz Steiner Verlag, 1983), pp. 1–2.
2. For a discussion of the use of medicine as a weapon of colonialism, see R. C. Keller, *Colonial Madness: Psychiatry in French North Africa* (Chicago, IL: University of Chicago Press, 2007).
3. C. Crawford, 'Legalizing Medicine: Early Modern Legal Systems and the Growth of Medico-legal Knowledge', in M. Clark and C. Crawford (eds), *Legal Medicine in History* (Cambridge: Cambridge University Press, 1994), pp. 89–116.
4. See Fisch, *Cheap Lives and Dear Limbs*, pp. 1–4.
5. I refer to the recent work of Q. Pearson, 'From "Inauspicious to "Suspicious" Death: Inquests in Turn of the Twentieth Century Bangkok', Presented at the History of Science Society Meeting, Philadelphia, 2012.
6. For a short review of the development of tropical medicine see, M. Yoeli, 'The Evolution of Tropical Medicine: A Historical Perspective', *Bull N Y Acad Med*, 48:10 (1972), pp. 1231–46. On the development of military medicine, see C. Kelly, *War and the Militarization of British Army Medicine, 1793–1830* (London: Pickering & Chatto, 2011).
7. See C. Crawford, 'Legalizing Medicine', in Clark and Crawford, *Legal Medicine in History*, pp. 89–116.
8. B. Shapiro, *A Culture of Fact: England, 1550–1720* (Ithaca, NY: Cornell University Press, 2000), p. 9. According to Shapiro three principles of the common law system were particularly important to the development of a competent legal system: the distinction between 'fact' and 'matters of fact' and 'matters of law', lay jurors as arbiters of fact, particularly in regard to witness testimony, and finally the value of public proceedings and unbiased judgments.
9. A. Burney, *Bodies of Evidence: Medicine and the Politics of the English Inquest, 1830–1926* (Baltimore, MD: Johns Hopkins University Press, 2000), p. 5.
10. R. F. Hunnisett, *The Medieval Coroner* (Cambridge: Cambridge University Press, 1961), p. 1.
11. Ibid, pp. 191–9. There were several reasons for the decline of the coroner: the number of appeals declined, the abolition of the murdrum fine decrease the amount of revenue to

be gained by the coroner's inquest, the cessation of the courts of the general eyre which the county connected with local and county law courts, the rapidly rise of the justices of the peace, p. 197.

12. J. M. Jentzen, *Death Investigation in America: Coroners, Medical Examiners and the Search for Medical Certainty* (Cambridge: Harvard University Press, 2009), p. 10–11.

13. F. Fukuyama, *The Origins of Political Order: From Prehuman Times to the French Revolution* (New York: Farrar, Straus & Giroux, 2011), p. 185.

14. Ibid, p. 155.

15. On the development of the dual legal system see J. Fisch, Cheap Lives and Dear Limbs, pp. 5–6.

16. On Islamic criminal law, refer to J. Fisch, Cheap Lives and Dear Limbs, pp. 14–15. The Islamic law traditionally identified five public crimes for which a fixed punishment (hadd) is provided: unlawful intercourse, slander of unlawful intercourse, drinking wine, theft and highway robbery. Hadd was possible for no other offenses. For unlawful intercourse can be punished with death. Otherwise it leads, as with slander and drinking, corporal punishment; for theft is the loss of one limb, for highway robbery of two and if attended with murder, death.

17. K. Raj, *Relocating Modern Science: Circulation and the Construction of Knowledge in South Asia and Europe, 1650–1900* (New York: Palgrave McMillan, 2007), p. 109.

18. Ibid., p. 132. The British sought a far more ambitious project. In March 1788 they laid out the plan to 'give the native of these Indian provinces permanent equity for the due administration of justice among them, similar to that which Justinian gave to his Greek and Roman subjects, a legal corpus' after the model of Justinian's inestimable Pandects on which English law was itself based, complied by the more learned of native lawyer, with an accurate verbal translation of it into English.

19. N. Cheevers, *A Manual of Medical Jurisprudence for Bengal and the Northwestern Provinces* (Calcutta: F. Carbery Bengal Military Orphan Press, 1856), p. 9.

20. Ibid, p. 2.

21. Ibid, p. 14.

22. Ibid, p. 15. Contained in the Nizamut Adawlut Reports, N.W. P. 24 March 1853.

23. Sati was eliminated by the British in 1825, see J. Fisch, *Cheap Lives, Dear Limbs*, p. 90.

24. J.R.B. Sánchez, 'Sensitivity and Expert Controversies: The Appropriation of the Marsh Test for Arsenic Research by French Toxicologists (1836–1845)', In: I Malaquias et al (eds), *Chemistry, Technology and Society*, 5th International Conference on History of Chemistry, Aviero, Sociedade Portequesa de Quimica, 2006, pp. 300–14.

25. N. Cheevers, *Manual of Medical Jurisprudence for Bengal*, p. 86.

26. Ibid, p. 191.

27. For a review of the use of indigenous Indian poisons see N. Cheevers, Manual of Medical Jurisprudence for Bengal, pp. 68–98.

28. Ibid, p. 168.

29. D. Arnold, *Colonizing the Body: State Medicine and Epidemic Disease in Nineteenth-Century India* (Berkeley, CA: University of California Press, 1993), p. 223.

30. Ibid, pp. 4–5.

31. Ibid, p. 58.

32. Ibid, p. 108.

33. Ibid, p. 217, p. 315.

34. S. Cole, *Suspect Identities: A History of Fingerprinting and Criminal Identification* (Cambridge: Harvard University Press, 2001), pp. 65–8. Herschel's letter to the Bengal

Inspector of Jails, generally known as the 'Hooghly Letter', proposed that fingerprinting be expanded to other geographical areas and explained the uniqueness and permanence of friction ridge skin. About the same time, another Englishman, Henry Faulds, while working in Japan became interested in fingerprints he observed on ancient Japanese pottery. Faulds was he first person to publish a journal on fingerprints that emphasized their value as evidence at crime scenes. Sir Francis Galton was Charles Darwin's cousin.

35. R. A. Stindler, 'The Case of the Mysterious Dum-Dum Bullets', *Am J For Med Path*, 4: 3 (1983), pp. 205–7. The dum-dum bullet was eventually outlawed for military purposes by the Convention of The Hague in 1902.
36. H. L. Bami and B. Knight, 'Forensic Sciences in India', *Am J For Pathol Med*, 3:3 (1982), pp. 265–70.
37. Ibid.
38. Ibid.
39. K. Fahmy, 'The Anatomy of Justice: Forensic Medicine and Criminal Law in Nineteenth-Century Egypt', *Islamic Law and Society*, 6:2 (1999), p. 225.
40. I. Gordon, R. Turner and T. W. Price, *Medical Jurisprudence*, 3rd edn (Edinburgh and London: E. & S. Linvingston, 1953), p. 1.
41. Ibid, p. 239.
42. See, G. Saayman and FFW van Oosten, 'Forensic Medicine in South Africa – Time for a Change', *Medicine and Law*, 13 (1994), pp. 129–32.
43. Gordon, Turner and Price, *Medical Jurisprudence*, p. 231. All criminal proceeding is carried out under Criminal Procedures and Evidence Act No 31 of 1917. Notification of deaths and inquest of any dead body of a person who appears to have come by his death from violence, criminal neglect, or otherwise non-natural causes to report the death to the magistrate of the district.
44. Ibid, p. 243.
45. Ibid, p. 238.
46. Ibid, p. 242.
47. G. Saayman and FFW van Oosten, 'Forensic Medicine in South Africa – Time for a Change', *Medicine and Law*, 13 (1994), pp. 129–32.
48. M. Dada and J. Clarke, 'Courting Disaster? A Survey of the Autopsy Service Provided by District Suergeons in Kwazulu-Natal', *Med Law*, 19 (2000), pp. 763–77. See also, G. Saayman, 'Forensic Medicine in South Africa – Time for Change?', *Med Law*, 13 (1994), pp. 129–32.

INDEX

African National Congress, 36
African Renaissance, 27
AIDS, 25–6, 33–9, 51
    pandemic, 33
Alipore Jail Committee, 135
All India Ayurvedic Mahasammelan, 18
All India Veterinary School, 72
Allderidge, Patricia, 143
American Gynecological Society, 118
Amritabazar Patrika, 117
antapur, 125
Anatomy Act, 13
Anderson, Clare, 133
Anglo-Boer War, 88, 90–1, 172
animal disease, 61–2, 64–9, 71–2
    and colonial knowledge, 64
    see also rinderpest
Annesley, James, 54
Apothecaries Act, 13
Arnold, David, 2, 16, 30–1, 54–5, 58, 67,
    102, 129–30, 140
Arogya Jiwan, 16
Arya Vaidya Samajam, 17–8
Asiatic Society, 20
Aturghar, 116
Astanga Ayurvedic College, 21
Ayurveda, 5, 12–4, 16, 19, 21–2, 96, 97, 168
    See also Ayurvedic movement
Ayurvedic Committee, 21
Ayurvedic movement, 17
    see also nationalism

Bainbridge, G., 99
Bala, Poonam, 30, 67
Bankim Chandra Chattopadhyay, 14
Belgatchia Veterinary College, 65

Bengal Chemical and Pharmaceutical
    Works, 16
Bengal Forceps, 119, 123
Bengal Social Science Association, 14
Bethlem Royal Hospital, 143–4
bhadralok, 5, 16, 62, 67–73
    and western knowledge, 71
    see also middle class
bhadramahila, 114–15
Bhisak Darpan, 69
Bhore Committee, 124
Blaauw, Jan, 56
Black Death, 75, 100–1, 105–10
black insane, 146–7, 150, 152
    and asylum, 157
Black Plague, 75
Boahen, Albert A., 2
bovine tuberculosis, 71
Brown, K., 71
bubonic plague, 76, 81, 86, 88, 97
Burrows, Edmund H., 2
Burton, Antoinette, 2

Carmichael Medical College, 118–19
Carroll, Lewis, 17
caste, 11–12, 14–17, 22, 75, 77, 79, 83–4,
    93, 96, 116–17, 121, 163, 168
    divisions and identities, 17
cattle disease, 63–5, 68, 71
    and plague, 61–2
    see also rinderpest
Census of 1901, 16–17
Central Advisory Board of Health, 20
Chaudhary, Shaukat Rai, 19
Chaudhuri, Kirti N., 2
chawls, 92
Chikitsa Sammilani, 69

childbirth, 7, 113, 118, 120–5
    and medical intervention, 119
    see also reproductive health
cholera, 54, 63, 105–6
Clarence-Smith, William G., 65
Clem, Sunter, 26
colonial asylum, 129, 143–4, 147–8, 153–4
    histories of, 156–7
colonial psychiatry, 8, 128–30, 136, 140–1,
    144–7
convicts, 8, 127–41,
Coolie Location 77–82, 89
Co-ordinating Committee for Traditional
    Health Practitioners, 35
Coroner's Act, 170
Corpus, 161
Countess of Dufferin's Fund, 15, 112, 118
Cranefield, P. F., 71
Criminal Tribes Act, 169
Cuvier, Georges, 53, 72

dai (s), 7, 113, 116–17, 120–3, 125
    see also Hindu midwives, 117
darogah, 165–6
Deacon, Harriet, 1, 7
Dharmasastras, 163
Digby, Anne, 2
Dirks, Nicholas B., 20
Dr Alfred Bull, 114
Dr C. Palmer, 63
Dr Charles Porter, 79
Dr Clara Swain, 117
Dr Dodds, 151
Dr Fleetwood Churchill, 113
Dr Godfrey, 81
Dr J. Dougall, 134
Dr J. Reid, 134
Dr John Gregory, 90
Dr Bernard Fuller, 90
Dr Kedarnath Das, 112, 118–19, 123
Dr Madhusudan Gupta, 112, 115–7
Dr Nthato Motlan, 29
Dr William Elmslier, 117
Dr William Godfrey, 78
Dr William Stephenson, 123
Dum Dum bullets, 170
Dutch East India Company, 4, 41, 57, 160
Dutch laws, 160
dyarchy, 19

East coast fever, 71–2
    see also rinderpest
East India Company, 12, 22, 160, 163
Echenberg, Myron, 6
Eden, Ashey, 137
Edgar, Robert, 144, 146
elites, 6, 11–12, 14, 18, 20, 22, 50, 53
    and patronage, 30
Engels, Dagmar, 1
English Law, 160, 165
epizootic, 61–3, 67–8, 72, 88–9, 99–100,
    104, 106–7
    see also veterinary services
Ernst, Waltraud, 128, 144
European Law, 159

Fahmy, Khaled, 171
Fanon, Franz, 144
Farrell, H., 65
forceps, 111–12, 118–20, 122–3
    see also Simpson Forceps
forensic medicine, 160
Fort William, 115

Gaudiya Sarvavidyayatana, 21
General Medical Council, 14
germ theory, 27, 71, 80, 101, 106, 110, 169
    see also Plague Research Commission
Ghosh, Durba, 1
Government of India Act, 20
Governmental Chemical Laboratory, 172
Govinda Sundari Ayurvedic College, 21
Gramsci, Antonio, 1

Haffkine, Waldemar, 86, 95, 97
Halbfass, Wilhelm, 20
Hallen, J. H. B., 64
Hankin, Ernst H., 102–3
Harrison, Mark, 3, 54, 58
Hassan, Narin, 14, 16
Hastings, Warren, 164
herbal medicine, 51
Herschel, William, 169
Hindu College, 13
Hindu intellectuals, 18
    and texts, 18, 99
Hirst, L. Fabian, 110, 105–6, 102
Hodgson, Marshall G. S., 3
Hopkins, Donald R., 47

Horrox, Rosemary, 100
Hunter, William, 102

India Academy of Forensic Sciences, 170
Indian Evidence Act, 170
Indian medicine, 15–16, 18, 22, 168
    see also Ayurveda
    see also Unani
Indian National Congress, 21
Indian Opinion, 92–3
Indian Penal Code, 170
Indian Plague Commission, 99–102, 104–5
Indian Science Congress, 20
indigenous healers, 26, 28–9, 31–4, 36, 38, 44
    and AIDS, 35
Indigenous Knowledge Systems Centre, 35
indigenous medicine, 17, 28, 121
    see also Ayurveda
    see also Unani
Ingutsheni Asylum, 147
insanity, 128, 130, 132, 136, 149, 153–5
International Congress of African Historians, 2

Jackson, Lynette, 130
Jacobs, Marisa, 26
Jeeves, Alan, 26
Jenner, Edward, 47
    see also small pox
Jones, William, 20
Journal of Hygiene, 102

Kapila, Shruti, 140
Kettner, Hans Jurgen, 57
Khanyile, Cyril, 35
Khoikhoi, 5, 41, 45, 46, 48–9, 54–9
    and white settlers, 44
    and public health, 49
Kilburn, 88
Klein, Ira, 4
Koch, Robert, 71, 81
kraals, 44–5, 48–9
    see also Khoikhoi
Ksatriyas, 163
Kuhn, Thomas, 100
Kwazulu-Natal Traditional Healers Council, 37

Laduries, Emmanuel LeRoy, 45
Lady Dufferin, 112
Laws of Manu, 163
legal medicine, 159, 161, 171
    see also medical jurisprudence
Leguat, Francis, 44
Locke, S., 22
London Vegetarian Society, 70, 72
Lopez, Abel Ricardo, 5
lunatic asylum archives, 157
lunatic asylums, 128–9, 140–1, 145, 154
lunatics, 128, 131–4, 137–40, 143, 148, 150
    and legislation, 151
lying-in hospitals, 113

McCulloch, J. M., 144
McKittrick, Meredith, 130
MacLeod, Kenneth, M., 62
MacLeod, Roy, 72
Madhusudan Gupta 118
Major J. M. Woolley, 127–8
makgoma, 34
Mallick, Manicklal, 69, 70
Mandela, Nelson, 25
Manu, 116
    Laws of, 163
Maritzburg Town Council, 95
Marks, Shula, 1, 145
maternal health, 123
Medical College Hospital, 116
Medical education, 12–14, 16–17, 167
    and reforms, 13–14
    see also Native Medical Institution
medical jurisprudence, 159
Medical Registration Act, 14
Medical Research Council, 35
Medical Women for India Fund, 15
medico-legal laboratories, 174
medico-legal treatises, 161
middle class, 5, 15–16, 18, 39, 62, 66, 70–2, 90, 94, 114–15
    see also elites
midwifery, 7, 114, 117–18, 120–1, 123
    and midwives, 50
    see also dais
Mills, James H., 128–29, 144
Mills, James, 144
Miss Fanny Butler, 117

Mitchell, Timothy, 73
Mitra, Kissory Chandra, 16
Montague-Chelmsford Reforms, 11, 19
Mughal empire, 160
Murti, G. Srinivas, 21

Nadar Mahajana Sangam, 17
Native Code (of 1928), 31
Native Doctors, 12
    see also Native Medical Institution
National Health Plan for South Africa, 36
National Health Service, 39
nationalism, 13, 18, 21, 160
    and Ayurveda, 22
Native Medical Institution, 12, 30, 168
    anatomical practices in, 13
    abolition of, 13
Native Strangers' Location Bill, 91
Naturopathy, 96
Ngwekezane Hospital, 35

panchayat, 163
Pandit Madhusudan Gupta, 168
Parle, Julie, 144–6, 156
Parsis, 93
Pasteurella pestis, 89
pastoralists, 43
    and medicine, 43
    see also Khoikhoi
plague science, 106
    see also Plague Research Commission
plague bacillus, 97, 108–9
    see also *Yersinia pestis*
plague epidemic, 75, 78, 97
    and pandemic 6, 100
    see also plague science
Plague Research Commission, 7, 95,
    99–101, 105, 106, 108–10
plague vaccine, 95
    see also Haffkine, Waldemar
pneumonic plague, 75–7, 80, 84, 97, 104
Pritchard, Edward Evans, 29
Professional Herbal Preparation Associa-
    tion, 37
public health, 20, 22, 31, 46, 48–9, 62,
    69–70, 72–3, 96, 124–5, 160, 169,
    171, 173–4
Public Health Acts, 173

Puranas, 72
purdah, 96
pardanashin, 118

Ramanna, Mridulla, 67
Ramasubban, Radhika, 4
Rattus rattus, 100, 107
Ray, Prafulla Chandra, 15, 19
Ray, Utsa, 67, 70
Reconstruction and Development Pro-
    gramme, 36
Regulating Act, 164
reproductive health, 111–13, 115–89,
    124–5
Riebeeck, Jan Van, 30
rinderpest, 61, 63–7, 68, 70–2
    see also cattle disease
Ripon College, 70
Ripon Hospital, 94

S. S. Kassala, 89
Sadowsky, Jonathan, 130, 144–5
Samuel Kwadi Traditional Hospital, 37
sanitary reforms, 103
Sanskrit College, 115, 168
Sapire, Hilary, 144, 146
Sarda Act, 124
sari'a law, 163–5
Satthianadhan, Krupabai, 15
Schuenemann,Verena, 108
Select Committee on the Treatment of
    Lunatics, 152
Sen, Chandra Kishore, 17
Sen, Satadru, 130
Sen, Kaviraj Chandra Kishore, 17
Shrewsbury, John F. D., 100, 107
Simond, Paul-Louis, 101
Simpson Forceps, 120
Simpson, James Young, 113
Simpson, W. J., 102–3
Sir Edward Henry, 169
Sir Francis Galton, 169
Sirkar, Mahendralal, 16
Slack, Paul, 100
small pox, 41, 45–9, 53, 56
Snow, P. C. H., 94
Soman, Krishna, 7

South African Medical and Dental Council, 32
South African Police Service, 173
Spencer, Herbert, 70
Stalkartt, John, 61
Stanford, Walter E., 90
Stoler, Ann, 144, 151
sugrihini, 114
sutikagriha, 116
swadeshi, 18
   see also nationalism
Swartz, Sally, 131
Swasthya Samachar, 69
syphilis, 33

Tait, Robert Lawson, 113
Tavernier, Jean-Baptiste, 43
Taylor, Sherman, 128
Thomas Babington Macaulay, 13, 165
Thomson, S. J., 99
Thomspon, J. Ashburton, 104
Thunberg, Carl, 41
Tortorici, Zeb, 7
Town Council, 82–3, 92, 95
traditional medicine, 121
   see also Ayurveda
   see also Unani
Tribedi, Ramendra Shundor, 70
Tutu, Desmond, 25–6
Twining, William, 54
typhus, 45

Unani, 5, 15, 18, 30, 123
Upanishads, 72

Vacaspati, Shyamadas, 21
vaids, 18, 72, 97
   and vaidyas, 30
Valkenberg Lunatic Asylum, 145
Varier, P. S., 17
Vaughan, Megan, 130, 144–6, 149
Vedas, 16, 72

veterinary education, 64
   and veterinary services, 61, 72–3
   see also epizootic
Vincent, R. H., 86
Voelkar, J. A., 64

Waddington, Keir, 71
Warburton, Henry, 13
Weinstein, Barbara, 5
white insane, 146, 148, 152
Willis, C. S., 66
women missionaries, 117
Woolley, J. M., 127–8, 131
Worboys, Michael, 71, 102
World Health Assembly, 36
World Health Organization, 27

Xenopsylla cheopsis, 100

Yang, A. Anand, 129
Yersin, Alexandre 89
Yersinia pestis, 76, 89, 100, 105, 108–10

Zande, 29
zenana, 113, 117
Zulu healers, 35